PAEDIATRIC RADIOLOGY: *Clinical Cases*

PRABHAKAR RAJIAH MBBS MD FRCR
Diagnostic Radiologist
Cleveland Clinic
USA

ABDUSAMEA G S SHABANI MBBch FRCR
Consultant Paediatric Radiologist
Department of Paediatric Radiology
Royal Manchester Children's University Hospital
UK

PasTest
Dedicated to your success

Egerton Court
Parkgate Estate
Knutsford
Cheshire
WA16 8DX
Telephone: 01565 752000

First Published 2008

ISBN: 1905 635 206
978 1905 635 207

A catalogue record for this book is available from the British Library.

Cover image: Studying CT scans PETER BOWATER/SCIENCE PHOTO LIBRARY
Text prepared by Carnegie Book Production, Lancaster
Printed and bound in the UK by Athenaeum Press, Gateshead

CONTENTS

FOREWORD

Radiology plays a vital role in the investigation of neonatal and childhood diseases and its correct interpretation can be fundamental to making a diagnosis. It is therefore relevant to both clinician and radiologist alike, and is often used, quite justifiably, as part of the examination process.

Over the past few years the range of imaging techniques has broadened considerably with magnetic resonance becoming increasingly available, often complementing ultrasound as a safe, non-invasive method of investigating children. Plain radiography still has an important role, and the 'humble' chest X-ray remains the most commonly requested radiological examination, and often the most difficult to interpret! Computed tomography is used less frequently because of the concerns regarding radiation exposure, but is still the best technique for imaging trauma, bony lesions and the lung parenchyma. The functional information obtained by nuclear medicine studies can also be crucial in decision making.

With all these imaging modalities available, the authors, Prabhakar Rajiah and Abdusamea Shabani, have pulled together a varied and interesting group of cases to test the reader. Some of the cases may seem straightforward, others rather more intellectually taxing, but behind the additional questions posed with each case, there is a wealth of extra information provided which helps to develop a more complete understanding of the clinical problem.

Clearly the aim of this book is to provide a challenge to the budding paediatrician, or established consultant for that matter, and to exercise their mind by solving the puzzle presented by the radiological images. There is also no doubt that paediatric radiologists, general radiologists or anyone having an interest in interpreting children's imaging will find this book helpful and rewarding.

Dr Neville Wright
Consultant Paediatric Radiologist &
Clinical Director of Children's Radiology
Booth Hall & Royal Manchester Children's Hospitals
May 2008

INTRODUCTION

Radiology is a rapidly evolving field with new technological developments every year. It has become an integral component of the diagnostic and therapeutic dimension of every speciality, including paediatrics, and plays a vital role in management of patients. Radiological pictures are also increasingly used in many postgraduate examinations. Hence it is essential for paediatricans and radiologists alike to be well informed in the appropriate investigation for any paediatric clinical case and to be aware of the typical and atypical findings of each clinical scenario.

Paediatric Radiology: Clinical Cases consists of 186 cases and approximately 325 images. The book is divided into five sections – Chest and cardiovascular radiology, gastrointestinal and hepatobiliary radiology, genitourinary radiology, musculoskeletal radiology and neuroradiology. Each case is presented with pertinent history, followed by radiological pictures and 5–6 questions. The second part of each chapter contains the case diagnosis, clinical features, radiological findings, imaging techniques, diagnostic algorithm, differential diagnosis and management.

The book covers almost the entire gamut of radiological findings in common pediatric conditions. The cases include pictures from multiple modalities such as X-rays, ultrasound, Doppler, CT scan, MRI and nuclear medicine. The cases range from the very common to the unusual and challenging.

It is hoped that the format of the book, images and discussion will be helpful not only for paediatric and radiology trainees preparing for postgraduate exams, but also for medical students intending to specialise in either of these fields. Paediatricians, paediatric surgeons and radiologists who wish to update their knowledge on the radiological aspects of paediatric diseases may also find this book useful.

Dr Prabhakar Rajiah
Dr Abdusamea G S Shabani

ACKNOWLEDGEMENTS

We would like to acknowledge the help of Dr Neville Wright, Dr Mussa Kaleen and staff of the Royal Manchester Children's Hospital for their contributions and suggestions in the preparation of this book.

1

CHEST AND CARDIOVASCULAR RADIOLOGY QUESTIONS

Case 1.1

A preterm neonate is being monitored in the intensive care unit (ICU) for multisystemic problems and is on a ventilator. There is sudden deterioration of her condition after a few days of stability. On examination, she is tachypnoeic and there are decreased breath sounds in the lungs.

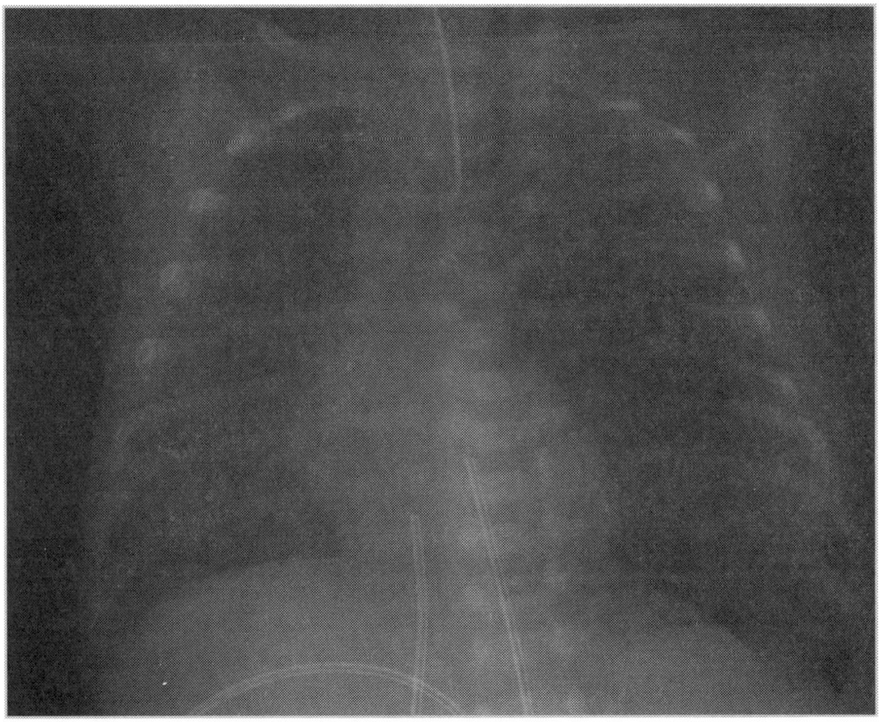

Fig 1.1

1. What are the findings on the chest X-ray?
2. What is the diagnosis?
3. What is the underlying disease?
4. What is the mechanism of development of this condition?
5. What are the radiological features?
6. What are the complications?

Answers *on pages 41–85*

Case 1.2

A 10-year-old boy presents with head and neck swelling, dyspnoea and hoarseness of voice. On examination there is oedema in the face and neck with prominent veins. There are multiple lymph nodes palpable in the axilla and groin. There are decreased breath sounds in both the lungs.

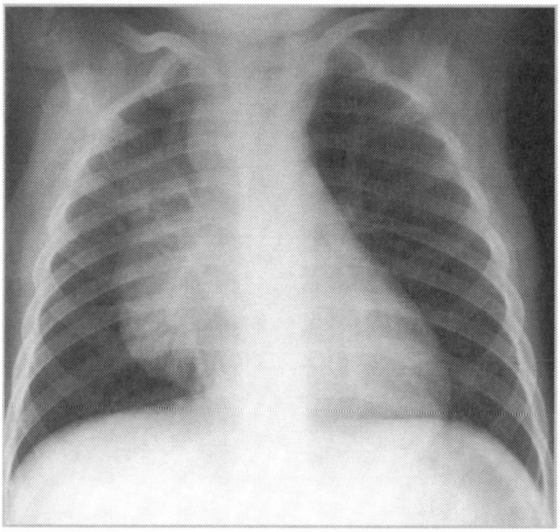

Fig 1.2a

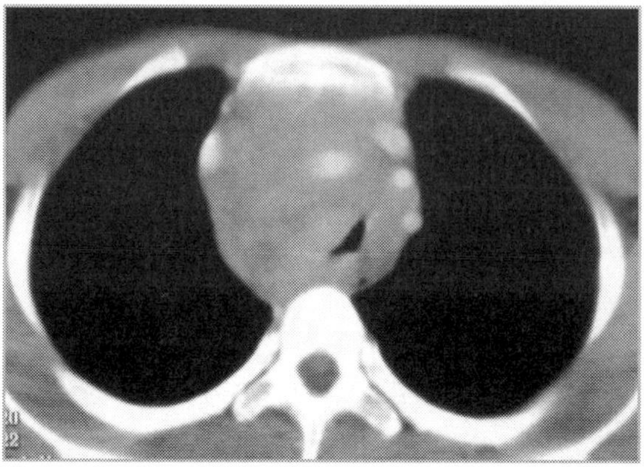

Fig 1.2b

1. What do you find on the X-ray and CT scan?
2. What is the diagnosis?
3. What are the types of disease?
4. What are the common locations?
5. What are the radiological features?
6. What is the differential diagnosis?

Answers *on pages 41–85*

Case 1.3

A 14-year-old boy presents with fever, coughing and difficulty breathing. On examination, he is febrile with tachypnoea. Bronchial breathing is heard on the right side.

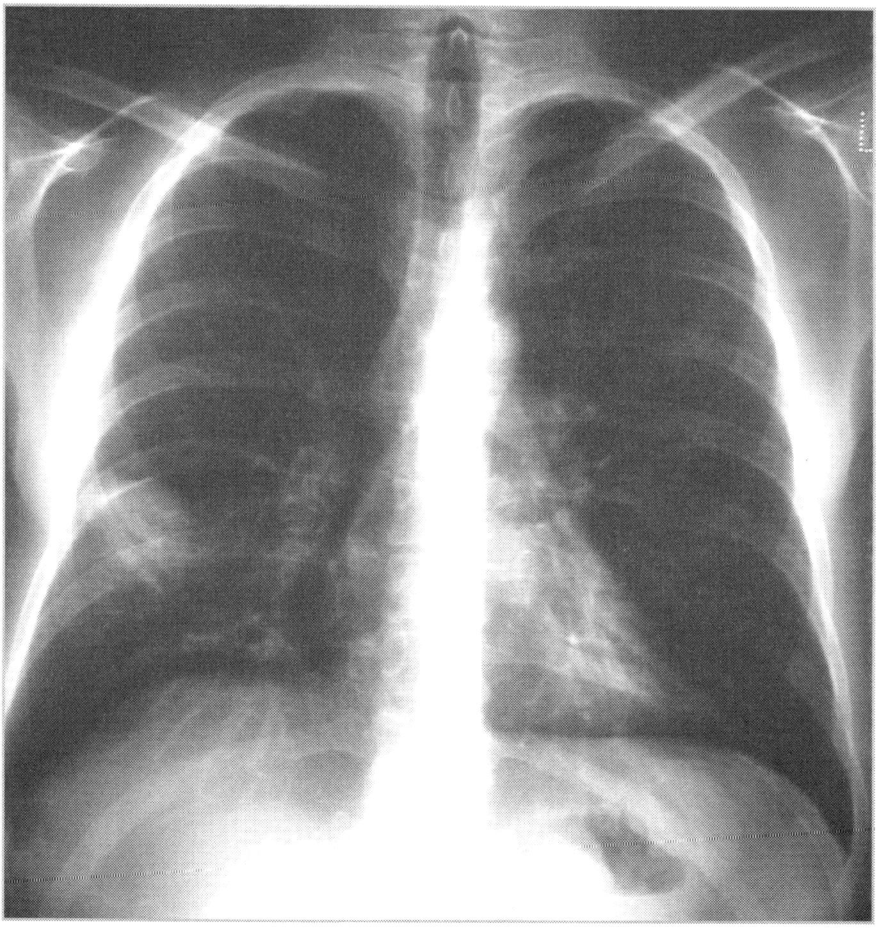

Fig 1.3

1. What can you see on the chest X-ray?
2. What is the diagnosis?
3. What are the causes of this disease?
4. What are the radiological features?
5. What is the differential diagnosis?

Answers *on pages 41–85*

Case 1.4

A 6-year-old girl with a chronic disease presents with dyspnoea and cough with productive sputum. On examination, bronchial breathing sounds are heard bilaterally, more on the right side. A chest X-ray and CT scan were done.

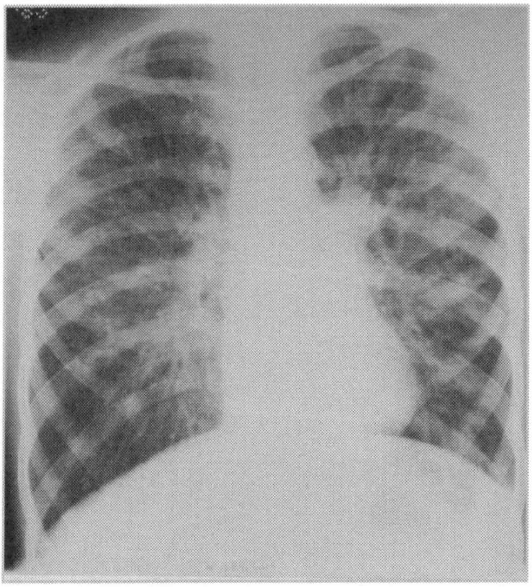

Fig 1.4a

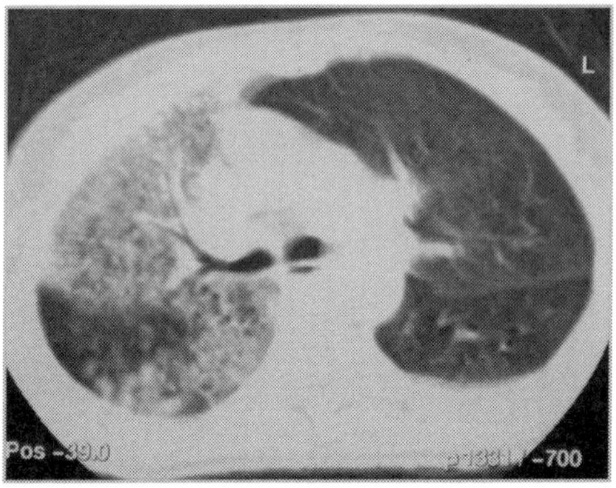

Fig 1.4b

1. What do you see on the chest X-ray and CT scan?
2. What chronic disease condition can you identify?
3. What are the causes and clinical features of this disease?
4. What are the complications of this disease?
5. What are the radiological features?
6. How is this disease scored?

Answers *on pages 41–85*

Case 1.5

A 12-year-old boy presents with frequent episodes of cough and fever. On examination, the patient is febrile and tachypnoeic. Bronchial breathing is heard on the right side.

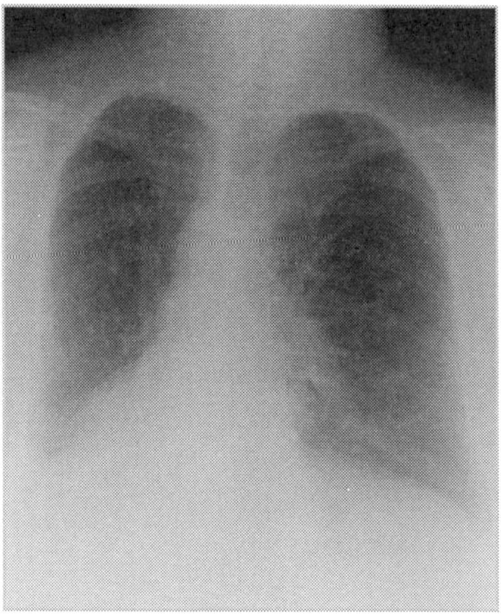

Fig 1.5a

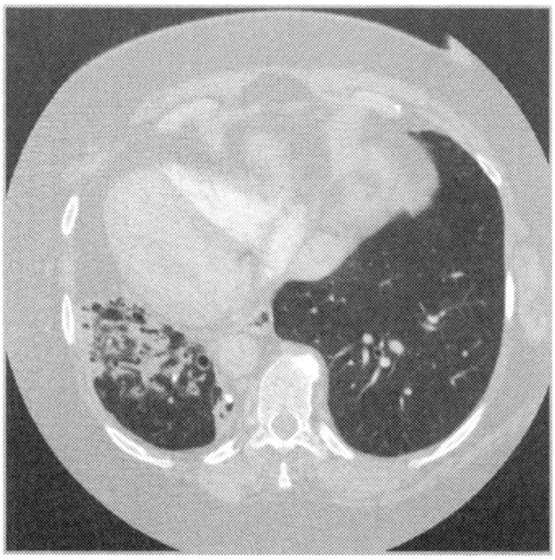

Fig 1.5b

1. What do you find on the chest X-ray?
2. What do you find on the chest CT scan?
3. What is the diagnosis?
4. What is the pathophysiology of this disease?
5. What are the radiological features and treatment?

Answers *on pages 41–85*

Case 1.6

An 8-year-old girl presents with dyspnoea, fever and cough. Clinical examination showed tachypnoea. The heart sounds are shifted to the right side and the breath sounds are decreased on the right side.

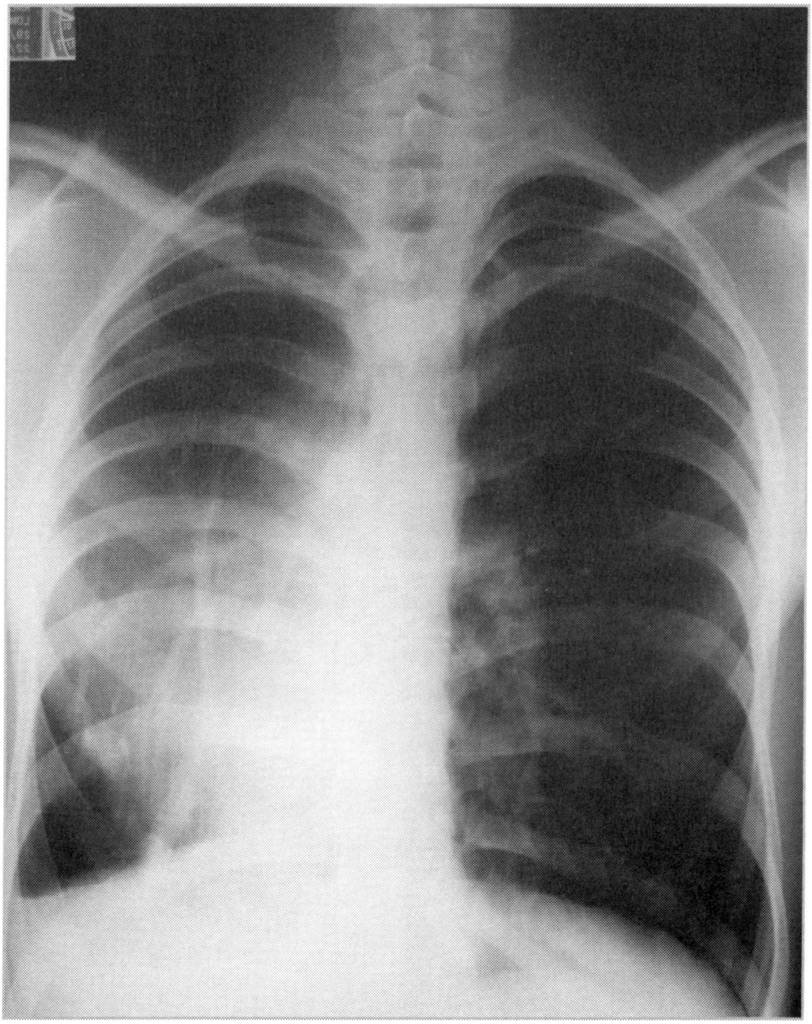

Fig 1.6

1. What do you see on the chest X-ray?
2. What is the diagnosis?
3. What are the causes and associations?
4. What are the clinical features?
5. What are the radiological features?

Answers *on pages 41–85*

Case 1.7

A 1-year-old child who is in the ICU for management of lymphoma develops an audible grunt. On examination she is afebrile, but tachypnoeic. There are decreased breath sounds on the left side and dullness on percussion.

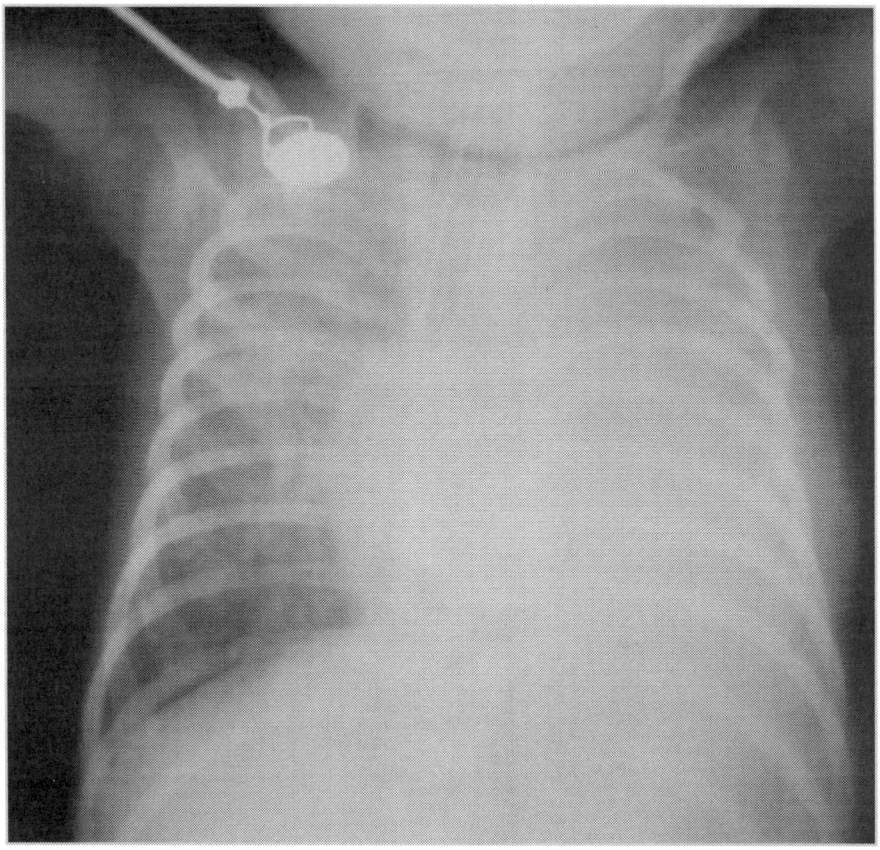

Fig 1.7

1. What do you observe on the chest film?
2. What is the cause of the patient's condition?
3. What should be the next step?
4. What are the common causes of this radiological appearance?
5. What are the radiological findings and what is the differential diagnosis?

Answers *on pages 41–85*

Case 1.8

A 10-year-old Asian girl presents to the accident and emergency department (A&E) with high fever, cough with sputum, dyspnoea, cyanosis, respiratory distress and fatigue. On examination, she is febrile, tachypnoeic, with bilateral bronchial breathing and intercostal recession. The chest X-ray was done for further evaluation.

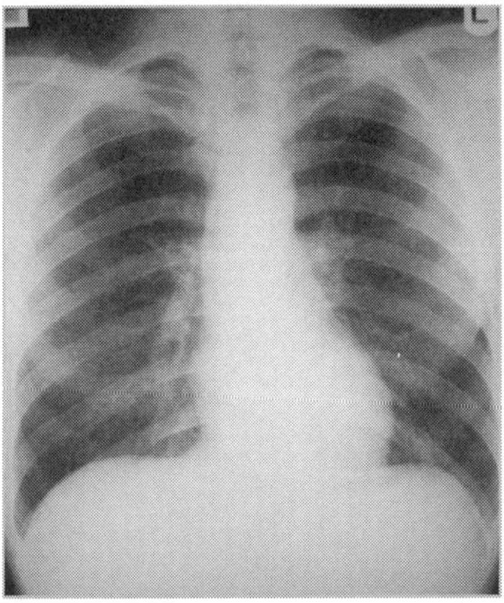

Fig 1.8a

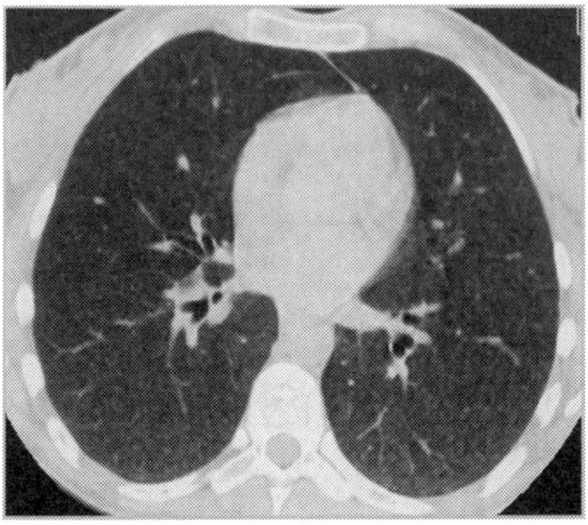

Fig 1.8b

1. What do you observe on the chest X-ray of the child?
2. What do you see on chest HRCT in this child?
3. What is the diagnosis?
4. What are the clinical features and what further tests are required for confirmation?
5. What are the radiological features and how will you manage this child?

Answers *on pages 41–85*

Case 1.9

A 13-year-old boy presents with severe throat pain and fever. On examination, there is severe tenderness in the neck and the patient is febrile.

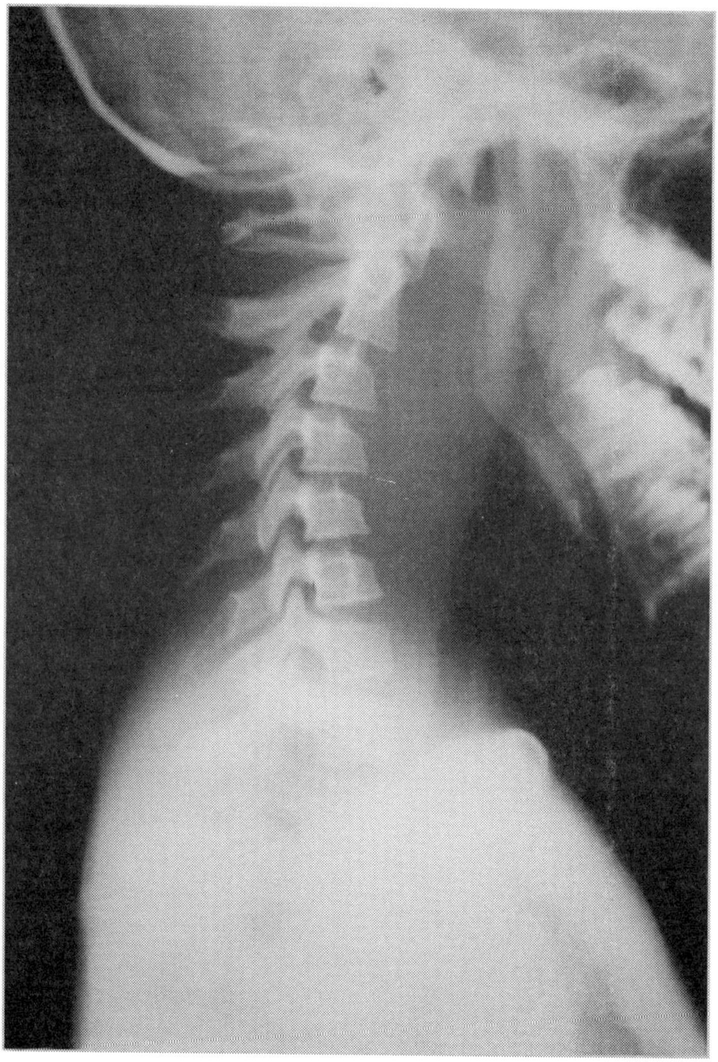

Fig 1.9

1. What do you find on this plain X-ray?
2. What is the diagnosis?
3. What are the causes of this disease?
4. What are the radiological features?
5. What is Grisel syndrome?

Answers *on pages 41–85*

Case 1.10

A 5-year-old boy presents with difficulty swallowing, an itching sensation in the throat and drooling. On examination his oropharynx appears normal. There is no tonsillar enlargement or neck node. There is no tachypnoea or features of respiratory distress.

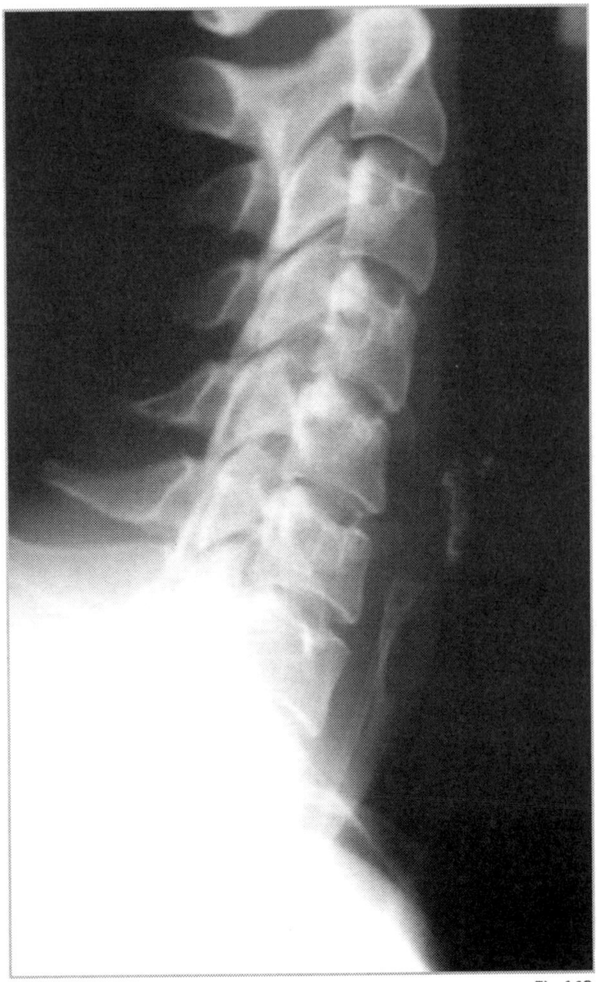

Fig 1.10

1. What do you observe on the lateral X-ray of the neck?
2. What is the diagnosis?
3. What are the predisposing factors and common locations?
4. What are the radiological features?
5. How is this condition managed and what are the complications?

Answers *on pages 41–85*

Case 1.11

A 2-year-old boy presents with recurrent respiratory infections. On examination, he is febrile, with tachypnoea. Breath sounds are decreased on the right side and there is hyperresonance on percussion.

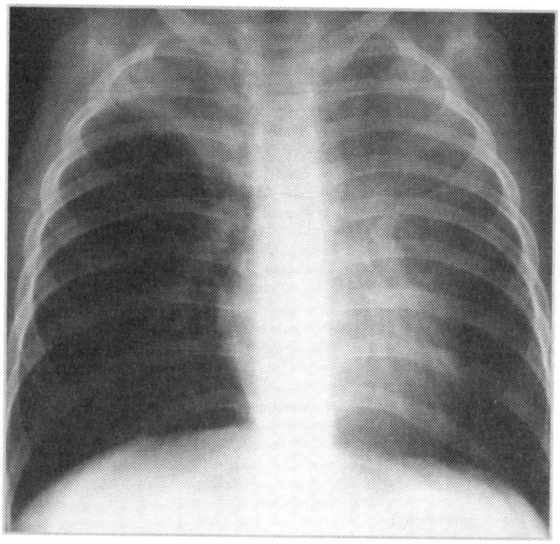

Fig 1.11a

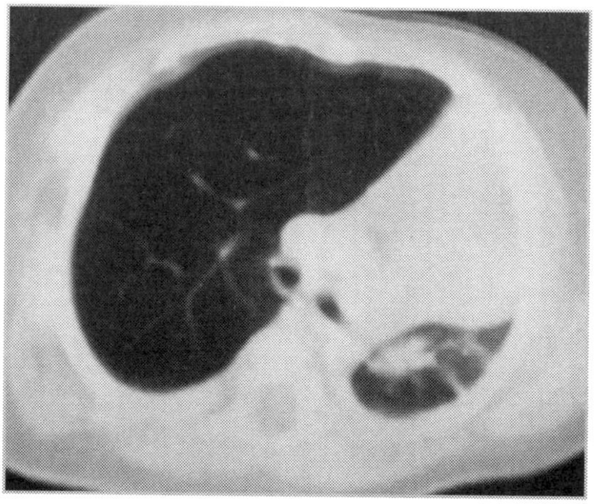

Fig 1.11b

1. What can you see on the chest X-ray and the CT scan?
2. What is the diagnosis?
3. What is the development of this disease?
4. What are the clinical presentations and treatment for this disease?
5. What are the common locations? What are the radiological features?
6. What is the differential diagnosis?

Answers *on pages 41–85*

Case 1.12

A 10-day-old neonate presents with severe respiratory distress and cyanosis. Decreased breath sounds and abnormal splashing sounds were heard on the left side. The chest was hyperresonant on percussion.

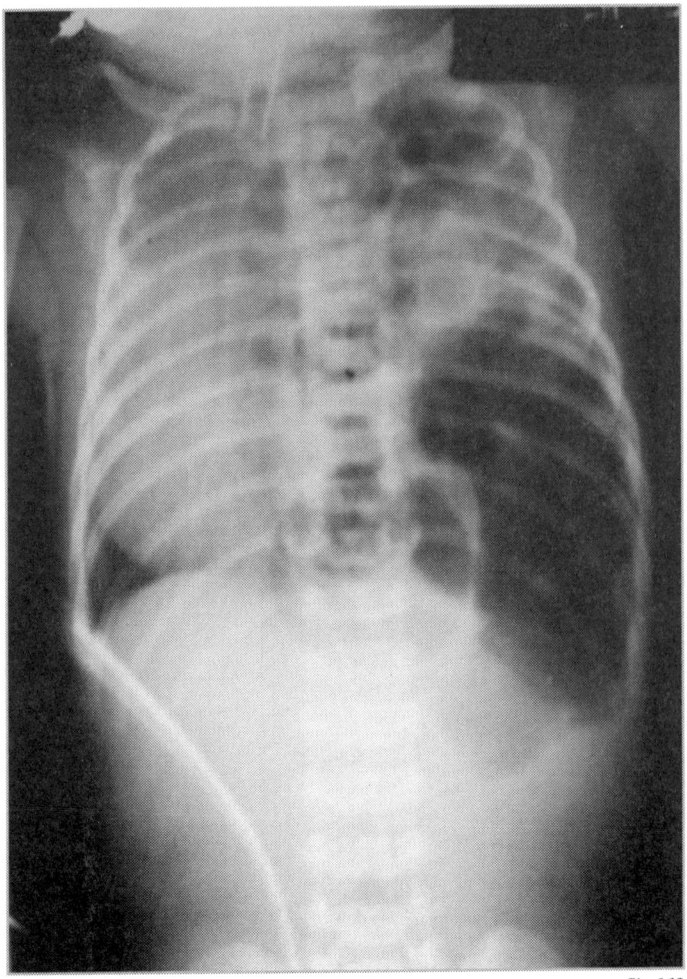

Fig 1.12

1. What can you see on the chest X-ray?
2. What is the diagnosis?
3. What is the development and what are the types of this disease?
4. What are the radiological findings? What is the differential diagnosis for this appearance?
5. What are the prognostic factors, complications and treatment?

Answers *on pages 41–85*

Case 1.13

A preterm girl, delivered at 30 weeks' gestation and weighing 900 g, developed cyanosis, expiratory grunting, intercostal recession and nasal flaring.

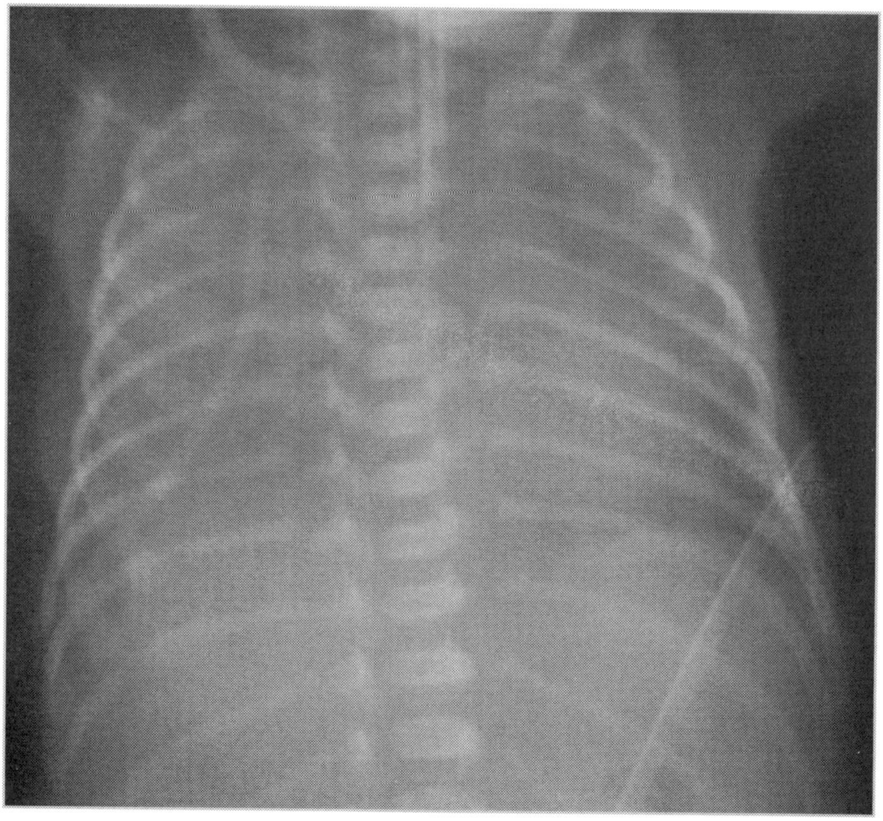

Fig 1.13

1. What can you see on the chest X-ray?
2. What is the diagnosis?
3. What are the predisposing factors and pathology of this disease?
4. What are diagnostic criteria and how is this managed?
5. What is the common differential diagnosis?

Answers *on pages 41–85*

Case 1.14

A 15-year-old girl presents with fever and dyspnoea. On examination the boy is febrile and has tachypnoea. Reduced breath sounds were heard on the right side.

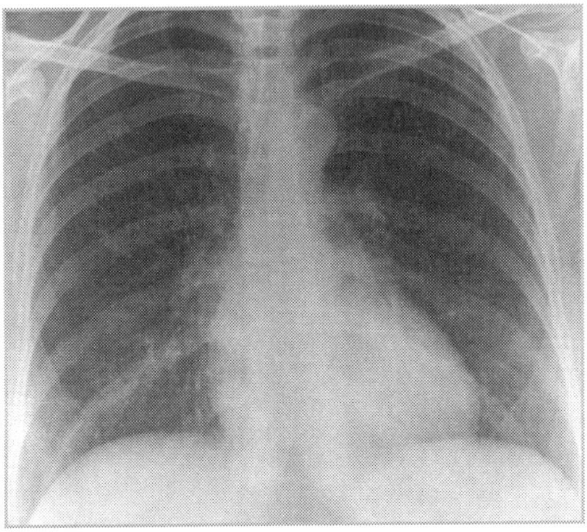

Fig 1.14a

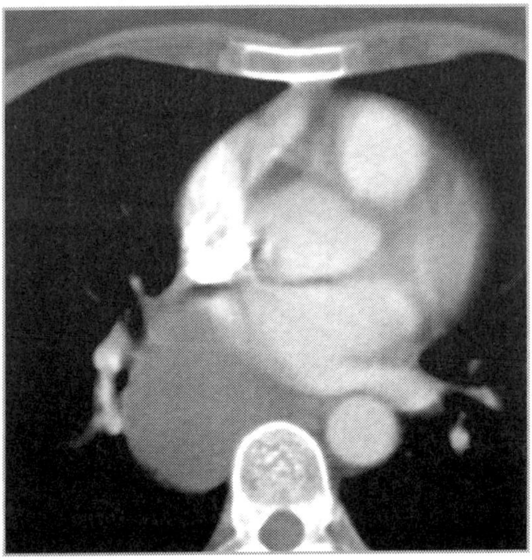

Fig 1.14b

1. What can you see on the chest X-ray?
2. What do you see on the chest CT scan?
3. What are the diagnosis and differential diagnosis?
4. What is the development of this disease?
5. What are the clinical presentations and course of this disease?

Answers *on pages 41–85*

Case 1.15

A 4-year-old girl presents with recurrent respiratory tract infections and dyspnoea. On examination, the girl is febrile and tachypnoeic. Bronchial breathing is heard on the right base. Percussion is normal. Lab tests show a high white blood cell (WBC) count. The X-ray showed a right lower lobar opacity on two X-rays done with a gap of 6 months.

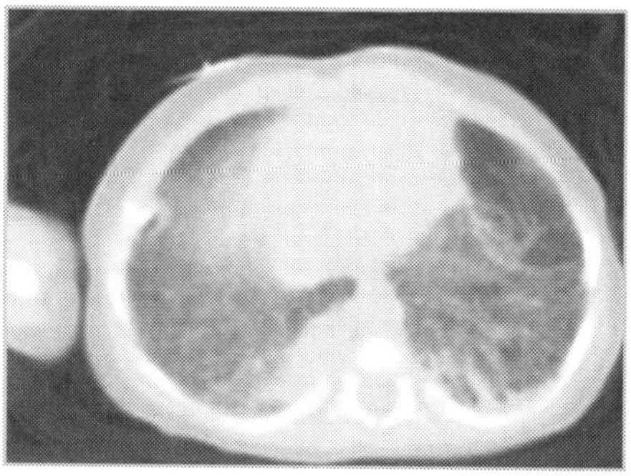

Fig 1.15a

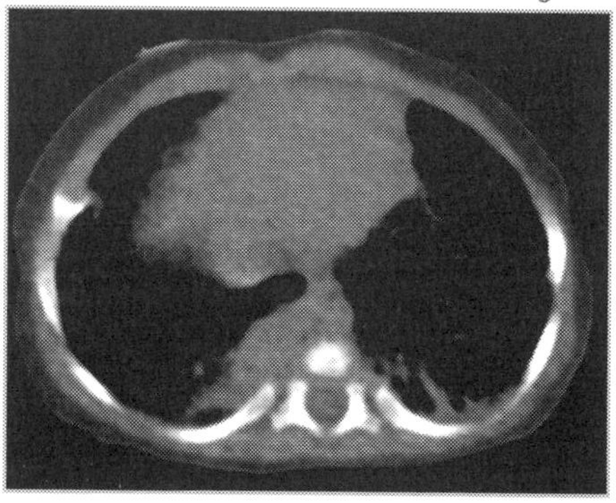

Fig 1.15b

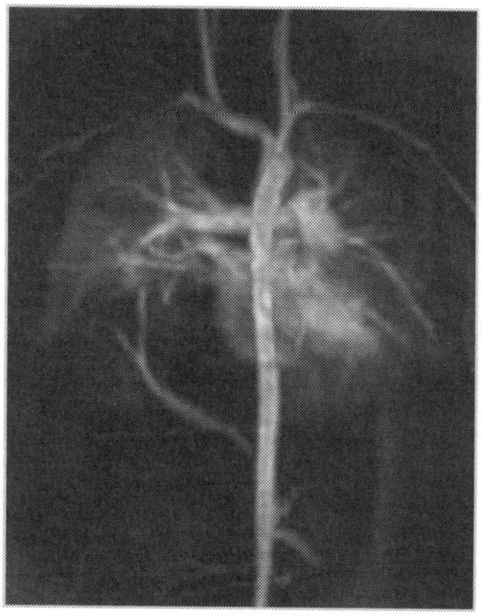

Fig 1.15c

1. What do you see in the CT scan and MR angiography?
2. What is the diagnosis?
3. What are the different types of this disease?
4. What are the clinical presentations and course of this disease?
5. What are the radiological features?

Answers *on pages 41–85*

Case 1.16

A 15-year-old girl with acute myeloid leukaemia underwent haematopoietic stem cell transplantation. On day 18 after transplantation, he presents with sudden onset of chest pain, dyspnoea and fever. On examination, he is febrile and tachypnoeic. There is bronchial breathing in the left upper lobe. Lab findings revealed neutropenia.

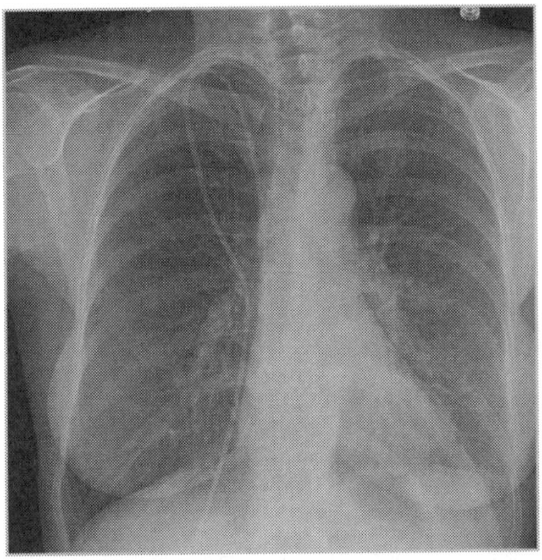
Fig 1.16a

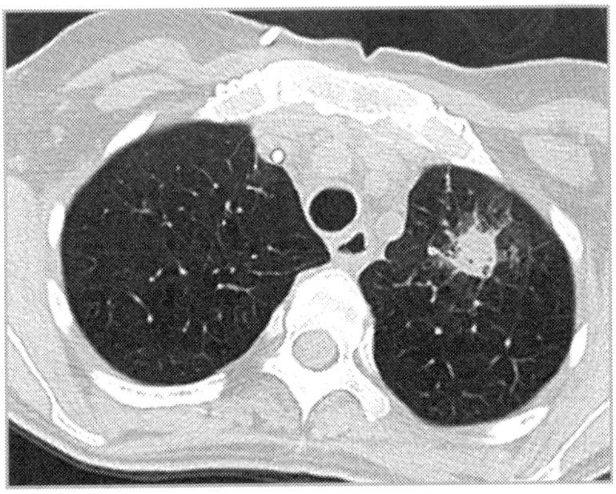
Fig 1.16b

1. What do you observe on the chest X-ray and CT scan?
2. What is the diagnosis?
3. What are the causes of this disease?
4. What are the other manifestations in patients who are bone marrow transplant recipients?
5. What are the radiological features and differential diagnosis?

Answers *on pages 41–85*

Case 1.17

A 4-year-old boy presents with sudden onset of chest pain, dyspnoea, fever and night sweats. On examination, he has intercostal recession, respiratory distress and tachypnoea, and he is febrile. There is no lymphadenopathy. Bronchial breathing is heard on the left side of the chest. Percussion was normal.

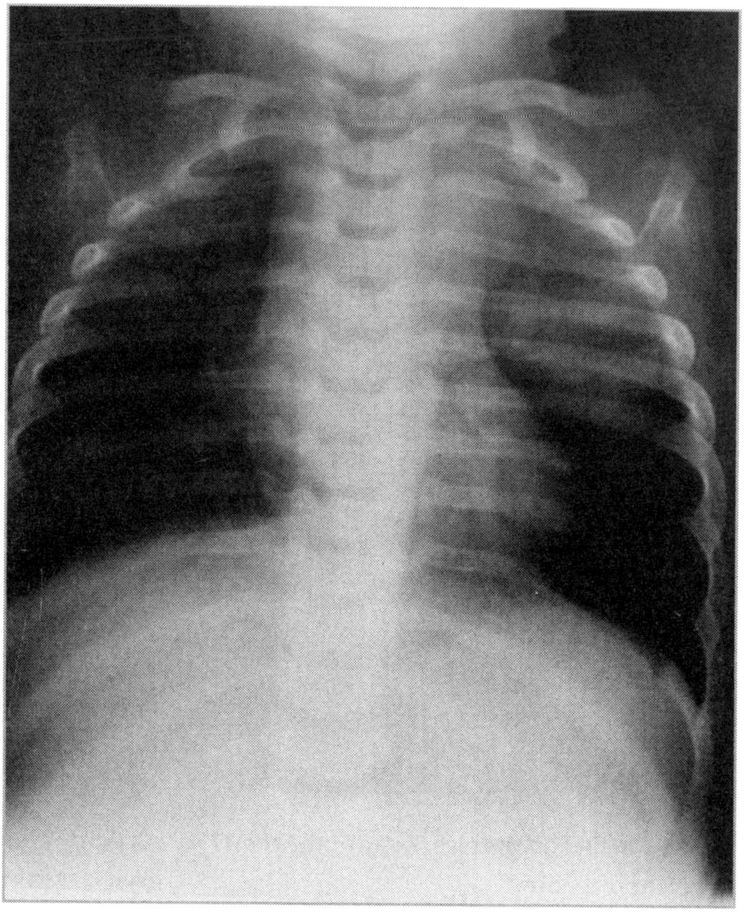

Fig 1.17

1. What do you observe on the chest X-ray?
2. What is the diagnosis?
3. What is the most common causative aetiology?
4. What are the predisposing factors?
5. What are the radiological features and differential diagnosis?
6. What are the complications and treatment?

Answers *on pages 41–85*

Case 1.18

A 7-year-old boy presents with fever, cough, night sweats, chest pain and failure to thrive. On examination, he is febrile and there are bronchial breath sounds in the right upper lobe.

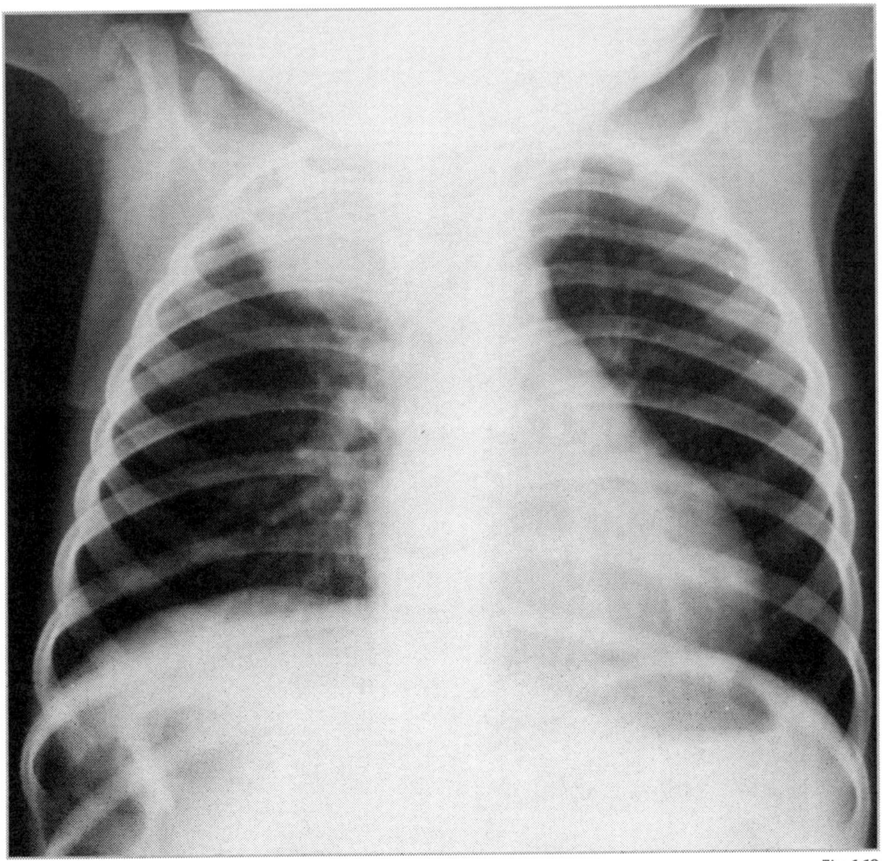

Fig 1.18

1. What do you find on the plain X-ray of the chest?
2. What is the diagnosis?
3. What are the causative organism and the pathophysiology?
4. What are the radiological features?
5. What is the differential diagnosis?
6. What are the variant lesions and complications?

Answers *on pages 41–85*

Case 1.19

A 15-year-old girl presents with chest pain, backache and weight loss. On examination, the chest appears normal. Tenderness was noted in the mid-thoracic vertebrae.

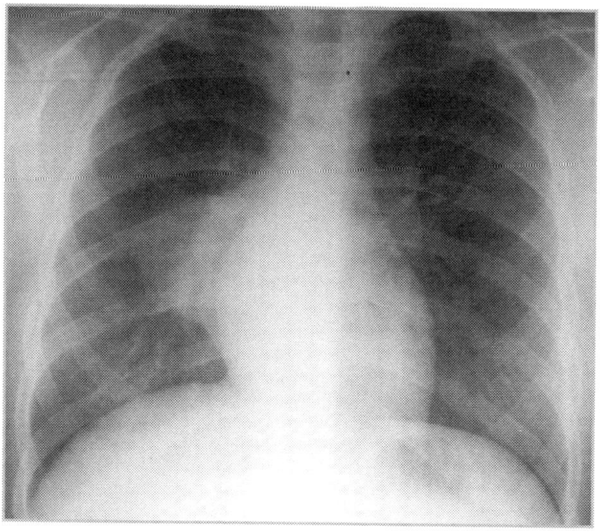

Fig 1.19a

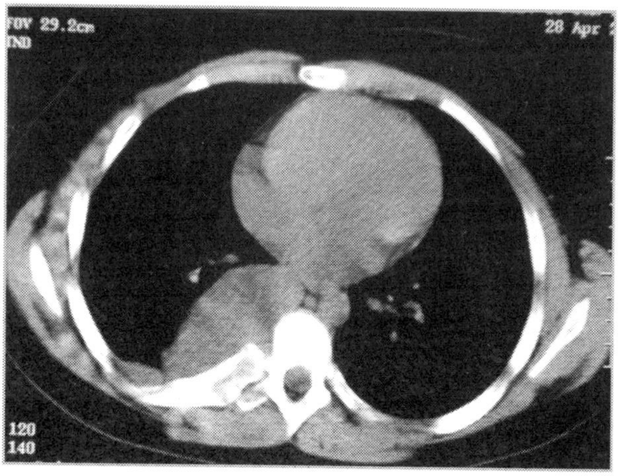

Fig 1.19b

1. What are the findings on the plain X-ray of the chest?
2. What are the findings on the CT scan of the chest?
3. What are the diagnosis and the most common association?
4. What are the clinical features?
5. What are the radiological features and differential diagnosis?

Answers *on pages 41–85*

Case 1.20

A 4-year-old boy presents with tachypnoea and a history of frequent respiratory infections. Clinical examination shows decreased breath sounds on the left side.

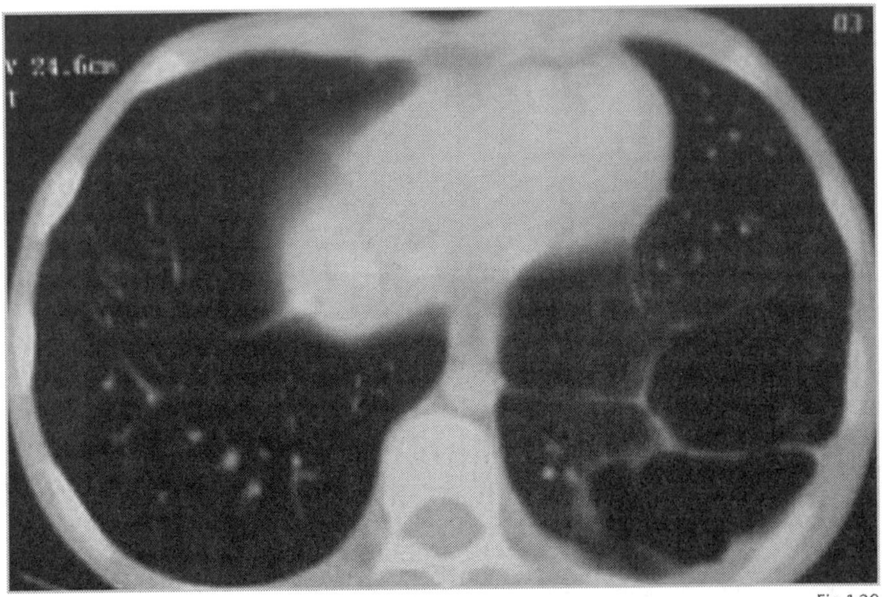

Fig 1.20

1. What do you see on the CT scan of the chest?
2. What is the diagnosis?
3. What is the development of this disease?
4. What are the clinical presentations and course of this disease?
5. What is the differential diagnosis for this disease?

Answers *on pages 41–85*

Case 1.21

A 7-year-old girl presents with fever and coughing. On examination she is febrile and tachypnoeic. A diagnosis of pneumonia was made and the patient was treated with antibiotics.

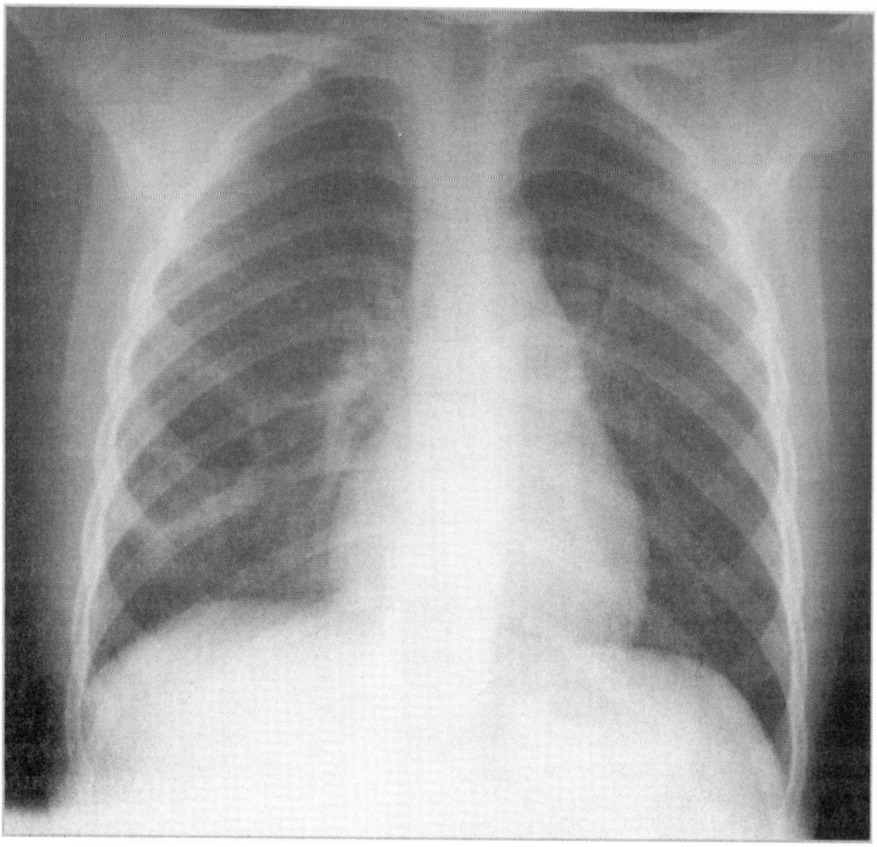

Fig 1.21

1. What can you see on the chest X-ray taken 3 months after the initial diagnosis of pneumonia?
2. What is the diagnosis?
3. What are the causative agents for this disease?
4. What are the mechanism of development and the clinical course?
5. What is the differential diagnosis?

Answers *on pages 41–85*

Case 1.22

An 11-year-old girl presents with sudden onset of chest pain, dyspnoea, fever and night sweats. On clinical examination, she is febrile and tachypnoeic. The breath sounds are decreased on the left side and there is a stony dull note on percussion.

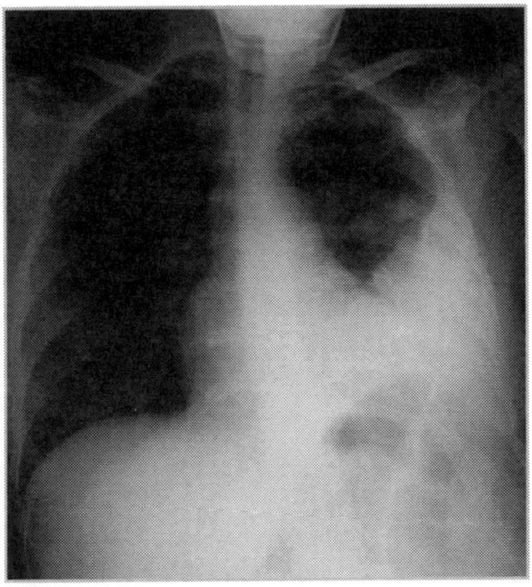

Fig 1.22a

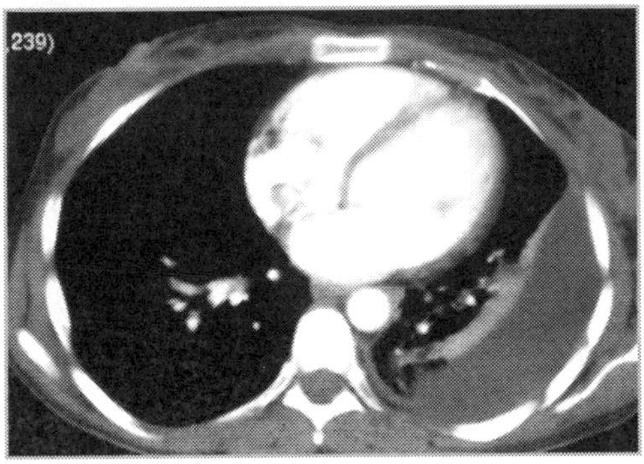

Fig 1.22b

1. What do you observe on the plain film of the chest?
2. What is the second investigation and what do you observe?
3. What is the diagnosis and the radiological differential diagnosis?
4. What are the causes?
5. What are the findings that are suspicious for an exudate than transudates?
6. What is the most sensitive method in the diagnosis of this condition and what are the radiological features?

Answers *on pages 41–85*

Case 1.23

A 3-month-old girl presents with fever, coughing, grunting and difficulty in feeding. On examination, she is febrile, with tachypnoea, nasal flaring, chest retraction and irritability. Bilateral bronchial breathing is heard.

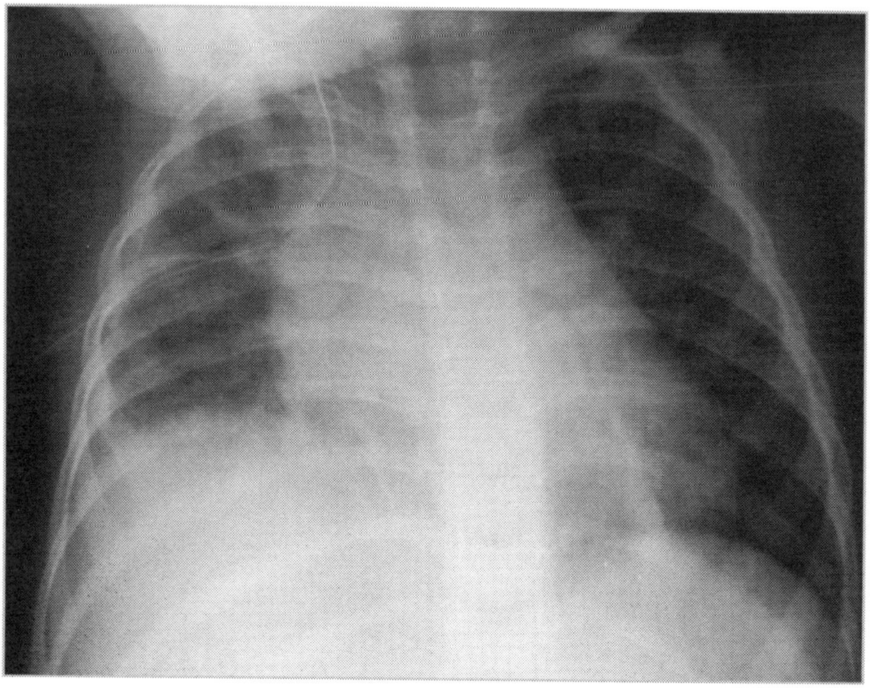

Fig 1.23

1. What can you see on the chest X-ray?
2. What is the diagnosis?
3. What is the aetiology of this disease?
4. What are the radiological features and differential diagnosis?
5. What are the clinical course and complications?

Answers *on pages 41–85*

Case 1.24

A 2-month-old child presented with recurrent cough. Clinical examination was unremarkable.

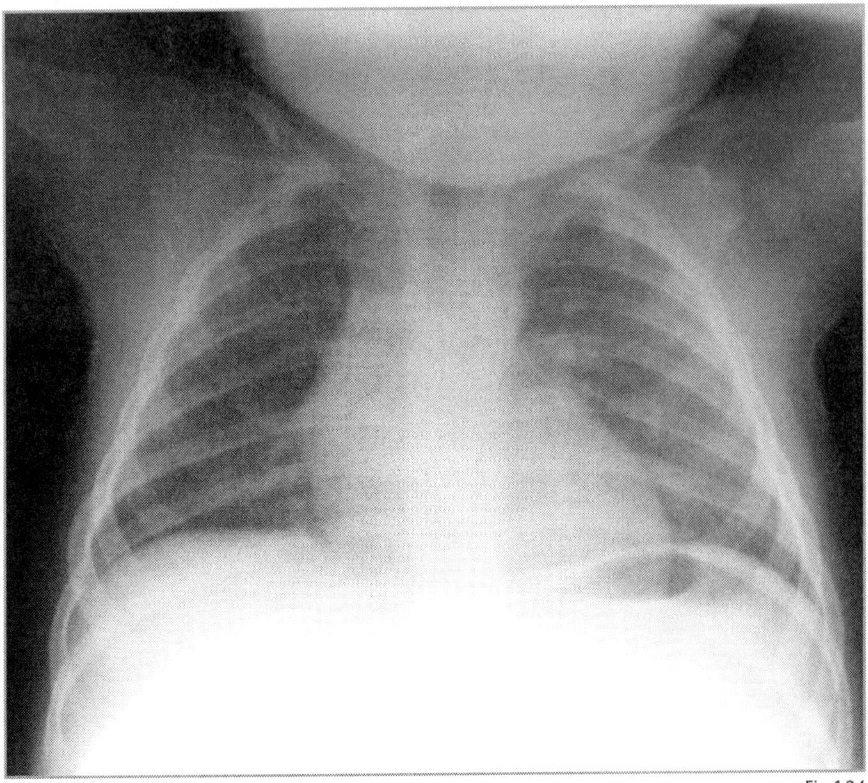

Fig 1.24

1. What do you observe on the chest X-ray?
2. What is the cause of this radiographic appearance?
3. What is the development of this condition?
4. What are the radiological features?
5. What are the complications associated with this structure?

Answers *on pages 41–85*

Case 1.25

A 15-year-old boy presents with recurrent bouts of productive cough and fever. On examination, he is febrile and had bronchial breathing and crackles in the bases.

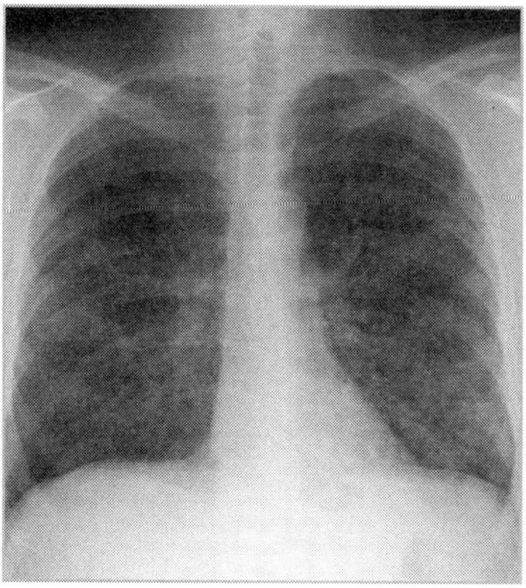

Fig 1.25a

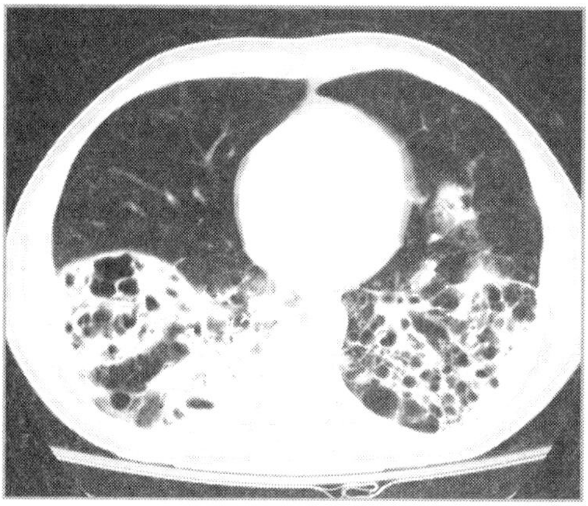

Fig 1.25b

1. What are the findings on the chest X-ray?
2. What is the second investigation and what do you note?
3. What is the diagnosis?
4. What is the classification of this disease?
5. What are the common causes?
6. What is the common radiological differential diagnosis?

Answers *on pages 41–85*

Case 1.26

A 2-month-old girl, born preterm, developed RDS, which was managed on an ICU with mechanical ventilation. She was showing good improvement in her condition but, at around 2 months, she showed sudden deterioration with increasing respiratory distress.

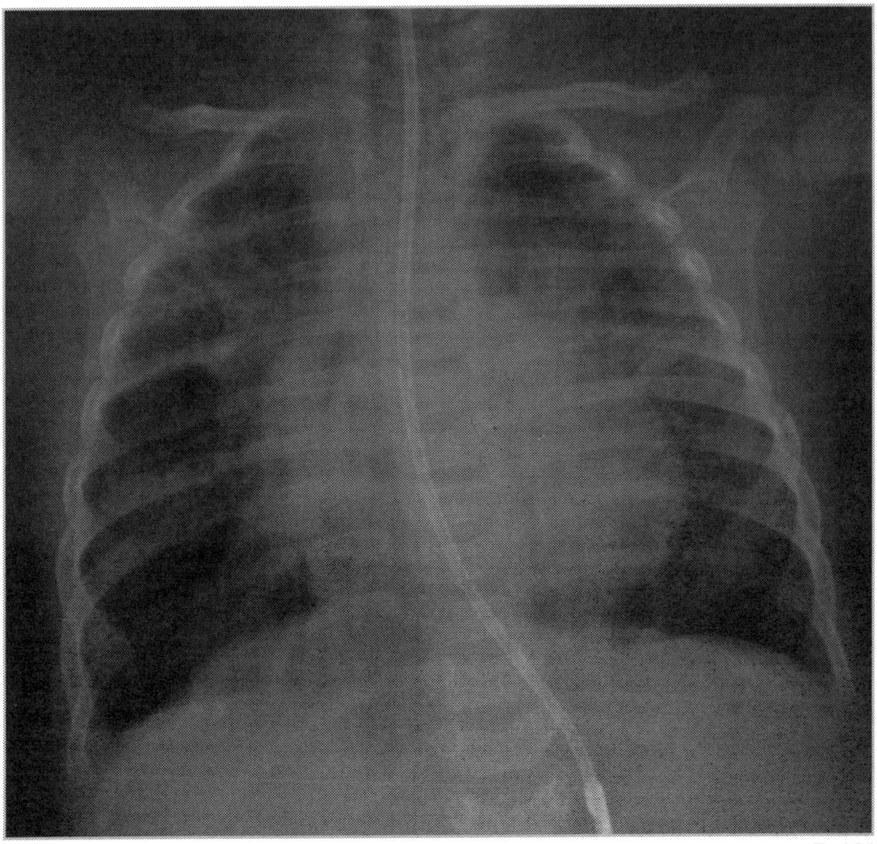

Fig 1.26

1. What can you see on the chest X-ray?
2. What is the diagnosis?
3. What are the predisposing factors for this condition?
4. What are the different stages and radiological features?
5. What are the complications and treatment of this disease?

Answers *on pages 41–85*

Case 1.27

A 4-month-old boy presents with low-grade fever, coughing and difficulty feeding. On examination, he is febrile and irritable, with tachypnoea, nasal flaring and chest retraction. Bilateral bronchial breath sounds are heard.

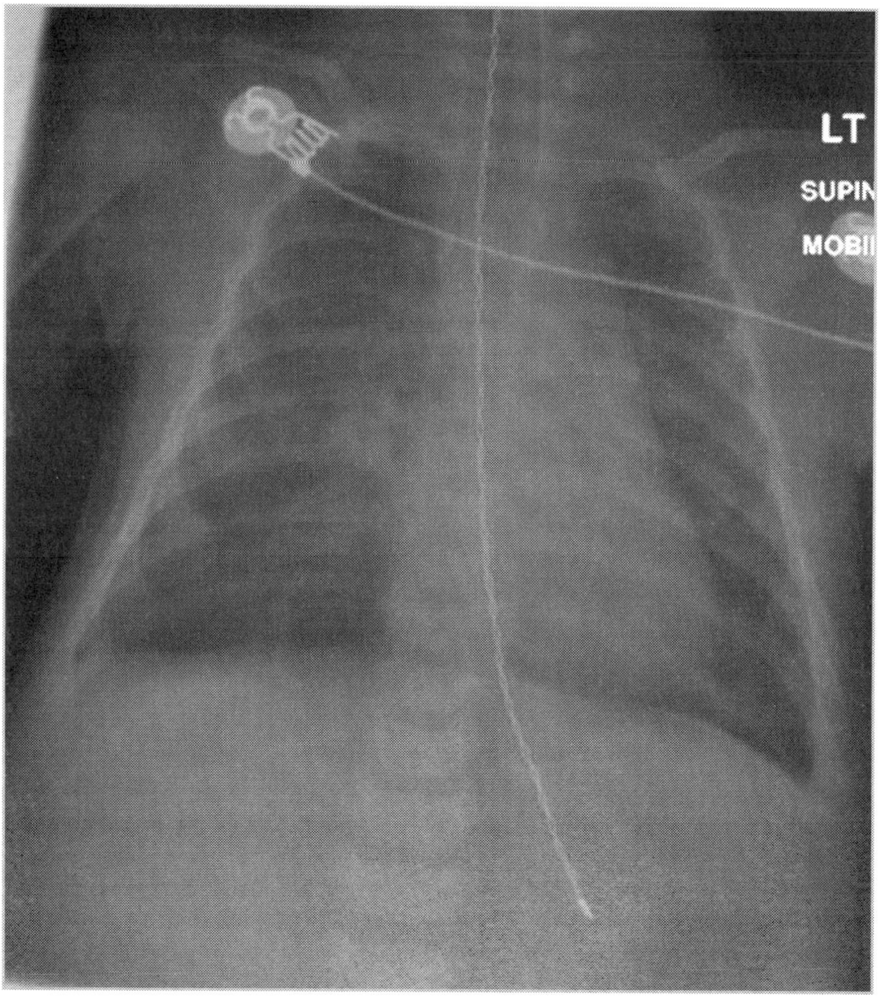

Fig 1.27

1. What can you see on the chest X-ray?
2. What is the diagnosis?
3. What is the differential diagnosis?
4. What is the aetiology of this disease?
5. What are the radiological features, clinical course and treatment?

Answers *on pages 41–85*

Case 1.28

An 8-year-old girl presents with a chronic problem and chest pain, difficulty breathing and fever. On examination there are crackles in both lungs. Breath sounds are normal.

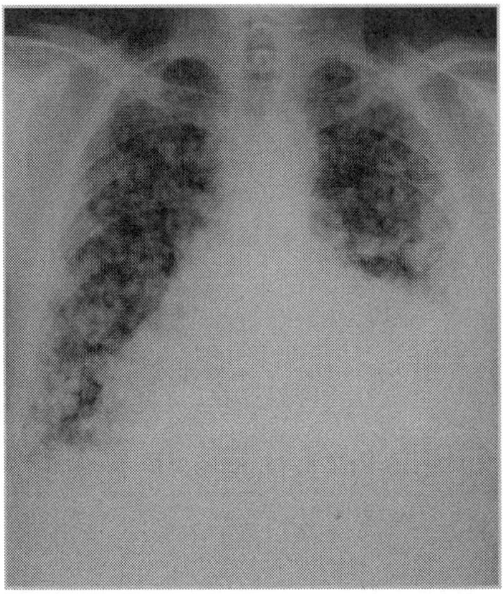

Fig 1.28a

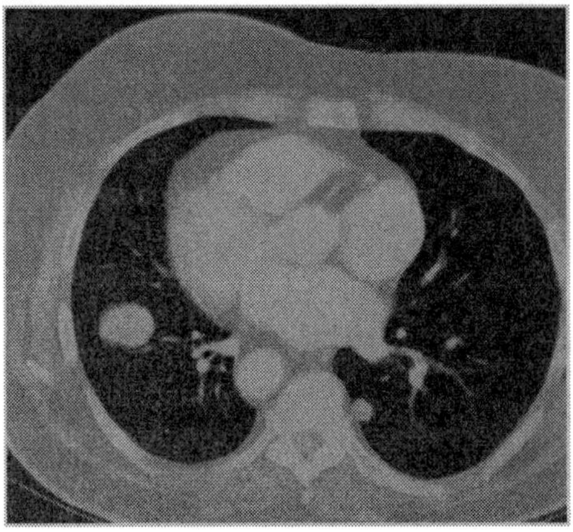

Fig 1.28b

1. What are the findings on the X-ray?
2. What are the findings on CT?
3. What is the diagnosis?
4. What are the aetiological factors?
5. What are the differential diagnosis and the variations in presentation of this disease?

Answers *on pages 41–85*

Case 1.29

A 9-year-old boy was involved in a road traffic accident and was brought to A&E with dyspnoea, chest pain, haemoptysis and respiratory distress. On examination he was haemodynamically stable and tachypnoeic, and had two rib fractures on the left side. Breath sounds were diminished on the left side.

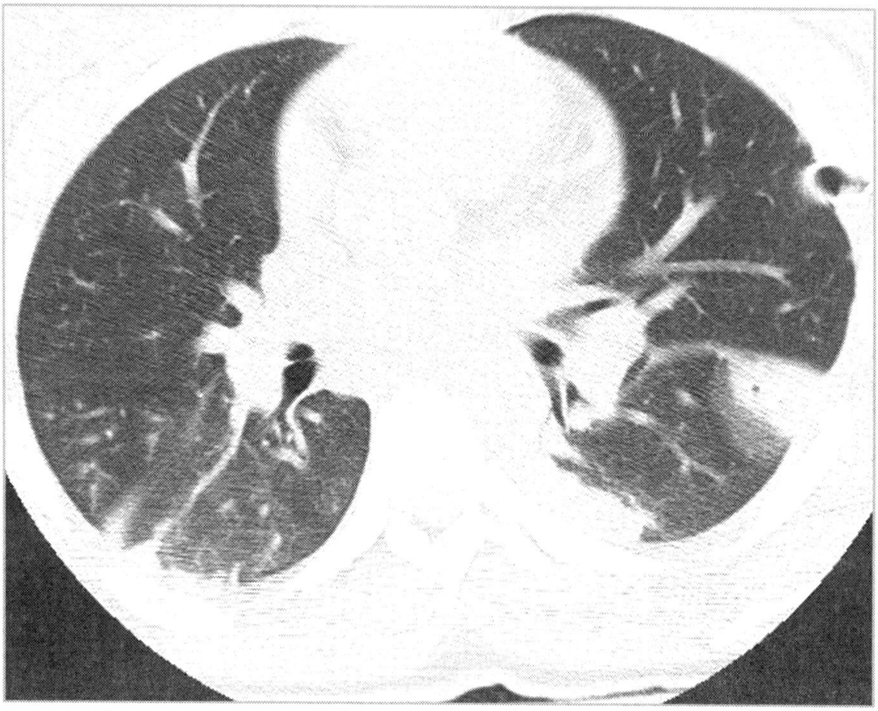

Fig 1.29

1. What do you see on the chest CT scan?
2. What is the diagnosis?
3. What is the differential diagnosis?
4. What are the radiological features and complications of this condition?

Answers *on pages 41–85*

Case 1.30

A 1-year-old girl presents with cyanosis, respiratory distress and failure to thrive. On clinical examination, the baby is cyanotic and tachypnoeic, and has features of cardiac failure.

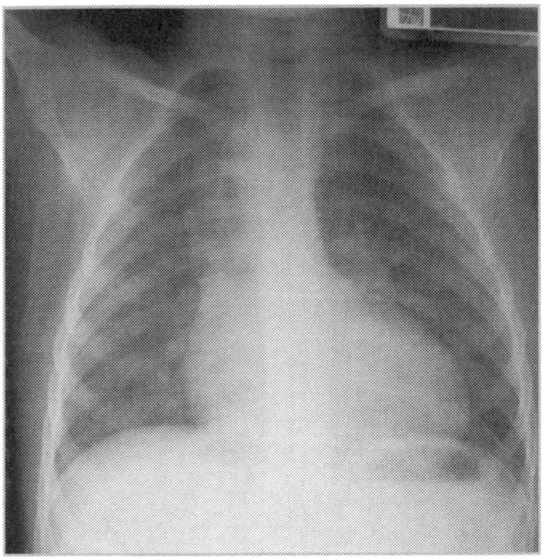

Fig 1.30a

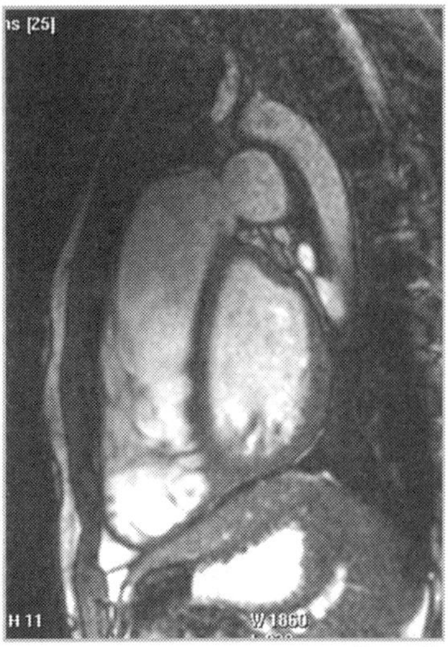

Fig 1.30b

1. What do you observe on the chest X-ray?
2. What is the diagnosis?
3. What is the second investigation and how does it help?
4. What are the physiology and clinical features of this condition?
5. What are the radiological features?
6. What are the associations and treatment?

Answers *on pages 41–85*

Case 1.31

An 11-year-old boy presents with intermittent dysphagia and frequent vomiting. Clinical examination was unremarkable.

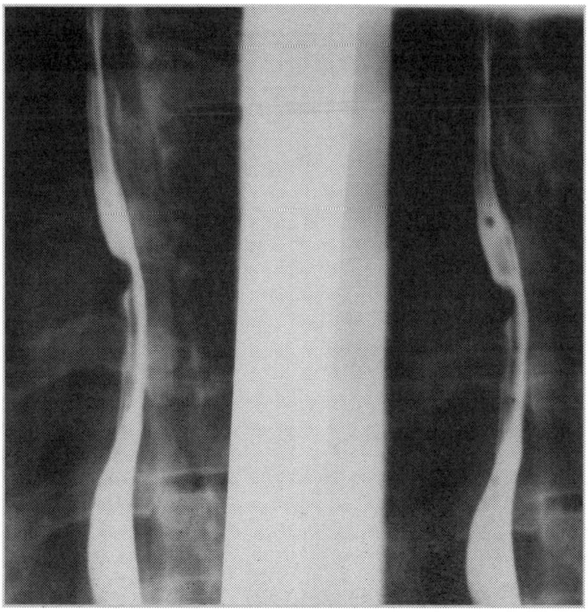

Fig 1.31a

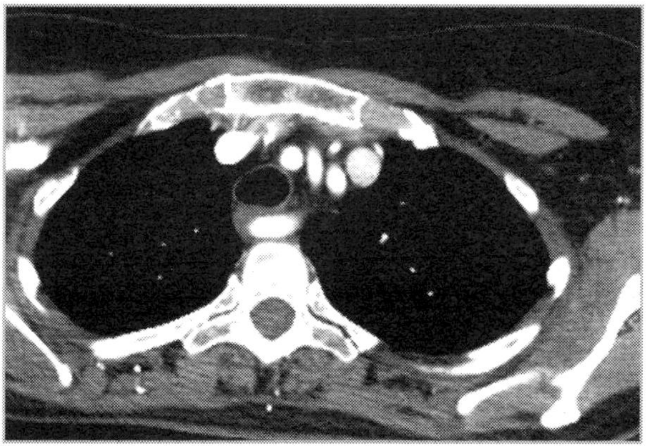

Fig 1.31b

1. What do you observe on the barium swallow and CT scan?
2. What is the diagnosis?
3. What is the development of this condition?
4. What are the types of this disease?
5. What are the clinical and radiological features?

Answers *on pages 41–85*

Case 1.32

A 10-year-old presents with chest pain, difficulty in breathing, haemoptysis and palpitations. On examination he had a palpable thrill and a loud S1. There were bilateral crackles in his lungs.

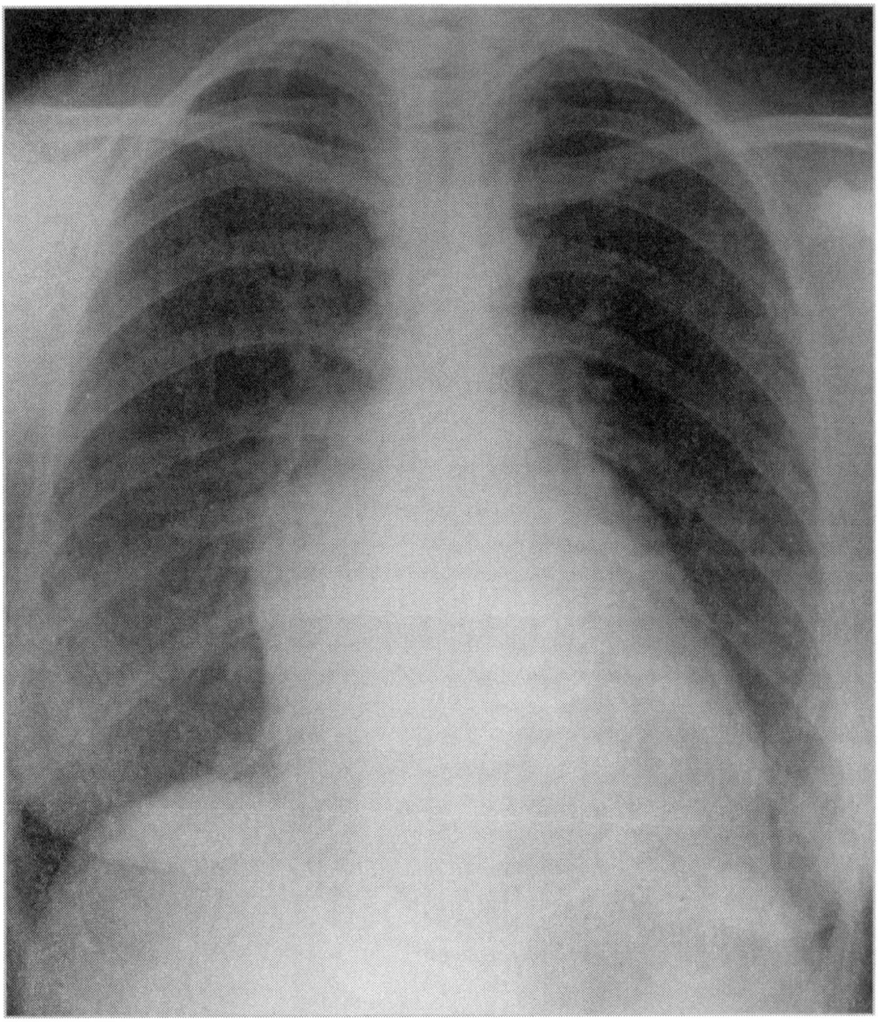

Fig 1.32

1. What do you observe on the chest X-ray?
2. What is the diagnosis?
3. What are the aetiology and clinical features of this condition?
4. What are the types and radiological features?
5. What are the complications and associations?

Answers *on pages 41–85*

Case 1.33

An 8-year-old boy presented with chest pain, headache and dyspnoea on exertion. Clinical examination revealed a systolic murmur in the cardiac apex. Blood pressure in the upper extremities was 150/110 mmHg and 140/78 mmHg in the lower extremities.

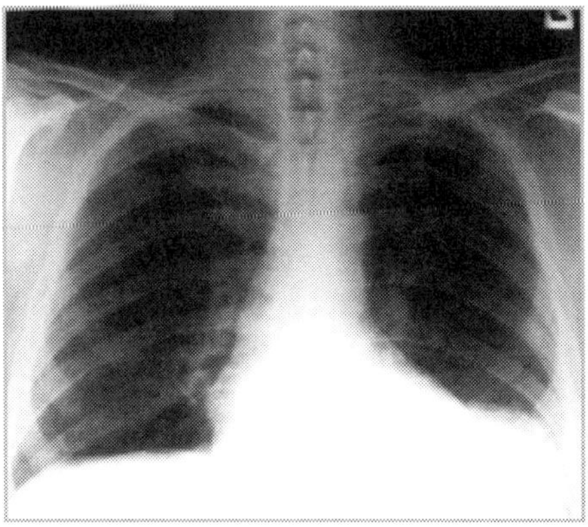

Fig 1.33a

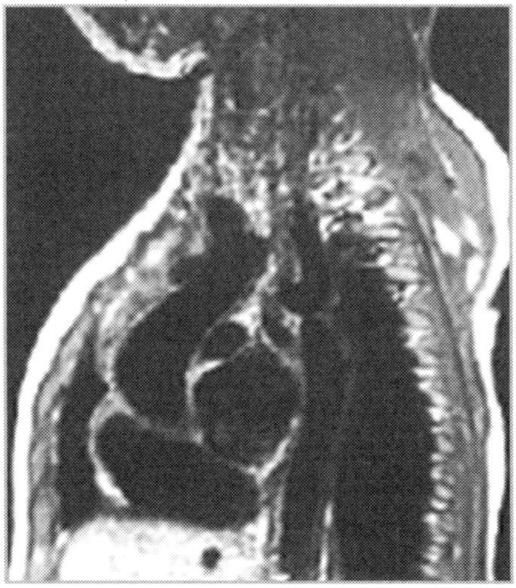

Fig 1.33b

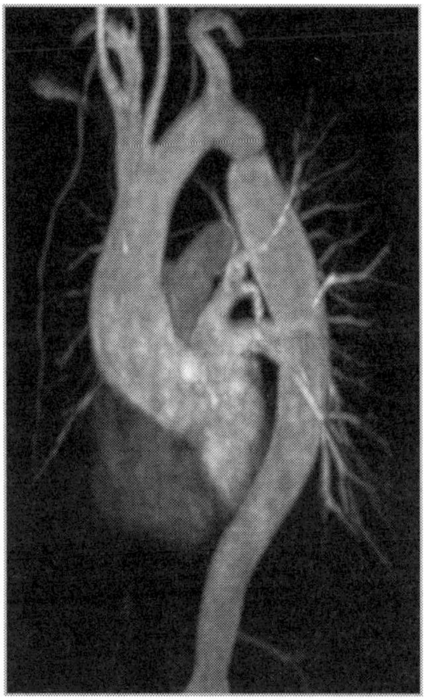

Fig 1.33c

1. What do you see on the plain film?
2. What does MRI show? What is the diagnosis?
3. What are the clinical features ad associations?
4. What are the radiological findings?
5. What is the management?

Answers *on pages 41–85*

Case 1.34

A 1-year-old girl presents with difficulty breathing, frequent respiratory infections, feeding difficulties and failure to thrive. Clinical examination revealed features of respiratory distress. A cardiac murmur was heard.

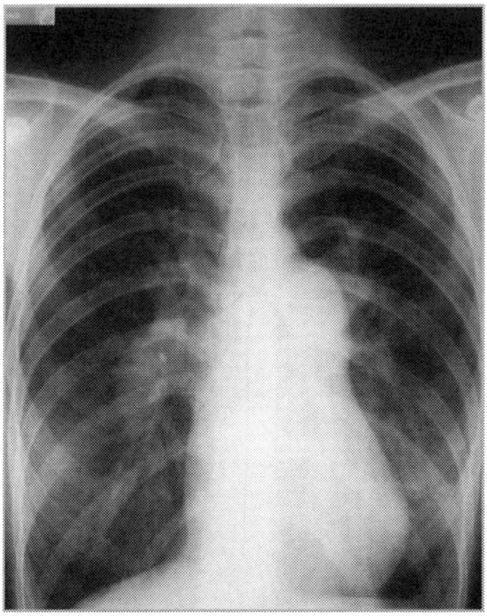

Fig 1.34a

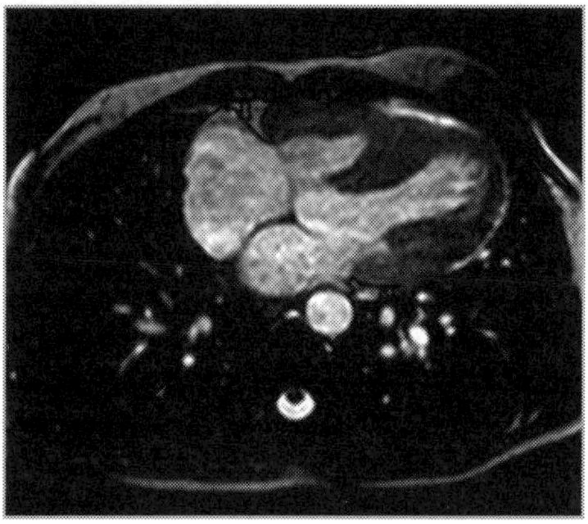

Fig 1.34b

1. What do you see on the plain X-ray of the chest?
2. What is the diagnosis? What do you see on the MR scan?
3. What are the pathophysiology and development of this condition?
4. What are the radiological features?
5. What are the clinical features and complications?

Answers *on pages 41–85*

Case 1.35

A 12-year-old girl presents with difficulty breathing and cyanosis on exertion, palpitations and frequent respiratory infections.

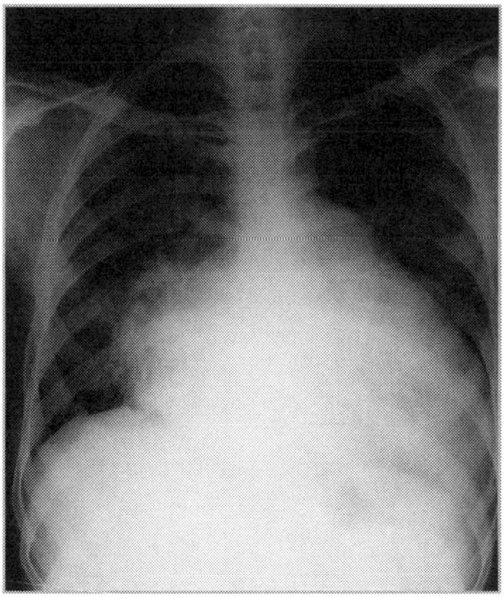

Fig 1.35a

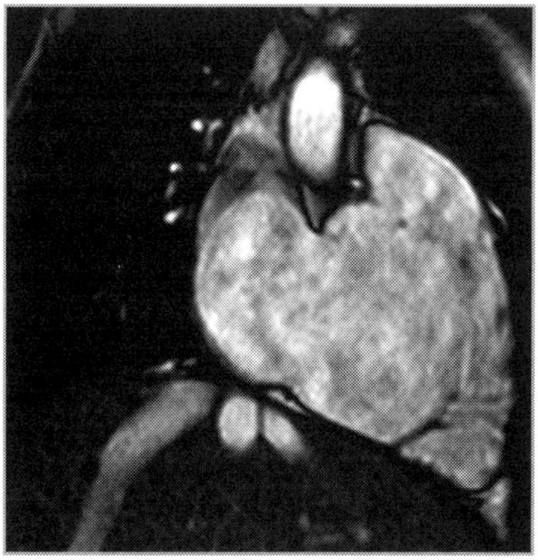

Fig 1.35b

1. What do you see on the plain X-ray of the chest?
2. What is the diagnosis? What do you see on the MR scan?
3. What is the pathophysiology and development of this condition?
4. What are the radiological features and differential diagnosis?
5. What are the clinical features and complications?

Answers *on pages 41–85*

Case 1.36

A 2-year-old girl presented with sudden onset of stridor, dyspnoea, cough and drooling of saliva. On examination, she is very tachypnoeic, pyrexial and cyanosed with severe retraction of the intercostal muscles.

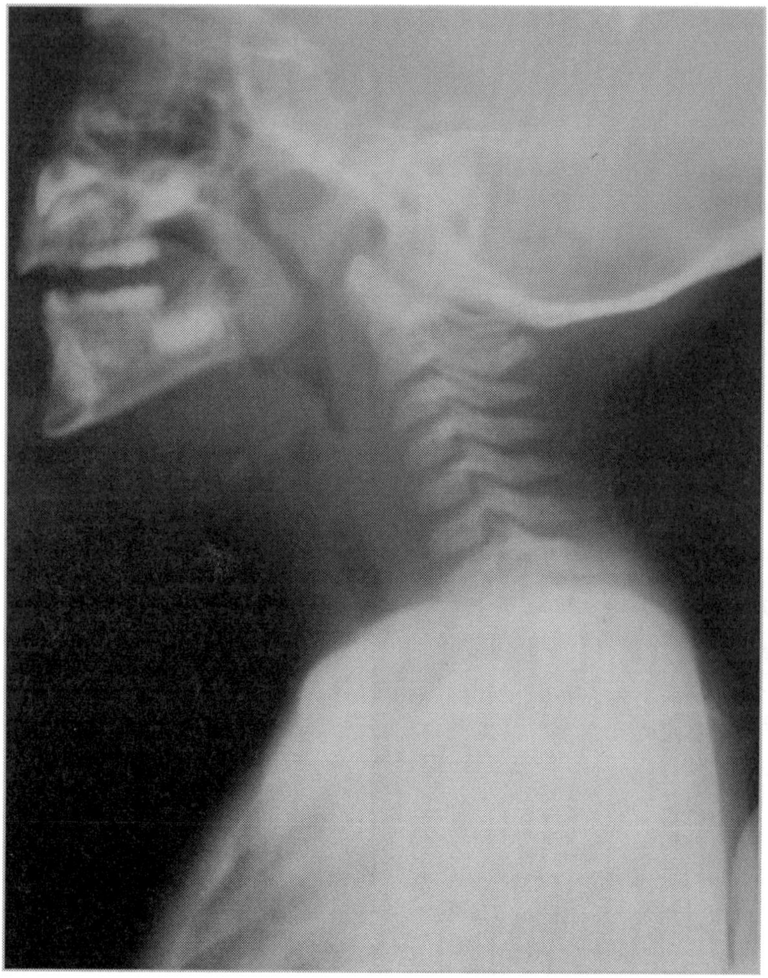

Fig 1.36

1. What do you observe on the lateral X-ray of the neck?
2. What is the diagnosis?
3. What is the cause of this condition?
4. What are the radiological features and what precautions should be taken for this patient?
5. How this condition managed and what are the complications?

Answers *on pages 41–85*

Case 1.37

A 6-year-old boy presents to A&E with sudden onset of cough, chest pain and a choking sensation. On examination, he is tachypnoeic and there are decreased breath sounds on the right side.

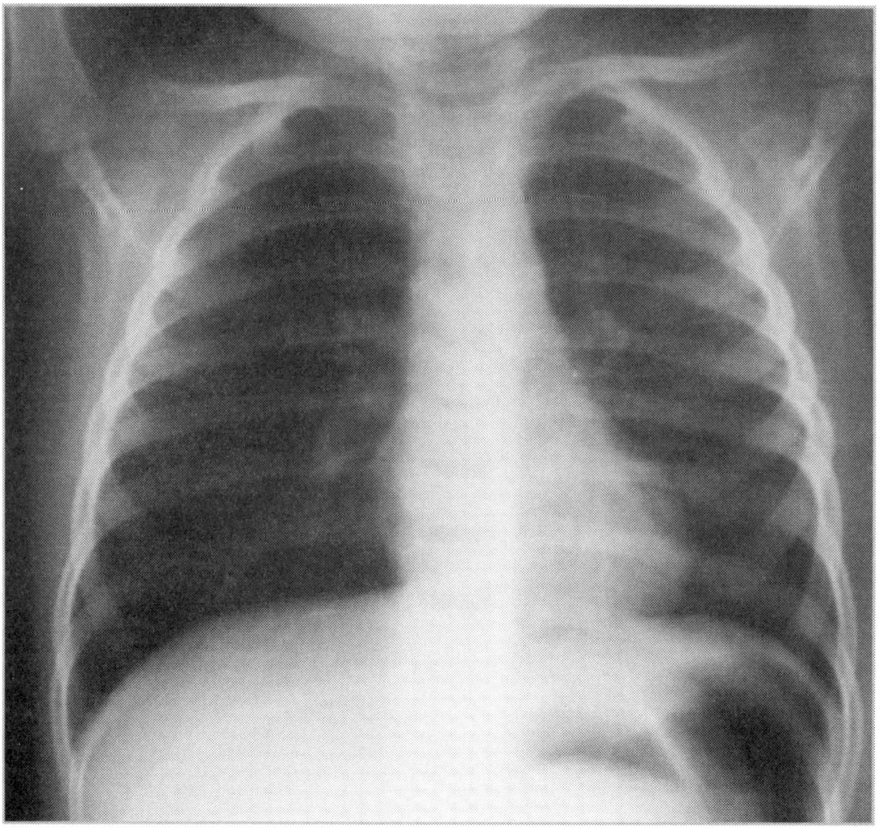

Fig 1.37

1. What do you observe on the chest X-ray?
2. What are the common causes for this appearance?
3. What are the clinical features?
4. What is the most common location?
5. What are the complications?

Answers *on pages 41–85*

Case 1.1: Answers

1. The lungs are hyperinflated and there are patchy airspace opacities scattered throughout them. In addition, there are peribronchovascular lucencies and small linear cystic areas in both lungs.

2. Pulmonary interstitial emphysema.

3. Respiratory distress syndrome (RDS).

4. Pulmonary interstitial emphysema is an accumulation of gas in the interstitial spaces, which develops as a complication of positive pressure ventilation. As a result of high pressure, the alveolar duct ruptures (usually at the junction of the bronchiole and alveolar duct) and the gas escapes into the perivascular sheath surrounding the arteries, veins and lymphatics, and tracks into the mediastinum, forming blebs. Pulmonary interstitial emphysema is bilaterally symmetrical and develops in a patient with RDS. It usually occurs early during ventilation and presents within 72 hours. It usually starts in one area of the lung and extends to involve multiple lobes, with hyperexpansion and worsening of the clinical condition. As a result of the use of surfactant, pulmonary interstitial emphysema is now less frequent. It is also seen in infants on long-term ventilator support with uneven aeration and bronchopulmonary dysplasia.

5. Pulmonary interstitial emphysema is seen as elongated, linear lucencies in the distribution of the peribronchovascular region. Subsequently these lesions become more cystic. Subpleural blebs are seen as cystic spaces. These cysts may rupture to produce pneumothorax. The lungs are hyperexpanded and the heart appears small as a result of increased intrathoracic pressure and decreased venous return. Usually it is bilateral but it can be unilateral or lobar. The differential diagnosis is bronchopulmonary dysplasia, which might present with focal areas of hyperaeration caused by partial bronchial obstruction, although the lucencies are less linear in this condition.

6. Complications are pneumothorax, pneumomediastinum, subcutaneous emphysema, pneumopericardium, pneumoperitoneum, pneumatosis intestinalis, intracardiac air and air-block phenomenon (cardiac tamponade caused by an obstruction to pulmonary venous return). Treatment is with high-frequency oscillatory ventilation with the rapid exchange of low volumes of gas at low pressure. Localised pulmonary interstitial emphysema is managed with selective intubation of the airway, bypassing the bronchus to the involved lobe.

Case 1.2: Answers

1. The X-ray shows a lobulated mass in the anterior mediastinum that is not obscuring the vascular structures, which are seen through the mass. There are also prominent masses in the parahilar region and in the right paratracheal region. The CT scan shows a lobulated mass in the anterior mediastinum, which is encasing the vascular structures, and compressing and displacing the trachea to the left side.

---

2. Lymphoma. The clinical symptoms of head and neck swelling and oedema are produced as a result of compression of the superior vena cava (SVC) by the tumour.

---

3. Lymphoma is divided into Hodgkin's and non-Hodgkin's types. Hodgkin's lymphoma is more common in the thorax than non-Hodgkin's lymphoma at presentation. There are four types of Hodgkin's lymphoma: **lymphocyte predominant**, **lymphocyte depleted**, **mixed** and **nodular sclerosing**. The nodular sclerosing type is common in the mediastinum. Non-Hodgkin's lymphoma is classified into low-, intermediate- and high-grade lesions, according to the Working classification. According to the WHO (World Health Organization) classification, they are classified into B-cell, T-cell and natural killer (NK) cell tumours, Hodgkin's lymphoma and other minor groups.

---

4. In the chest, lymphoma commonly affects the anterior mediastinum, and the pretracheal, hilar, subcarinal, axillary, perioesophageal, paracardiac, superior diaphragmatic and internal mammary nodes. Hodgkin's lymphoma affects the anterior mediastinum more whereas non-Hodgkin's lymphoma affects the posterior mediastinum more.

---

5. As mentioned above, the X-ray shows a lobulated anterior mediastinal mass. Mediastinal masses produce mediastinal widening. The location in the mediastinum can be determined by the relationship with the pulmonary vasculature and adjacent structures. If pulmonary vasculature is seen through the lesion, it is either in the anterior or the posterior mediastinum. Middle mediastinal tumours obliterate the pulmonary vasculature. In posterior mediastinal lesions, the paravertebral spinal line is obliterated. A CT scan shows homogeneous, lobulated, lymph nodal masses. Calcification and necrosis are uncommon before treatment with radio- or chemotherapy. A CT scan of the chest, abdomen and pelvis is indicated for staging the disease.

6. Germ cell tumours, thymoma, metastasis, retrosternal thyroid and aneurysm are the differential diagnoses of anterior mediastinal disorders.

Case 1.3: Answers

1. The X-ray shows a well-defined, round, soft-tissue density lesion in the right midzone.

2. Round pneumonia.

3. Round pneumonia is usually seen at age < 8 years. The most common causative organism is *Streptococcus pneumoniae*. Other organisms are *Klebsiella pneumoniae, Haemophilus influenzae, Coxiella burnetii, Myocbacterium tuberculosis, Legionella pneumophila* and *Staphylococcus aureus.*

4. The pneumonia appears well defined and rounded, unlike the usual heterogeneous pattern with air bronchogram and ill-defined margins. This is a result of the pneumonia being in the early consolidative phase, which appears round because of poorly developed collateral pathways (pores of Kuhn and channels of Lambert) and closely apposed connective tissue septa and smaller alveoli. These factors work together to produce more compact confluent areas of pulmonary consolidation, without the softer margins that are evident in the typical infiltrates of pneumonia seen in adults. It is more common in the lower lobes and posterior segments. As it occurs in the early stages of infection, patients are usually asymptomatic or present with mild symptoms. Air bronchogram is occasionally seen. No calcification or cavitation is seen. With time, the round pneumonia evolves into a more typical consolidation and eventually resolves after treatment with antibiotics.

5. Most of the pulmonary masses in children are benign, such as round pneumonia and plasma cell granuloma. Round pneumonia is a common cause of pulmonary mass in children. Differential diagnoses for a well-defined mass include neoplasms (lymphoma, metastasis, hamartoma, carcinoid), inflammatory (tuberculosis [TB], histoplasmosis, coccidioidomycosis, hydatid cyst, lung abscess), congenital (sequestration, bronchogenic cyst, bronchial atresia, arteriovenous [AV] malformation), pulmonary infarct, mucoid impaction and round atelectasis.

Case 1.4: Answers

1. The chest X-ray shows bilateral diffuse reticular changes, which are predominantly seen in the central portions of the lung. There is bronchial wall thickening and dilatation, and also bilateral hilar enlargement. The CT scan shows patchy, reticular changes in the right lung.

---

2. Cystic fibrosis.

---

3. Cystic fibrosis is an autosomal recessive disease, affecting chromosome 7, which has an incidence of 1/3000 in the white population. It is caused by an abnormality of the cystic fibrosis transmembrane regulator (CFTR), which causes abnormal transmembrane transport of Na^+ and Cl^-. It is diagnosed by the sweat test when the $Cl^- > 60$ mmol/l (40–60 mmol/l is equivocal, < 40 mmol/l is negative).

---

4. Infection, inflammation, airway obstruction, bronchiectasis and cor pulmonale are the respiratory complications of cystic fibrosis.

---

5. The lungs are normal initially, but abnormal Cl^- secretion results in viscid airway mucus. Infection, inflammation and airway obstruction cause progressive small and large airway disease. Bronchial wall thickening progresses to bronchiectasis and chronic airway disease causes hyperinflation. Initial changes are hyperinflation and peribronchial thickening. Progressive air trapping with bronchiectasis may be apparent in the upper lobes. With advancing pulmonary disease, there is development of pulmonary nodules resulting from abscesses, infiltrates with or without lobar atelectasis, marked hyperinflation with flattened domes of the diaphragm, thoracic kyphosis and bowing of the sternum. Pulmonary artery dilatation and right ventricular hypertrophy associated with cor pulmonale are usually masked by marked hyperinflation. Hilar enlargement can be caused by adenopathy or pulmonary hypertension with dilated central pulmonary arteries. Increasing cardiac size indicates cor pulmonale and the prognosis is poor without transplantation. Pneumomediastinum and pneumothorax can occur. Lobar pneumonia is very rare in established cases and the chest X-ray does not reflect clinical changes in acute exacerbations.

6. There are many scoring systems. A commonly used scoring system is the Northern score. The lung is divided into upper and lower zones. Each zone is scored 0–4 based on radiological findings (1 minimal increase in linear markings and/or nodular cystic lesions < 0.5 cm; 2 more pronounced linear markings and/or more widespread nodular cystic lesions; 3 prominent increase in linear markings, profuse nodular cystic lesions, large areas of collapse/consolidation; 4 little or no area of normal lung). A further 0–4 points are allocated according to overall perception of severity. The maximum score is 20. This allows assessment of both acute changes and additional complications such as hilar adenopathy, cardiac size, hyperinflation and pneumothorax.

Case 1.5: Answers

1. On the chest X-ray, the heart is located on the right side. There is also opacification of the right lower zone. The left lung appears normal.

2. High resolution CT (HRCT) confirms the presence of dextrocardia. There are dilated bronchi in the right lower lobe. The bronchi are also thickened with mucus plugging within them, and there are patchy opacities in the right lower lobe.

3. Kartagener syndrome.

4. Kartagener syndrome, also called immotile cilia syndrome, is caused by deficiency of dynein arms of cilia, which causes immobility of respiratory auditory and sperm cilia, and is inherited in an autosomal recessive fashion. It is characterised by the triad of situs inversus, chronic sinusitis and bronchiectasis. The typical ciliary axoneme consists of two central microtubules surrounded by nine microtubular doublets. Each doublet has an A subunit and a B subunit attached as a semicircle. A central sheath envelops the two central microtubules, which attach to the outer doublets by radial spokes. The outer doublets are interconnected by nexin links, and each A subunit is attached to two dynein arms that contain adenosine triphosphatase (ATPase) – one inner arm and one outer arm. The primary function of the central sheath, radial spokes and nexin links is to maintain the structural integrity of the cilium, whereas the dynein arms are responsible for ciliary motion. Clinically, the patients have chronic mucoid rhinorrhoea, recurrent chronic sinusitis, recurrent otitis media, chronic bronchitis, recurrent pneumonia, bronchiectasis, obstructive lung disease, digital clubbing and infertility.

5. The X-ray shows thoracic and abdominal situs inversus, bronchiectasis, sinus hypoplasia and mucosal thickening. Saccharine test and biopsy can be done for confirming the ciliary dysmotility. Antibiotics are given for infections. Tympanostomy is done for otitis media. Functional endoscopic sinus surgery is done for chronic sinus problems. Bronchodilators are given for obstructive lung disease.

Case 1.6: Answers

1. The chest X-ray shows opacification and volume reduction of the right lung. The heart and mediastinum are displaced to the right side and there is herniation of overinflated left lung to the right side. There is a long, linear band extending in a vertical direction in the right middle and lower lobes.

2. Scimitar syndrome. This is a combination of pulmonary hypoplasia and partial anomalous pulmonary venous drainage. In these patients, both the right pulmonary veins (superior and inferior) drain to the inferior vena cava (IVC) via a descending vein coursing parallel to the right heart border. This condition is commonly associated with right lung hypoplasia of variable degree.

3. Pulmonary hypoplasia contributes to 15–20% of neonatal deaths. It can be primary (10%) or associated with conditions causing restricted lung growth or reduced breathing as a result of primary pulmonary malformation. Common causes include **oligohydramnios** (renal agenesis, urinary obstruction, prolonged rupture of membranes), **abnormalities causing compression of developing lung** (diaphragmatic hernia, pleural effusions or chondrodysplasia) or **disorders impairing fetal breathing** (anencephaly, neuromuscular disorders). It can be seen on antenatal ultrasonography. In bilateral pulmonary hypoplasia, the chest is bell shaped. The lungs may have a normal appearance or there can be associated generalised lung shadowing. Primary unilateral hypoplasia, also called hypogenetic lung, is often isolated and asymptomatic. Secondary hypoplasias are associated with diaphragmatic hernia/cystic adenomatoid malformation/oesophageal atresia/tracheo-oesophageal fistula.

4. Scimitar syndrome has a variable presentation. Common presentations are dyspnoea, tachypnoea, respiratory distress, cyanosis, failure to thrive or cardiac failure. It can be asymptomatic. Clinical findings are a shift in heart sounds and cardiac impulse to the right side and a systolic murmur. Breath sounds may be diminished on the right side.

5. On X-rays, the normal lung is normally aerated and herniates with the mediastinum to the opposite side, with no evidence of aerated lung in the opposite side. The CT scan confirms the appearance. In scimitar syndrome, there is hypoplasia of the right lower lobe with an associated abnormal pulmonary venous drainage that drains into the IVC. This abnormal vein has the appearance of a scimitar on a chest X-ray. Differential diagnoses for this appearance are total collapse/consolidation of the left lung, pneumonectomy, hypoplasia and agenesis.

Case 1.7: Answers

1. There is a homogeneous opacity in the left lung. There is volume reduction on the left side and tracheal deviation to the left side.

2. The tip of the endotracheal tube is positioned within the right main bronchus, instead of its normal position, which is 2 cm proximal to the carina. The right lung is inflated, but the left lung has collapsed because it is not being aerated.

3. The endotracheal tube should be repositioned to 2 cm proximal to the carina.

4. Atelectasis can be caused by intrinsic or extrinsic airway obstruction or compression of the lung. Intrinsic airway obstruction is the most common cause. Asthma, bronchiolitis, aspiration, endobronchial TB, aspiration from gastro-oesophageal reflux, foreign bodies, cystic fibrosis and increased airway secretions are the common causes of intrinsic obstruction. This is most common in the right middle lobe because it is the narrowest and surrounded by lymphoid tissue. Extrinsic compression is caused by enlarged lymph nodes such as TB, lymphoma and other tumours, or an

enlarged heart compressing the left main or left lower lobe bronchus, and left-to-right cardiac shunts that increase blood flow through pulmonary arteries. Hypoventilation for prolonged periods such as those with surgery, neuromuscular disease or dysmorphic chest walls also results in lung collapse. Compressed lung tissue occurs in pleural effusion, pneumothorax, empyema, chest wall masses, cardiomegaly or intrathoracic abdominal contents. In children, when the airways are obstructed, atelectasis develops because the interairway canals of Lambert or pores of Kuhn are not fully developed.

5. The X-ray shows volume reduction, mediastinal deviation and increased opacification in the lung or the lobe or segment involved. A CT scan can be used to find the cause of obstruction. Bronchoscopy is useful for distinguishing intrinsic and extrinsic obstruction and to take a tissue biopsy. Differential diagnosis for opacification with volume loss include atelectasis, hypoplasia, agenesis and pneumonectomy. Pneumonia, pleural effusion and tumour can produce opacity without volume loss.

Case 1.8: Answers

1. The chest X-ray shows multiple small nodules in both lungs. There is no pleural effusion. The heart is normal.

2. An HRCT scan shows multiple, well-defined, tiny nodules in all the lobes.

3. Miliary TB. This is the widespread dissemination of *Mycobacterium tuberculosis* from haematogenous spread and is better described as acute disseminated TB. Following exposure and inhalation of TB bacilli into the lung, a primary pulmonary complex is established and pulmonary lymphangitis and hilar lymphadenopathy develop. Mycobacteraemia and haematogenous seeding occur after the primary infection. After initial inhalation of TB bacilli, miliary TB may occur as primary TB or it may occur years after the initial infection.

4. Classic miliary TB is defined as millet-like (1–5 mm) seeding of TB bacilli in the lung. This pattern is seen in 1–3% of all TB cases. Miliary TB may occur in an individual organ (very rare, < 5%), in several organs, or throughout the whole body (> 90%), including the brain. The infection is characterised by a large number of TB bacilli, although it may easily be missed and is fatal if untreated. On postmortem examination, multiple TB lesions are detected throughout the body in organs such as the lungs, liver, spleen, brain and others. Up to 25% of patients with miliary TB may have meningeal involvement. In addition, miliary TB may mimic many diseases, so a high index of clinical suspicion is important to obtain an early diagnosis and ensure improved clinical outcomes. Signs and symptoms include weakness, fatigue, weight loss, headache, fever, cough, lymphadenoapthy, hepatomegaly, splenomegaly and malaise. The erythrocyte sedimentation rate (ESR) is elevated and there can be leukopenia or leukocytosis. Cultures for mycobacteria are positive. Tuberculin testing is usually negative. Sputum for acid-fast bacilli and culture, tuberculin skin test and blood culture are needed for confirmation.

5. Classically, it appears as multiple, small, well-defined nodular opacities, 2–3 mm in size, throughout both lungs, but it may also show patchy consolidation or reticulonodular opacities. An HRCT scan also shows tiny nodules diffusely scattered in the lung. Successful treatment allows the lung changes to resolve completely with no residual abnormality. Early empirical treatment is required to avoid mortality. For susceptible organisms, this is carried out for 6–9 months and for meningeal involvement for 9–12 months. Steroids are given for hypotension caused by adrenocortical insufficiency.

Case 1.9: Answers

1. The X-ray shows enlargement of the soft-tissue space anterior to the cervical spinal vertebrae, with anterior displacement of the vertebrae.

2. Acute retropharyngeal abscess.

3. Retropharyngeal abscess forms in the retropharyngeal space, which is posterior to the pharynx, and bound by the buccopharyngeal fascia anteriorly, prevertebral space posteriorly and carotid sheaths laterally. It extends superiorly to the base of the skull and inferiorly to the mediastinum. Infection develops secondary to lymphatic drainage or continuous spread of upper respiratory or oral infections. Pharyngeal trauma from endotracheal intubation, endoscopy, foreign body ingestion and removal causes an abscess. It is more common in those who are immunocompromised or chronically ill. An abscess in this space is caused by *Staphylococcus aureus*, *Haemophilus* spp., β-haemolytic streptococci, *Bacteroides* spp., peptostreptococci, *Fusobacterium* and *Prevotella* spp., and coagulase-negative staphylococci. Clinical features are sore throat, fever, neck stiffness, odynophagia and cough. In infants, fever, neck swelling, poor oral intake, rhinorrhoea, lethargy and cough are seen. Complications are airway obstruction, mediastinitis, aspiration pneumonia, epidural abscess, jugular venous thrombosis and erosion into the carotid artery

4. In the lateral view of the neck, there is enlargement of the retropharyngeal space (> 7 mm at C2 and > 22 mm at C6). Gas or a foreign body can be seen. On a CT scan, a hypodense lesion with rim enhancement is seen in the retropharyngeal space, with mass effect on adjacent structures. Similar appearances are seen on MRI. A chest X-ray may show aspiration pneumonia.

5. In patients presenting with airway obstruction, oxygen is given and endotracheal intubation/cricothyrotomy performed. Definitive treatment is drainage. Antibiotics are used. Grisel syndrome is a non-traumatic rotatory subluxation of C1 over C2, caused by inflammation in the pharyngeal or retropharyngeal space. The inflammatory process leads to hyperaemia in the paravertebral tissues, causing progressive decalcification of C1 and C2, and subsequent weakening of ligamentous insertions of the transverse ligament into C1. Infection spreads through the pharyngovertebral veins that drain the pharynx into the periodontal venous plexus.

Case 1.10: Answers

1. The lateral view of the X-ray shows a radio-opaque foreign body in the throat.

2. Foreign body in the throat: part of a wishbone of a chicken.

3. Foreign body ingestion is common in children, with most children being in the 18–48 month age group. Children typically ingest objects that they pick up and place in their mouths such as coins, buttons, marbles, crayons and similar items. The oesophagus has three areas of narrowing: the upper oesophageal sphincter (cricopharyngeus), the crossover of the aorta at the level of the T4 vertebra and the lower oesophageal sphincter.

Seventy per cent of children have entrapment of foreign bodies at the level of the upper oesophageal sphincter. Older children present with foreign body sensation (scratches or abrasions to the mucosal surface of the oropharynx create a foreign body sensation), discomfort, dysphagia or drooling. Gagging, vomiting and throat pain are seen if the foreign body moves down into oesophagus. Chronic foreign bodies can present with poor feeding, irritability, failure to thrive, fever, stridor or pulmonary symptoms.

4. The X-ray of the neck is very useful in diagnosis of a foreign body and localising the site of entrapment. X-rays are not useful if the foreign body is not radio-opaque. Of swallowed bones 20–50% are visualised on X-rays. Coins are usually seen in a coronal alignment in an anteroposterior (AP) radiograph. If the foreign body is in the trachea, it is oriented in the sagittal plane because the tracheal rings are incomplete in the posterior aspect. A barium swallow or CT scan can be done if there is ingestion of non-opaque foreign bodies, such as plastic objects, toothpicks or aluminium drink can tabs.

5. Complications of oropharyngeal foreign bodies are abrasions, lacerations, punctures, abscesses, perforations and soft-tissue infections. Oesophageal foreign bodies can produce similar complications with pneumomediastinum, mediastinitis, pneumothorax, pericarditis or tamponade, fistulae or vascular injuries. In stable patients, direct and indirect oropharyngeal examination and fibreoptic nasopharyngoscopy are performed and foreign bodies removed. If a foreign body is sharp, elongated or multiple, endoscopic removal is done. Airway management is indicated when patients present with airway compromise, drooling, inability to tolerate fluids or with sepsis, perforation or active bleeding. Button battery ingestion is an emergency, because necrosis of the oesophageal wall can occur in hours and hence should be removed at the earliest. If the foreign body is located in the stomach, it can be allowed to pass with follow-up radiographs in 24–48 hours.

Case 1.11: Answers

1. The X-ray shows hyperexpanded right lung, with a large lucent area in the lower lobe. The trachea is shifted to the left side. The CT scan shows hyperlucent, avascular area with a very thin wall in the right lower lobe, with displacement of the mediastinal structures to the left side.

2. Congenital lobar emphysema.

3. Congenital lobar emphysema is caused by progressive overdistension of one or more pulmonary lobes but usually not the entire lung. It is idiopathic in 50%, but can be caused by airway obstruction with a valve mechanism (bronchial cartilage deficiency or immaturity, mucus, web, stenosis or extrinsic compression). Congenital lobar emphysema has two forms: **hypoalveolar** (fewer than expected number of alveoli) and **polyalveolar** (greater than expected number of alveoli). It is associated with patent ductus arteriosus (PDA) and ventricular septal defect (VSD) in 10%. In the first few days of life it can be seen as alveolar opacification because there is no clearance of lung fluid through the bronchi. It maybe asymptomatic in neonates, but becomes symptomatic later in life. It can be detected on antenatal ultrasonography, with an overdistended fluid-filled lung lobe. Children present with respiratory distress or recurrent respiratory infections. Surgical resection is the definitive treatment.

4. The common locations are: left upper lobe (40%), right middle lobe (35%) and right upper lobe (20%). X-rays show a hyperlucent lobe with contralateral mediastinal shift. Attenuated vasculature is noted. Compression of the remaining lung, flattened diaphragm and widened intercostal spaces are noted. Contralateral mediastinal shift or lung herniation is seen. The appearance of the lobe is unchanged on expiration (unlike foreign body inhalation) or in the decubitus position.

5. Differential diagnoses for this appearance are cystic adenomatoid malformation, congenital diaphragmatic hernia (bowel loops can be traced going into abdomen), pneumothorax (no vascular markings seen), Swyer–James syndrome (secondary to viral infection, small hyperlucent lung, pruning of peripheral pulmonary vasculature) and inhaled foreign body (change in appearance in expiration and inspiration).

Case 1.12: Answers

1. The X-ray shows multiple lucencies in the left thoracic cavity with shift of the mediastinum to the right side. There is a paucity of bowel loops in the abdomen.

2. Congenital diaphragmatic hernia.

3. The types are:

Bochdalek's hernia (90%), with a defect in the pleuroperitoneal canal, seen posteriorly; 75% are left sided; contains stomach/colon/small intestine/spleen/pancreas/kidneys. Right-sided hernias are difficult to detect because of echogenicity of the liver and lung. The herniated bowel loop frequently malrotates.

Morgagni's hernia (10%): seen on anterior and right side, at costophrenic angle; contains omentum or colon; associated with accompanying anomalies.

Eventration: caused by absence of muscle in the dome of the diaphragm.

Associated with trisomies 13, 18, congenital cytomegalovirus (CMV), rubella, arthrogryposis multiplex congenita and pulmonary hypoplasia. Rarely congenital **hiatus herniation** of the stomach can be seen. There is an association with De Lange syndrome and familial cases have been reported. The incidence of diaphragmatic hernia is 1 in 2000–3000 births. Children present with respiratory distress.

4. On the X-ray, the lungs are multicystic and the hemidiaphragm is not visualised. Mediastinal shift is seen to the opposite side. There is a paucity of bowel loops in the abdomen. The stomach is more centrally placed than normal. Diagnosis becomes difficult when there is no gas in bowel loops or herniation of liver or solid viscera, in which case there will be homogeneous opacification that needs to be differentiated from fluid or mass. Herniation of bowel loops can be confirmed by contrast examination, which opacifies the bowel loops in the chest. Differential diagnosis for this appearance are congenital lobar emphysema (hyperexpansion of single lobe, attenuated vascular markings), cystic adenomatoid malformation, congenital diaphragmatic hernia (bowel loops can be traced going into the abdomen), pneumothorax (no vascular markings seen), Swyer–James syndrome (secondary to viral infection, small hyperlucent lung, pruning of peripheral pulmonary vasculature) and inhaled foreign body (change in appearance in expiration and inspiration).

5. The mortality rate is 60% and higher when associated with other abnormalities, such as neural tube defects and pulmonary hypoplasia. Poor outcomes are seen when the stomach herniates (indicates herniation at earlier stage of gestation and hence more pulmonary hypoplasia), there is associated pneumothorax or it is right sided. Aerated ipsilateral lung and aerated contralateral lung > 50% are favourable features. Complications are pulmonary hypoplasia, gastric volvulus, midgut malrotation and volvulus, gastric or intestinal perforations, hypoplastic left ventricle, pleural effusion and lateral renal hypertrophy. Treatment is by surgery. Fetal surgery can be performed to reduce the development of pulmonary hypoplasia. Emergency postnatal surgical reduction can be performed. Surgery can also be performed with a delay of 24 hours to 10 days, during which time the baby is stabilised and a nasogastric tube is used for decompression of the bowel. Some surgeons prefer to operate on these neonates when normal pulmonary artery pressure is maintained for at least 24–48 hours based on echocardiography. Postoperative pneumothorax is common and occasionally a chest tube is required.

Case 1.13: Answers

1. The X-ray shows low-volume lungs with heterogeneous granular opacities and air bronchogram. There is no pleural effusion or pneumothorax.

2. Respiratory distress syndrome.

3. RDS/hyaline membrane disease/surfactant deficiency disorder is an acute lung disease of the newborn preterm infant as a result of a deficiency of surfactant, which causes poor pulmonary compliance, atelectasis, decreased gas exchange, and severe hypoxia and acidosis. The lack of surfactant and the resultant poor compliance of the lungs produce debris, consisting of damaged or desquamated cells, exudative necrosis and leaked protein, which lines the alveolar sacs. Symptoms occur within 2 hours of life. The incidence depends on the gestational age at birth. HMD (hyaline membrane disease) tends to occur in neonates younger than 32 weeks' gestational age and weighing < 1200 g, of mothers with diabetes, after caesarean delivery, second born of twins or with a family history. Secondary surfactant deficiency is seen in intrapartum asphyxia, pulmonary infection, haemorrhage, meconium aspiration and oxygen toxicity to the lungs.

4. Radiological findings: any opacity in the chest of a preterm infant is considered an RDS, unless proved otherwise. The lungs are ground-glass opaque or reticulogranular, which is the characteristic appearance. Lung volumes are low as a result of atelectasis. A bell-shaped thorax is seen if not intubated. Air bronchograms are seen within the opacities. There is no consolidation or pleural effusion. In RDS, symptoms of respiratory distress appear shortly after birth and always within the first 8 hours of life. Increased pulmonary vascular resistance develops because of a non-compliant lung, hypoxia and acidosis, which increases right-to-left shunt through a PDA. The symptoms of RDS usually peak by the third day, and may resolve quickly when diuresis starts and infants begin to need less oxygen and mechanical ventilation. Complications are seen in those who receive mechanical ventilation. The complications are pulmonary interstitial emphysema, acquired lobar emphysema. bronchopulmonary dysplasia and PDA (normally closes within 1–2 days after birth). The role of the radiologist is to follow the X-rays serially and detect the development of complications.

5. Differential diagnoses for neonatal respiratory distress are RDS, transient tachypnoea of the newborn (TTN), meconium aspiration syndrome and neonatal pneumonia.

Disease	Time course	X-ray	Lung volume
RDS	4–6 days	Granular	Low
TTN	< 48 hours	Linear, streaky	High or normal
Meconium aspiration	At birth	Coarse, patchy	Hyperinflation
Neonatal pneumonia	Variable	Granular	High or low

Case 1.14: Answers

1. The X-ray of the chest shows a round mass in the right parahilar region, behind the right atrial shadow. The lungs are normal.

2. The CT scan shows a well-defined, hypodense, mediastinal cyst that is seen just inferior to the carina and posterior to the left atrium. The margins of this lesion are well defined and there is no invasion of adjacent structures. There is no wall calcification.

3. Bronchogenic cyst. Differential diagnoses for a cystic lesion include pericardial cyst, necrotic lymph node and lung abscess. Differential diagnoses for a solid lesion include lymphoma and TB.

4. Bronchogenic cyst is a type of bronchopulmonary foregut malformation in which a supernumerary lung bud develops below the normal lung bud in between week 26 and week 40 of gestation. Other diseases in this spectrum are sequestration, congenital cystic adenomatoid malformation and congenital lobar emphysema. The location and communication with the gastrointestinal tract depends on when in embryonic life the bud develops. Most malformations present clinically when they become infected.

5. The cysts are well defined, lined by columnar respiratory epithelium and filled with mucoid material. They are seen in the mediastinum in 85% (posterior > middle > anterior mediastinum) and in the lungs in 15%. The classic appearance is a well-defined round mass in the subcarinal or parahilar region. Intrapulmonary bronchogenic cysts are usually seen in the medial third of the lung. The cysts are thin walled and can be fluid or air filled. Most of the cysts are asymptomatic, but they can produce fever and dyspnoea if infected and stridor or dysphagia caused by mediastinal compression. CT shows a well-defined, non-enhancing cystic lesion. It can be seen as a well-defined non-enhancing solid lesion if the contents are mucoid. Calcification can be seen. On MRI, the cyst is usually bright on T2, but can be dark or bright on T1, depending on the content.

Case 1.15: Answers

1. The CT scan shows a well-defined area of consolidation in the right lower lobe, adjacent to the paravertebral region. This is well seen in the mediastinal and lung windows. Coronal view from an MR angiography shows a blood vessel arising from the right side of the distal abdominal aorta and coursing superiorly and laterally above the level of the diaphragm to supply posteromedial segment of the right lower lobe.

2. Intralobar sequestration.

3. Sequestration can be intralobar or extralobar.

4. Pulmonary sequestration is an embryonic mass of lung tissue that has no identifiable bronchial communication and receives its blood supply from one or more anomalous systemic arteries. Multiple feeding vessels may be present. This congenital anomaly can be classified as extralobar sequestration (ELS) or intralobar sequestration (ILS). ILS is seen in older children or adults and is located within the pleura. It usually presents as an airless consolidation type or an air-containing cystic type. It is supplied by the thoracic or abdominal aorta and drained by the pulmonary vein. It is associated in 10% with skeletal anomalies, foregut anomalies and diaphragmatic anomalies. ELS is seen in neonates, is located outside the lung and has its own pleural covering. It is always airless unless it communicates with the gastrointestinal tract. It can be seen in the abdomen. It is supplied by the thoracic or abdominal aorta and has systemic venous drainage to the IVC, azygos or portal vein. Associated anomalies are seen in 65% and can be diaphragmatic defect, pulmonary hypoplasia, bronchogenic cyst or cardiac anomalies. They present earlier, as a result of the presence of associated anomalies. Clinically it presents with recurrent infection, lung abscess, bronchiectasis or haemoptysis.

5. Sequestrations are usually seen in the posteromedial segment of the lower lobe and are more common on the left side than the right. The X-ray shows a well-defined mass or cyst if the sequestration is uninfected. When infected, the sequestration is seen as an ill-defined consolidation with or without air–fluid levels and parapneumonic effusion. CT or magnetic resonance angiography (MRA) is used to define the arterial and venous drainage. Differential diagnoses for the radiological appearance include lung abscess, empyema. Bochdalek's hernia, neurogenic tumour, meningocele, pleural tumour and extramedullary haematopoiesis.

Case 1.16: Answers

1. The X-ray of the chest shows an area of heterogeneous opacification in the medial aspect of the left upper lobe. There are also patchy opacities. The CT scan of the left upper lobe shows an area of consolidation in the left upper lobe, with areas of ground-glass opacity surrounding it.

2. Fungal infection.

3. Fungal infections account for 25–30% of all pneumonias in bone marrow transplant recipients. Aspergillus infection is seen in 10% of all allogeneic bone marrow transplants. It can occur at any time after transplantation, but is one of the most common infections in the early period. Risk factors for development are neutropenia in the early stages and steroid treatment for graft-versus-host disease (GVDH) in the later stages. Complications after bone marrow transplantation occur in specific phases. The pre-engraftment period (first 15–30 days), between stem cell transfusion and restoration of haematopoiesis, is characterised by severe pancytopenia. The early post-transplantation phase (30–100

days) begins after successful engraftment of donor stem cells and resumption of haematopoiesis Although neutropenia resolves by this time, lymphocyte recovery lags behind. The late post-transplantation period (> 100 days) is characterised by normal lymphocyte levels, but recovery of humoral immunity lags behind. Early complications in the lung are interstitial pneumonitis (infective and non-infective), infection, oedema, haemorrhage, thromboembolism, calcification and bronchiolitis obliterans.

4. Complications in other systems are:

Gastrointestinal tract: GVDH, neutropenic colitis, hepatic veno-occlusive disease, abscesses, post-transplantation lymphoproliferative disorder, hepatic regenerative nodules

Genitourinary tract: abscesses, haemolytic uraemic syndrome, papillary necrosis, renal vein thrombosis, nephrolithiasis, haematoma and haemorrhagic cystitis

Musculoskeletal system and kidney: bone infarction, avascular necrosis

Central nervous system (CNS): infection, infarction, haemorrhage, therapy-induced toxic effects and recurrent malignancy.

On the X-ray and CT scan, aspergillus infections are seen as peripheral pulmonary nodules. One of the characteristic signs is a hazy ground-glass opacity surrounding the nodule, which is caused by haemorrhage around a central infarction as a result of vascular invasion of *Aspergillus* spp. The nodules cavitate when the neutrophil count recovers. Pleural effusions and lymphadenopathy are uncommon findings. Differential diagnoses are bacterial pneumonias (unusual in the early phase in spite of bacteraemia as a result of the empirical use of broad-spectrum antibiotics), pulmonary oedema (prominent pulmonary vasculature, increased interstitial markings, and peribronchial thickening, perihilar shadowing, pleural effusions and airspace opacification), diffuse alveolar haemorrhage (patchy or diffuse airspace consolidation and ground-glass opacification) and interstitial pneumonias (CMV, *Pneumocystis jirovec*, adenovirus, idiopathic causes – interstitial septal thickening, nodules, ground-glass opacities, patchy opacification).

Case 1.17: Answers

1. The X-ray shows a homogeneous consolidation in the left upper zone, with an air bronchogram within it. There is no mediastinal shift and there is no blunting of the costophrenic angle.

2. Lobar consolidation with pneumonia.

3. In children, 30% of pneumonias are caused by *Mycoplasma pneumoniae.* Viral infections account for 65% and are more common in those aged > 3 years. Bacterial pneumonias account for less than 5%. Bacterial pneumonias are caused by *Haemophilus influenzae* (infancy), pneumococci (1–3 years) and staphylococci (infancy).

4. Recurrent infections in children indicate underlying causes such as cystic fibrosis, recurrent aspirations, immunodeficiencies, sequestration, bronchogenic cysts, hypogammaglobulinaemia, hyperimmunoglobulinaemia E and Kartagener syndrome.

5. The usual radiological findings are an alveolar opacity, which has ill-defined margins with an air bronchogram. The consolidation can be segmental or lobar. Effusions can be associated. *Mycoplasma pneumoniae* has four patterns:

(a) bronchopneumonia in single lower lobe (lobar consolidation is rare)

(b) plate-like atelectasis

(c) nodular infiltration

(d) hilar adenopathy and pleural effusions.

HRCT can be used when the diagnosis is in doubt. Pneumatoceles are seen in staphylococcal infection. Viral infections can present as bronchiolitis with a normal X-ray or bronchiolitis with parahilar or peribronchial opacities, atelectasis, reticulonodular interstitial opacities or hazy lungs. Differential diagnoses of consolidation are pulmonary oedema, pulmonary haemorrhage, aspiration and lymphoma. Aspiration pneumonia has a characteristic distribution. In the supine position, it is seen in the upper lobe and superior segments of the lower lobes. In the upright position, it is seen in both lower lobes and associated with segmental and subsegmental atelectasis, interstitial fibrosis or inflammatory bronchial thickening. In pulmonary oedema, the heart is enlarged with prominent septal thickening and pleural effusions. Haemorrhage is difficult to differentiate from the other conditions.

6. Complications of pneumonia are pneumothorax, bronchiectasis, bronchiolitis. obliterans, necrotising pneumonia, abscess, acute respiratory distress syndrome (ARDS), respiratory failure and Swyer–James syndrome (small, hyperlucent lungs with decreased vascular markings). Extrapulmonary complications of *Mycoplasma* spp. include pericarditis, arthritis, Stevens–Johnson syndrome, haemolytic anaemia, thrombocytopenia, CNS infections, Guillain–Barré syndrome and peripheral neuropathy. Antibiotics are administered depending on the organism. *Mycoplasma pneumoniae* is confirmed by a cold agglutination test or the polymerase chain reaction (PCR). Erythromycin, azithromycin, clarithromycin and tetracycline are used for treatment of mycoplasma infection.

Case 1.18: Answers

1. The plain X-ray of the chest shows a large area of homogeneous consolidation in the right upper lobe and there is prominent right upper paratracheal and hilar lymph nodes.

2. Primary complex.

3. Primary complex is caused by *Mycobacterium tuberculosis* and is commonly seen in infants and children. Most of these patients are asymptomatic. Symptoms include fever, chest pain, cough and haemoptysis. Pathologically, primary complex is characterised by a small area of peripheral consolidation from which bacteria drain to the regional nodes. Normally immunological changes lead to arrest of the progress of infection and healing by fibrosis with or without calcification. If immunity fails, an extensive area of consolidation develops. Tuberculomas are caused by recurrent attacks of progression and arrest. Pleural effusion is produced by a subpleural focus and might be the only feature of this disease.

4. If the disease is arrested in the early stages, there are no radiological findings. A skin test is positive. Scarring and calcifications in the lungs and nodes can be seen. Active consolidation is usually located in the middle lobe, but can also be seen in the lower lobes and anterior segment of the upper lobes. The characteristic appearance is a focal, well-defined,

homogeneous, dense consolidation associated with hilar, paratracheal or subcarinal lymphadenopathy (80% are located on the right side). The consolidation can range from 10 mm to lobar. Cavitation is rare in primary TB, unlike post-primary TB. Atelectasis is seen in the anterior segment of the upper lobe or medial segment of the middle lobe as a result of endobronchial TB or extrinsic compression by lymph nodes. Pleural effusion can be seen. Enlarged nodes can be seen without underlying lung changes. The nodes can be unilateral hilar, unilateral hilar with right paratracheal, right paratracheal only or bilateral asymmetrical hilar nodes. The nodes can narrow airways, causing obstructive overinflation or collapse. Miliary TB is seen with haematogenous dissemination. Erosion of the node into the pericardium produces pericarditis and effusion. Erosion into the pleura produces pleural effusion, which might be an isolated finding. Involvement of the phrenic and recurrent laryngeal nerves produces paresis. Large nodes can cause SVC obstruction. Tuberculomas are well defined, round and nodular, and may show calcification.

5. The combination of an area of consolidation and a mediastinal/hilar node in a child is fairly specific for TB. Differential diagnoses for lung nodules in children are histoplasmosis, varicella and haemosiderosis. Differential diagnoses for lymph nodes are metastasis, lymphoma and histoplasmosis. Differential diagnoses for consolidations are pneumonias and lymphoma.

6. Variant lesions are: **ghon focus** – calcified lung lesion/scar < 5 mm; **Ranke's complex** – ghon lesion and calcified node; and **Simon's focus** – healed site of primary infection at apex. Multiple discrete nodules can also be seen. Complications are bronchopleural fistula, empyema and fibrosing mediastinitis. Progressive primary TB is seen if the immune reaction is inadequate. Miliary TB can be seen. Post-primary TB is reactivation TB after years of dormancy.

Case 1.19: Answers

1. The X-ray shows a mass in the right side. The pulmonary vasculature can be seen through the mass and there is silhouetting of the paravertebral stripe, indicating that the lesion is in the posterior mediastinum. In the CT scan, there is a large hypodense mass in the posterior mediastinum and right paravertebral region. The underlying posterior rib is expanded and dysplastic. The mass appears homogeneous with deformity of the ribs.

2. The CT scan confirms the mass to be located in the posterior mediastinum. In addition, the mass appears well defined and cystic, and there are deformed posterior ribs.

3. Neurofibroma. This is a nerve sheath tumour that is made up of neuronal elements containing Schwann cells, nerve fibres, fibroblasts and collagen. It is commonly seen at age 20–30 years in the spine and in an intradural extramedullary location. It is more common at the cervical and thoracic levels. Other locations are in the peripheral nerves. Neurofibroma is associated with neurofibromatosis type 1. Spinal neurofibroma is a sign of neurofibromatosis 1.

4. A large neurofibroma is seen as a paraspinal mass on an X-ray. In the chest, the ribs are dysplastic and ribbon shaped. MRI shows a well-defined mass with a dumb-bell configuration, which widens the intervertebral foramen with scalloping or erosion of the pedicles. On MRI the lesion is a homogeneous mass, isointense to muscle in T1 and hyperintense in T2. A target sign is characterised by a low signal centre in T2 as a result of collagen and condensed Schwann cells. There is not much contrast enhancement. CT shows a homogeneous, hypodense, dumb-bell lesion that does not show contrast enhancement. Occasionally soft-tissue nodules are seen in the subcutaneous plane.

5. Cord compression can be seen in large tumours and malignant transformation is rare. The most common differential diagnoses are meningioma (not dumb-bell, hyperdense, contrast enhancement), metastasis, dermoid, lipoma, ependymoma and neurenteric cyst.

Case 1.20: Answers

1. The CT scan shows a well-defined, multilocular, cystic lesion in the periphery of the left lower lobe.

2. Congenital cystic adenomatoid malformation.

3. Congenital cystic adenomatoid malformation is the proliferation of polypoid glandular lung tissue without normal alveolar differentiation. There is no bronchial cartilage or glands. The types are:

Type 1: one or more, 2–10 cm, large cysts accompanied by small cysts, with walls containing muscle, elastic or fibrous tissue, lined by mucin-producing pseudostratified columnar cells

Type 2: small cysts, 0.5–2.0 cm, uniform, with cuboidal columnar cell lining and thin fibromuscular wall. They are usually confined to one hemithorax and have a better prognosis

Type 3: microscopic adenomatoid cysts – seen as homogeneous echogenic mass without discernible individual cysts. This can be confused with pulmonary sequestration or diaphragmatic hernia and is less common.

Congenital cystic adenomatoid malformation is believed to result from focal arrest in fetal lung development before week 7 of gestation secondary to a variety of pulmonary insults. Depending on the time and type of insult, 4–26% of cases can be associated with other congenital abnormalities. Congenital cystic adenomatoid malformation differs from normal lung tissue because of a combination of increased cell proliferation and decreased apoptosis. A well-defined intrapulmonary bronchial system is lacking, and normally formed bronchi supplying the mass are absent. They receive their blood supply from the pulmonary circulation. The lobes are enlarged with displacement of structures to the opposite side.

---

4. Congenital cystic adenomatoid malformation can be diagnosed on antenatal ultrasonography. On plain X-rays, it is seen as multiple cystic pulmonary lesions of varying sizes, which shift the mediastinum to the opposite side. Air–fluid levels are seen in the cysts, which show variable thickness. Most cases present in the newborn period with respiratory distress. In older children, congenital cystic adenomatoid malformation can present with recurrent infections, and occasionally is seen in early stages as a homogeneous fluid-filled mass, which clears to leave an air-filled cystic lesion. The cysts are separated from each other with strands of normal pulmonary tissue. Air trapping in the cyst can cause rapid enlargement and respiratory distress. The CT scan shows small or large multiple cysts, which can show an air–fluid level. Low attenuation cysts indicate microcysts. Surgical resection is done for treatment. Bilateral lesions result in severe pulmonary dysfunction. Removal of all lesions may not occur if multiple segments are involved.

---

5. Differential diagnoses for this appearance are congenital lobar emphysema (usually in left upper lobe, large cyst, without discernible wall), congenital diaphragmatic hernia (bowel loops can be traced going into abdomen) and pneumothorax (no vascular markings seen)

Case 1.21: Answers

1. The chest X-ray shows a well-defined, thin-walled, lucent lesion in the right middle zone. There are no other changes in the lung or heart.

2. Pneumatocele.

3. The common cause for a pneumatocele in a child is *Staphylococcus aureus*. Other causative organisms are *Streptococcus pneumoniae*, *Haemophilus influenzae*, *Klebsiella pneumoniae*, *Serratia marcescens*, *Escherichia coli*, group A streptococci, *Mycobacterium tuberculosis*, *Pseudomonas aeruginosa* and adenovirus. Non-infectious aetiologies include hydrocarbon ingestion, trauma and secondary to positive pressure ventilation. There is increased association with Job syndrome.

4. Pneumatoceles are thin-walled, air-filled cysts developing within the lung parenchyma. They are usually seen after development of consolidation in the lungs (5–7 days), but occasionally they are the first radiological finding. Initially, pneumatoceles were thought to be caused by a ball-valve mechanism in the bronchi as a result of inflammation and narrowing of bronchus or rupture or a peribronchial abscess into the lumen, which leads to distal dilatation of bronchi; alveoli pneumatoceles are caused by bronchial inflammation rupturing the bronchiolar walls, resulting in the formation of 'air corridors'. Air dissects down these corridors to the pleura and forms pneumatoceles – a form of subpleural emphysema. It is common in infants and children < 3 years. Clinical features are cough, fever and respiratory distress. Fever, respiratory distress, grunting, nasal flaring and retractions are noted. Decreased breath sounds and crackles are heard. Treatment of the underlying pneumonia with antibiotics is the first line of therapy. Close observation in the early stages of the infection and periodic follow-up care until resolution of the pneumatocele are usually adequate treatment. The natural course of a pneumatocele is slow resolution with no further clinical sequelae. Complications are tension pneumatocele, pneumothorax and secondary infection.

5. Differential diagnoses for a thin-walled cystic lesion in a child include loculated pneumothorax, congenital diaphragmatic hernia, congenital lobar emphysema, cystic adenomatoid malformation, congenital cyst and bronchogenic cyst.

Case 1.22: Answers

1. There is homogeneous opacification of the left side of chest, which appears completely white. There is mediastinal shift to the right. The right lung is normal.

2. The second investigation is a CT scan. There is a fluid density in the left hemithorax, with a fluid level. There is no air in the pleural cavity.

3. Pleural effusion. The differential diagnoses for a homogeneous opacification of lung are consolidation (no mediastinal shift), collapse (mediastinal shift to same side), agenesis (mediastinal shift, compensatory inflation on opposite side), mass and radiation.

4. Causes include:

Increased hydrostatic pressure: congestive cardiac failure, constrictive pericarditis

Decreased colloid oncotic pressure: cirrhosis, nephritic syndrome, hypothyroidism

Chylous effusion: infections, empyema, parapneumonic effusion, TB, *Actinomyces* spp., hydatid, amoebiasis, *Mycoplasma* spp.

Tumours: metastasis, lymphoma

Vascular: pulmonary embolus (PE)

Abdominal diseases: pancreatitis, oesophageal perforation, subphrenic abscess, abdominal tumour with ascites, bile fistula

Collagen vascular diseases: juvenile rheumatoid arthritis (JRA), systemic lupus erythematosus (SLE), Wegener's granulomatosis, mixed connective tissue disease

Miscellaneous: trauma, drugs, uraemia.

5. Causes of exudates:

Pleural fluid protein/serum total protein > 0.5

Pleural fluid/serum lactate dehydrogenase (LDH) > 0.6

Pleural fluid LDH > two-thirds of upper limit of normal, for serum LDH

Pleural fluid protein > 3 g/dl

Pleural fluid specific gravity > 1.016

Effusion has internal septations or loculations

CT split pleural sign: enhancement of thickened pleural layers separated by fluid

Extrapleural fat thickening > 2 mm, with high density in the fat.

6. X-rays detect effusions when there is 300 ml fluid. Initially fluid collects in the subpulmonic space, which might not be well seen on the X-ray. The lateral decubitus view can detect 25 ml fluid. Ultrasonography can detect even smaller amounts and differentiate exudates from transudates, or effusion from consolidation. Guided aspiration of fluid can be done for diagnosis or treatment. Subpulmonic effusions can be identified by a lateral peak of the dome of the diaphragm, increased distance between the stomach bubble and lung, blunted posterior costophrenic angle, acute angled costophrenic angle, thin triangular mediastinal opacity. With increasing size of effusion, the costophrenic angles are blunted and there is homogeneous opacification of the lower lobes, with effacement of the dome of the diaphragm. There is a meniscus-shaped upper surface and associated collapse of the underlying lung. In massive effusion, the entire chest may be white and there is mediastinal shift to the opposite side along with depression, flattening or inversion of the diaphragmatic dome. Loculated effusions can be drained under ultrasonic guidance.

Case 1.23: Answers

1. The X-ray shows patchy alveolar opacities in the right lower lobe, including the right costophrenic angle. There is no hyperinflation or pneumothorax.

2. Bronchopneumonia.

3. Bronchopneumonia is a patchy consolidation involving one or more lobes, and usually the dependent lung zones, a pattern attributable to aspiration of oropharyngeal contents. The neutrophilic exudate is centred in the bronchi and bronchioles, with centrifugal spread to the adjacent alveoli. Bronchopneumonia is caused by bacteria. *Staphylococcus aureus* is the most common organism in infancy. *Haemophilus influenzae* is common in late infancy and pneumococci are the cause between age 1 and 3 years. Other infectious agents in the neonatal period include *E. coli*, *Chlamydia trachomatis* and group B streptococci. At age 1–3 months, *Strep. pneumoniae*, *Staph. aureus* and *H. influenzae* are the most common organisms. *Listeria monocytogenes* and other neonatal infectious agents are also seen. Atypical organisms include *C. trachomatis*, *Bordetella pertussis*, *Ureaplasma urealyticum*, cytomegalovirus (CMV) and *Pneumocystis jirovec* infection.

4. X-rays show patchy alveolar opacities in the peribronchovascular distribution. The HRCT scan confirms the distribution of these opacities. The differential diagnosis includes **viral infections** – bronchiolitis is the common pattern. In bronchiolitis the lungs are hyperinflated and there may be peribronchial and perihilar infiltrates and hilar adenopathy with areas of atelectasis. Reticulonodular interstitial pattern or hazy lungs can be seen. *Mycoplasma pneumoniae* presents with peribronchial and perivascular infiltrates, patchy consolidation or homogeneous acinar consolidation.

5. The child presents with tachypnoea and signs of respiratory distress, such as grunting, flaring and retraction, with lethargy, poor feeding or irritability. Fever may not be present in newborns; however, hypothermia and temperature instability may be observed. Cyanosis is seen in severe cases. Non-specific complaints such as irritability or poor feeding can be seen. Cough is unusual in the newborn period. Fine crackles and wheeze are heard. Lab tests are usually negative. Children are treated with oral antibiotics.

Case 1.24: Answers

1. The chest X-ray shows normal lungs. There is a triangular density in the superior mediastinum extending to the right side. No hilar adenopathy is visualised.

2. The plain X-ray findings are those of a normal thymus.

3. The thymus is formed along with the inferior parathyroid gland from the third and possibly fourth pharyngeal pouch at 4–5 weeks of gestation. Subsequently they separate from the pharyngeal wall and migrate caudally and medially with the thymus pulling the inferior parathyroid glands along the thymopharyngeal tract. The thymic primordium fuses with its contralateral thymus, inferior to the thyroid gland. The thymic tail thins and disappears by 8 weeks. Normal thymus increases in size from birth to puberty, after which it involutes and eventually shows fatty replacement after age 60 years.

4. The chest X-ray of a neonate often shows a prominent thymus, which should not be mistaken for a mediastinal tumour. It is seen in more than 50% of children up to the age of 2 years. The X-ray shows various signs:

Sail **sign**: a triangular density extending from superior mediastinum, to the right side

Notch **sign**: indentation at junction of the thymus and heart

Wave **sign**: rippled, undulated, lateral border resulting from indentation by the ribs. The shape of the normal thymus changes during respiration, becoming smaller in inspiration and larger in expiration. The CT scan of a normal thymus has muscular density before puberty and an increasingly fatty density after that. A normal thymus has flat or concave borders. It has an arrowhead shape in 62%, bilobed in 32% and single lobed in 6%. It measures < 18 mm before 20 years and < 13 mm after that.

5. The thymus can undergo thymic hyperplasia, atrophy and neoplasia (carcinoid, carcinoma, thymoma) and can be ectopically situated in the neck. Differential diagnoses of thymic shadow include thymic neoplasms/ hyperplasia, mediastinal mass, upper lobe pneumonia and atelectasis.

Case 1.25: Answers

1. The chest X-ray shows dilated tubular structures with thick walls in both the bases.

2. This is an HRCT scan. The HRCT imaging technique consists of obtaining 1- to 2-mm collimation scans at 10-mm intervals through the chest with a window level (WL) of −700 hounsfield units (HU) and a window width (WW) of −1000 HU. Thick-walled, dilated bronchi are seen. Note that the bronchi are larger than the corresponding vessels, which is the characteristic signet-ring appearance.

3. Bronchiectasis.

4. Bronchiectasis is localised, irreversible dilatation of part of the bronchial tree. The three main types are **cylindrical**, **varicose** and **cystic**. In the cylindrical type, there is fusiform dilatation and tramlines (parallel lines corresponding to thickened, dilated bronchi). The varicose type is seen in destroyed lung and has a varicose tortuous appearance. The cystic type is seen in destroyed lung and has a saccular dilatation, with a string-of-cysts appearance. An air–fluid level can be seen as a result of secondary infection. Bronchial thickening is seen in end-on views. Indistinct central vessels are seen as a result of peribronchovascular inflammation/fibrosis. Atelectasis is also noted. Crowding of vasculature can be seen because of volume loss caused by mucus obstruction of peripheral bronchi. Oligaemia can be seen as a result of hypoperfusion and compensatory hypertrophy can be seen in uninvolved segments. On HRCT, the internal bronchial diameter is greater than that of the adjacent artery. There is lack of bronchial tapering (the same diameter as the parent branch for > 2 cm). The bronchi are seen within 1 cm of the costal pleura or abut the mediastinal pleura. Bronchial wall thickening is seen. A cystic cluster of thin-walled cystic spaces can be present, often with air–fluid levels. In cylindrical bronchiectasis, bronchi coursing horizontally are seen as parallel lines, and vertically oriented bronchi are seen as circular lucencies that are larger than the adjacent pulmonary artery (signet-ring appearances). Varicose bronchiectasis is seen as non-uniform bronchial dilatation. Bronchial walls are thick with signet-ring sign. Areas of increased and decreased perfusion and attenuation are seen. Less common findings are tracheomegaly and enlarged mediastinal nodes. Fluid-filled bronchi are revealed as tubular or branching structures when they course horizontally or as nodules when they are perpendicular to the plane of the CT scan section.

5. Causes of bronchiectasis: postinfective (childhood infections such as TB, atypical mycobacterial infection, measles, *Klebsiella* spp., *Staph. aureus, M. pneumoniae*, pertussis, influenza, respiratory syncytial virus (RSV), herpes simplex virus [HSV], adenovirus, acute bronchopulmonary aspergillosis or ABPA), cystic fibrosis, sequestration, neoplasm, inflammatory nodes, foreign body, aspiration, William–Campbell syndrome, Mounier–Kuhn syndrome, Kartagener syndrome, Young syndrome, Swyer–James syndrome, yellow-nail syndrome, immunodeficiency, α_1-antitrypsin deficiency, traction secondary to fibrosis, lung and bone marrow transplants.

6. Differentiation of cystic bronchiectasis from the cystic spaces of honeycomb lung can be difficult. Honeycombing does not have air–fluid levels. Emphysematous changes can be differentiated from bronchiectasis because they demonstrate expiratory air trapping.

Case 1.26: Answers

1. Chest X-ray shows hyperexpansion of both the lungs. In addition, there are multiple, patchy areas of scarring in the upper lobes and cystic changes seen more on the right side.

2. Bronchopulmonary dysplasia.

3 Bronchopulmonary dysplasia is a chronic pulmonary disorder that results from the use of high positive-pressure mechanical ventilation and high-concentration oxygen in neonates with RDS. It is defined as oxygen dependence at 28 days. Bronchopulmonary dysplasia is pathologically characterised by inflammation, mucosal necrosis, fibrosis and smooth muscle hypertrophy of the airways. It is now uncommon in larger and more mature infants, gestational age > 30 weeks or weighting > 1200 g at birth. Predisposing factors are preterm delivery, high oxygen concentration, mechanical ventilation, RDS that requires mechanical ventilation, atopy, allergy, asthma, *Ureaplasma urealyticum*, air leaks, PDA, vitamin A or E deficiency, bacterial pneumonias, fluid overload and low indigenous steroid levels.

4. There are four classic stages in development, which are rarely seen now.

Stage	Time (days)	Pathology	X-ray	CT
I	< 4	Mucosal necrosis, hyaline membranes	Similar to RDS	RDS, pneumothorax, PIE
II	4–10	Necrosis, oedema, exudates, obliterative bronchiolitis	Diffuse opacities	Septal thickening, air trapping, atelectasis, consolidation, prominent pulmonary arteries, cardiomegaly
III	11–20	Bronchial metaplasia, compensatory hypertrophy, air trapping	Honeycombing, linear densities, hyperaeration	Linear atelectasis, fibrotic changes, honeycombing
IV	> 30 days	Fibrosis, emphysematous alveoli, pulmonary hypertension	Honeycombing, linear densities, hyperaeration (bubbly lungs)	Fibrotic changes, air trapping, triangular opacities, distorted architecture, bronchiectasis, bronchial thickening, tracheomegaly, pulmonary oedema

5. Cor pulmonale and recurrent respiratory infections are complications. Patients with mild bronchopulmonary dysplasia require only a few weeks of oxygenation with high concentrations. The disease resolves slowly and the clinical features progressively improve. Some patients may need prolonged oxygen therapy

Case 1.27: Answers

1. The X-ray shows hyperinflated lungs and bilateral parahilar and peribronchial opacities.

2. Bronchiolitis. This is an acute, infectious, inflammatory disease of the upper and lower respiratory tracts that results in obstruction of the small airways. Pathologically, necrosis of the airway epithelium, proliferation of goblet cells, epithelial regeneration with non-ciliated cells and lymphocytic infiltration are seen. The pathology results in obstruction of bronchioles from inflammation, oedema and debris, leading to hyperinflation, increased airway resistance, atelectasis and ventilation–perfusion mismatching.

3. Bronchopneumonia. Patchy alveolar peribronchial opacities are seen and there is no hyperinflation.

4. Bronchiolitis is caused by RSV (75%). Other organisms that may cause bronchiolitis are parainfluenza, influenza, adenovirus, *Mycoplasma pneumoniae* and human metapneumovirus. Infants are affected most often because of their small airways, high closing volumes and insufficient collateral ventilation. Recovery begins with regeneration of bronchiolar epithelium after 3–4 days, but cilia do not appear for up to 2 weeks. Predisposing factors are low birthweight, lower socioeconomic group, crowded living conditions, daycare, parental smoking, chronic lung disease (particularly bronchopulmonary dysplasia), severe congenital or acquired neurological disease, congenital heart disease with pulmonary hypertension, and congenital or acquired immune deficiency diseases. Virtually all children experience RSV infection within the first 3 years of life, but previous infection does not convey complete immunity. Boys are more commonly affected. Infants may become increasingly fussy, with difficult feeding, low-grade fever, coryza and congestion. Of primary RSV infections 60% are confined to the upper airway. Development of cough, dyspnoea, wheezing and feeding difficulties occurs with lower respiratory involvement. When the patient is brought to medical attention, the fever has usually resolved. Infants < 1 month may present as hypothermic. Severe cases progress to respiratory distress with tachypnoea, nasal flaring, retractions, irritability and, possibly, cyanosis.

5. Bronchiolitis can present with a normal chest X-ray or just overinflated lungs with flattening of the diaphragmatic domes. Occasionally parahilar and peribronchial opacities can be seen as a result of peribronchial cuffing and hilar adenopathy. Atelectasis can be seen. The WBC count is elevated. The virus can be isolated with cultures. Immunological tests such as ELISA (enzyme-linked immunosorbent assay) or IFA (immunofluorescence assay) can confirm. Bronchodilators should not be routinely used. If a trial of an α- or β-adrenergic medication is an option, it should be continued only if a positive (and continued) response is documented. Corticosteroids should not routinely be used and nor should ribavirin. Antibacterials should be used only on proven coexistence of bacterial infection. Assess hydration and the ability to take oral fluids. Supplemental oxygen should be supplied for $SpO_2 < 90\%$; saturation measurement is otherwise unnecessary. Palivizumab prophylaxis should be administered to selective children. Hand decontamination prevents nosocomial spread.

Case 1.28: Answers

1. The chest X-ray shows multiple nodules in both lungs, of various sizes.

2. The CT scan shows multiple pulmonary nodules

3. Multiple metastases

4. The common tumours that metastasise children's to lungs are osteosarcoma, Wilms' tumour, Ewing's sarcoma and rhabdomyosarcoma, testicular tumour, choriocarcinoma

5. Nodules are > 3 cm, and masses > 5 cm. **Differential diagnoses** for multiple pulmonary nodules in children:

Infective: TB, histoplasmosis, coccidioidomycosis, cryptococcosis, nocardia infection, measles, hydatid, inflammatory pseudotumour, pseudolymphoma

Tumours: metastasis, lymphoma, hamartoma

Vascular: AV malformations, pulmonary emboli, septic emboli

Collagen vascular: Wegener's disease, rheumatoid arthritis.

The following are **variations** in metastatic presentation:

Solitary pulmonary nodule: single nodule in lung

Calcifying metastasis: osteosarcoma, testicular

Cavitating: osteosarcoma; can present with pneumothorax

Haemorrhagic: fuzzy margins, choriocarcinoma

Endobronchial metastasis: lymphoma

Airspace pattern: like infection – lymphoma

Sterilised metastasis: no change in size even after adequate chemotherapy, choriocarcinoma, testicular cancer

Benign tumours with lung metastasis: chondroblastoma, giant cell tumour

Pleural metastasis: lymphoma.

Case 1.29: Answers

1. The chest CT shows an irregular area of consolidation in the periphery of the left lower lobe. A chest tube is also noted.

2. Lung contusion. This is the most common manifestation of blunt trauma to the chest. Pathologically it is characterised by oedema and blood in the airspace and interstitium. Clinically it presents with haemoptysis and is seen as early as 6 hours after trauma.

3. Pulmonary haemorrhage (larger area), infection, oedema (bilateral, batwing pattern), respiratory distress (diffuse) and fat embolism (takes 1–2 days) are the differential diagnoses.

4. The contusions are usually seen deep to the site of impact or contre coup. The X-rays show irregular patchy or diffuse homogeneous consolidation. CT is more sensitive and shows non-segmental, coarse, ill-defined, amorphous opacification. There is no cavitation. There is subpleural sparing of the 1–2 mm rim of lung tissue. Overlying rib fractures are seen. The opacity can enlarge for 48–72 hours and resolution begins from 48 hours. Complete resolution occurs in 2–10 days. Pneumothorax is a complication.

Case 1.30: Answers

1. The X-ray shows a boot-shaped heart with prominent aorta on the right side.

2. Tetralogy of Fallot with right-sided aortic arch.

3. This is MRI after surgery. MRI shows wide right ventricular (RV) outflow tract (RVOT), secondary to surgery. This patient has pulmonary regurgitation, which is a common complication after RV surgery.

4. Tetralogy of Fallot consists of infundibular pulmonary stenosis, VSD, overriding of arch of aorta and RV hypertrophy (RVH). If there is an associated atrial septal defect (ASD) as well, it is called pentalogy of Fallot. It accounts for 10% of congenital heart diseases and is the most common cause of cyanosis after 1 year. The infants usually present with cyanosis by age 3–4 months (PDA conceals cyanosis at birth). The other features are dyspnoea, cyanosis, clubbing, episodic spells of unconsciousness, squatting position when fatigued, polycythaemia, lowered PO_2 and systolic murmur in pulmonic area.

5. The radiological features of tetralogy are a boot-shaped heart as a result of the uplifting of the cardiac apex secondary to RVH and absence of a normal main pulmonary artery segment, which results in a concavity in the region of the pulmonary artery. Heart size is normal as a result of a lack of pulmonary blood flow or congestive heart failure. A decreased number and calibre of pulmonary vessels are seen. Pulmonary oligaemia is seen, which is noted as increased lucency in the lungs. Reticular opacities in horizontal distribution are seen in the periphery as a result of prominent bronchopulmonary collaterals. A right-sided aortic arch is seen in 20–25% of these patients, which indent the leftward-positioned tracheobronchial shadow. The X-ray can be normal in acyanotic tetralogy of Fallot and there may be findings of small- to moderate-sized VSD with mild RVH, right atrial enlargement and increased pulmonary vascular markings.

6. The associations are bicuspid pulmonic valve, pulmonary artery stenosis, right aortic arch, tracheo-oesophageal fistula, Down syndrome, forked ribs, scoliosis, coronary artery anomalies (single right coronary artery [RCA] or left anterior descending [LAD] artery arising from the RCA).

Treatments include palliative shunts such as the Blalock–Taussig shunt in which the subclavian and pulmonary arteries are anastomosed opposite to the aortic arch. Corrective cardiac surgery includes closure of the VSD and reconstruction of the RVOT by excision of obstructing tissue.

Case 1.31: Answers

1. The barium swallow lateral view shows a large indentation in the posterior aspect of the oesophagus. The indentation is smooth and clearly extrinsic. The mucosal surface is smooth. The CT scan shows an aberrant vascular structure extending behind the oesophagus.

2. Left-sided aortic arch with aberrant right subclavian artery and right ligamentum arteriosum, which is one of the types of vascular rings.

3. Vascular rings are unusual congenital anomalies that occur as a result of abnormalities in the development of the aortic arch and great vessels. These produce symptoms by compressing the structures encircled by them, such as the oesophagus and trachea. Symptoms include chronic stridor, wheezing, recurrent pneumonia, dysphagia and failure to thrive. A combination of X-rays and barium swallow is usually helpful in diagnosis. Direct visualisation of the aberrant vasculature is best assessed with CT and MRI with angiography. The various forms of this anomaly occur as a result of abnormal or incomplete regression of one of the six embryonic branchial arches.

4. Lesions with characteristic appearances are:

Anterior **tracheal and posterior oesophageal impression**: double aortic arch, right aortic arch with aberrant left subclavian/ductus/ligamentum, left aortic arch with aberrant right subclavian + right ductus/ligamentum

Small **posterior oesophageal impression**: left aortic arch with aberrant right subclavian artery, right aortic arch with aberrant left subclavian artery

Anterior **tracheal indentation**: innominate origin more distal along arch, left common carotid artery origin more proximal on arch, common origin of left common carotid and innominate artery

Posterior **tracheal and anterior oesophageal**: aberrant left pulmonary artery.

5. Left aortic arch with aberrant right subclavian artery is the most common congenital anomaly of the aorta. In this, the right subclavian artery arises as the fourth branch from the aorta (following the right common carotid artery, left carotid and left subclavian), crosses behind the oesophagus to the left side. It is associated with Down syndrome, absent recurrent laryngeal nerve and congenital heart disease. Although the aberrant artery usually courses behind the oesophagus, it can course between the oesophagus and trachea or anterior to the trachea. It is usually asymptomatic, but can produce dysphagia (dysphagia lusoria). A soft-tissue opacity crossing the oesophagus, obliquely upward towards the right shoulder, is pathognomonic. A mass-like opacity is seen in the right paratracheal region. A lateral X-ray may show a round opacity arising from the superior aortic margin posterior to the trachea and oesophagus. A dilated origin of the artery may be seen (Kommerell's diverticulum). Unilateral left-sided rib notching can be seen if the aberrant artery arises distal to coarctation. Only symptomatic vascular rings are treated surgically.

Case 1.32: Answers

1. The X-ray shows cardiomegaly with straightening of the left heart border and a shadow within the shadow on the right side of the cardiac contour.

2. Mitral stenosis.

3. Rheumatic fever is the most common cause of mitral stenosis. Other causes include infective endocarditis, carcinoid, eosinophilic endocarditis, rheumatoid arthritis, SLE, mucopolysaccharidosis, left atrial myxoma, thrombus congenital, Fabry's disease, Whipple's disease and methysergide therapy. Lutimbachir syndrome is a combination of mitral stenosis and ASD. Mitral stenosis leads to elevated left atrial pressure, which results in increased pulmonary vascular pressure, dilatation of the left atrium, pulmonary venous hypertension, postcapillary pulmonary arterial hypertension, RVH, tricuspid regurgitation, RV dilatation and right heart failure.

4. The X-ray shows features of left atrial enlargement – dilated left atrial appendage resulting in straight left cardiac border, **shadow within shadow**, which is double density of the left atrium within the right cardiac shadow (normal left atrium is not visualised on X-rays), splaying of the carina, displacement of the oesophagus posteriorly and to the right, and bulge of the posterior superior cardiac border below the carina. Calcification of valve leaflets is seen in 60%. The aorta can be small as a result of low cardiac output. The increased resistance results in the following stages:

Pulmonary venous hypertension (upper lobar diversion) at pressures of 16–19 mmHg

Interstitial pulmonary oedema (20–25 mmHg), which is seen as septal lines, reticular opacities and pleural effusion

Alveolar oedema (25–30 mmHg), which is seen as patchy alveolar opacities. Pulmonary arterial hypertension manifests as enlarged pulmonary arteries and peripheral arterial pruning with subsequent RVH and secondary tricuspid insufficiency

Pulmonary haemosiderosis is seen as 1- to 3-mm ill-defined nodules in the middle and lower lobes

Pulmonary ossification is seen as calcified 1- to 3-mm nodules in the middle and lower lungs.

Echocardiography is useful for assessing the morphology of the mitral valve, measuring orifice, mobility, thickness and calcification. Doppler ultrasonography is useful for quantifying haemodynamic severity.

5. Patients are asymptomatic or present with chest pain, dyspnoea, orthopnoea, paroxysmal nocturnal dyspnoea (PND), haemoptysis (rupture of anastomosis between bronchial veins) and Ortner syndrome (hoarseness of voice as a result of impingement on the left recurrent laryngeal nerve). Complications include atrial fibrillation, systemic embolism and infective endocarditis. Clinical examination reveals a palpable diastolic thrill, a loud S1 followed by S2 and opening snap and a characteristic low-pitched, mid-diastolic, rumbling murmur with presystolic accentuation, which is augmented by expiration, coughing, exercise, squatting and nitrite. Features of cardiac failure may also be seen. Definitive treatment is commissurotomy if the valves are pliable and valve replacement if not.

Case 1.33: Answers

1. The plain X-ray shows bilateral, inferior rib notching. The aorta has an abnormal configuration. The '3' sign is present with a central notch and protrusions on either side of it.

2. Sagittal black blood MR scan shows a notch in the isthmus of the aorta, just distal to the left subclavian artery origin. MRI after contrast administration shows a narrowing in the aortic isthmus. These findings reflect the plain film findings and confirm coarctation of the aorta.

3. Coarctation of the aorta is a part of a spectrum of abnormalities ranging from discrete narrowing at one end to an interrupted aortic arch at the other. Discrete coarctation is the most common type, seen in older children. The abnormalities are usually juxtaductal and postductal, depending on the relationship of the narrowing to the insertion of the ductus or ligamentum arteriosum. They are most commonly seen distal to the left subclavian artery and at (juxta) or just beyond (post) the ligamentum arteriosum. Very rarely they are seen proximal to the left subclavian artery. The most common presentation is with hypertension. Complications of hypertension ensue if left untreated. Associated berry aneurysms can rupture and cause subarachnoid haemorrhage; associated bicuspid aortic valve can cause infective endocarditis, and associated cardiovascular conditions include VSD, mitral valve abnormalities and bicuspid aortic valve, and right-sided and double aortic arch. Usually they are symptomatic and discovered as an incidental finding of hypertension, which may be very severe, or a murmur. Coarctation is also associated with an increased incidence of berry aneurysms.

4. On the chest X-ray, the heart is usually normal in size. The aortic arch is prominent if there is an associated bicuspid aortic valve. Classically, a notch is seen between the prestenotic dilatation of the distal transverse arch and the poststenotic dilatation of the descending thoracic aorta. (Figure of '3' sign – midportion of '3' represents notch at site of narrowing.) The reverse '3' sign is the corresponding finding on a barium swallow. Rib notching caused by pressure erosion from collateral vessels on the adjacent ribs is rarely seen before age 7–8 years. It is classically seen posteriorly from ribs 4 to 8. Dilated internal mammary arteries cause retrosternal notching. An echocardiogram is more useful in neonates. MRI gives qualitative and quantitative information. The site and extent of the stenosis, and the relationship to subclavian arteries and collateral vessels are all demonstrated. Information can also be obtained on peak pressure gradient and LV function. It is very useful in postoperative cases

5. Coarctation is treated by balloon angioplasty, stenting or surgical repair, depending on the severity and complexity of the lesion. Postoperative complications include restenosis and aneurysm formation. Balloon angioplasty is the preferred method for restenosis.

Case 1.34: Answers

1. The X-ray of the chest shows a large heart with an enlarged left atrium, left ventricle and pulmonary arterial segment. Both the pulmonary arteries are enlarged. There is pulmonary plethora with prominent pulmonary vessels.

2. VSD. MRI confirms the presence of a defect in the ventricular septum between the right and left ventricles.

3. VSD is the most common congenital heart disease. The septal defect can be **membranous** (most common type), **muscular**, **supracristal** (muscular ridge posteroinferior to pulmonary valve) or **AV canal type** (adjacent to anterior mitral leaflet). As a result of the septal defect, there is a flow of oxygenated blood from the left into the right ventricle, which increases the pulmonary vascular flow, and in turn increases the pulmonary venous return to the left atrium and ultimately into the left ventricle; this results in LV dilatation and hypertrophy. This elevates the end-diastolic pressure and LA pressure, resulting in pulmonary venous hypertension. Increased pulmonary flow raises capillary pressure, resulting in pulmonary oedema. As a result of the shunting, the cardiac output is reduced. The degree of left-to-right shunt determines the changes. The size of the VSD and pulmonary vascular resistance are important factors in determining the prognosis of VSD. Maladie de Roger is a small restrictive VSD, with no haemodynamic significance. In a large shunt, eventually Eisenmenger syndrome develops. As a result of increased pulmonary vascular resistance, there is reversal of the shunt in the right-to-left direction

4. The radiological features depend on the size of the shunt and pulmonary vascular resistance. No changes are seen in a small maladie de Roger shunt. In a moderate shunt, the heart is enlarged, with prominent left atrium and ventricle. The main pulmonary artery and pulmonary vessels can be normal or prominent. In a non-restrictive large shunt, the heart is enlarged with prominent left atrium and ventricle, and plethoric pulmonary vasculature. When Eisenmenger syndrome develops, the heart is enlarged, with enlarged right atrium, right ventricle and pulmonary artery. The left atrium and ventricle are normal or increased, and pulmonary vasculature can be pruned or prominent. There can be RVH with the cardiac apex rotated slightly upwards, to the left and posteriorly. Eventually the left atrium and ventricle decrease in size with decrease in size of pulmonary vasculature. Two-dimensional echocardiography, with Doppler echocardiography and colour flow imaging, can be used to determine the size and location of virtually all VSDs. The VSD can be demonstrated and shunt volume calculated using modern MRI techniques.

5. Small VSDs are asymptomatic. Moderate defects present with sweating, fatigue with feeding, failure to thrive and frequent infections. In a large VSDS, symptoms are more severe and may be delayed. In severe defects and Eisenmenger syndrome, dyspnoea, cyanosis, chest pain, syncope and haemoptysis are seen. The features of cardiac failure, harsh holosystolic murmur with a mid-diastolic rumble and loud P2, are present. Small shunts undergo spontaneous closure. Large shunts are closed surgically.

Case 1.35: Answers

1. The X-ray shows an enlarged, box-shaped heart. There is decreased vascularity in both lungs.

2. Ebstein's anomaly. In the MRI, the right atrium is enlarged. The septal leaflet of the tricuspid valve is not where it should be, but situated far inferiorly into the right ventricle.

3. Ebstein's anomaly is a congenital malformation in which the septal and posterior tricuspid leaflets of the tricuspid valve are displaced apically, leading to atrialisation of the right ventricle. Tricuspid regurgitation is caused by a leaflet anomaly. The regurgitation may be mild or severe depending on the extent of the leaflet displacement. Although the atrialised portion of the right ventricle is anatomically part of the right atrium, it contracts and relaxes with the right ventricle. This discordant contraction leads to stagnation of blood in the right atrium. During ventricular systole, the atrialised portion of the right ventricle contracts with the right ventricle, causing backward flow of blood into the right atrium, making the tricuspid regurgitation worse. Maternal lithium, benzodiazepine, varnishing substance and previous fetal loss are associated.

4. In infants, the heart can occupy up to 60% of the chest. The presence of pulmonary vasculature in the peripheral third of the lungs indicates plethora. Absence of vasculature in the central portions indicates oligaemia and peripheral pruning indicates pulmonary arterial hypertension. In Ebstein's anomaly, the heart is enlarged with a huge right atrium. The classic appearance is a squared-off/boxed-off heart. There is decreased pulmonary vasculature (right-to-left shunt at the atrial level) with a small aortic root and main pulmonary artery. On the lateral chest radiograph, distortion of the RV outflow or displacement by the atrialised segment of the right ventricle may cause abnormal filling of the retrosternal space. This finding is of use in older children and adults. Differential diagnoses for enormously enlarged heart are pericardial effusion, valvular heart disease, cardiomyopathy, cardiac failure and giant right atrial aneurysm. Echocardiogram or MRI can diagnose the condition. There is apical displacement of the septal leaflet of the tricuspid valve, > 20 mm or 8 mm/m^2. The right ventricle is dilated with decreased contractility. Associated anomalies can be found.

5. Clinical features are cyanosis, heart failure, fatigue, exertional dyspnoea and palpitations. Auscultation may reveal a triple or quadruple gallop rhythm and a split S2. A pansystolic murmur of tricuspid regurgitation or an ejection murmur of PS may be heard. The ECG shows a right bundle-branch block (RBBB) pattern, giant P waves and sometimes first-degree AV block or Wolff–Parkinson–White (WPW) syndrome (delta wave). Brain abscesses caused by a right-to-left shunt, bacterial endocarditis and paradoxical embolism are other complications. Ebstein's anomaly should be suspected in patients with WPW syndrome, cyanotic congenital heart disease, ASD, severe right heart failure, severe tricuspid regurgitation and left transposition of the great arteries. Antibiotic prophylaxis for endocarditis and treatment for heart failure and arrhythmia are given.

Radiofrequency ablation is used for treating supraventricular tachycardia. Surgical care includes correction of the underlying tricuspid valve and RV abnormalities and of any associated intracardiac defects. Surgery is done when there is severe heart failure, paradoxical embolism, refractory arrhythmias and significant cyanosis.

Case 1.36: Answers

1. The lateral view of the X-ray shows a swollen epiglottis and aryepiglottic folds like a thumbprint. The hypopharynx is also ballooned, but the subglottic structures are normal.

2. Acute epiglottitis.

3. Acute epiglottitis is acute inflammation of the supraglottic structures (epiglottis, arytenoids, aryepiglottic folds, valleculae) resulting in severe airway obstruction, caused by *Haemophilus influenzae* type b (Hib), *Strep. pneumoniae* or *Staph. aureus*. HIV, *Candida* spp., hot liquids and cocaine are other causes. It is seen between age 2 and 7 years and is more common in boys. Dysphagia, sore throat and fever are common symptoms. Patients are seated with their elbows on their knees, leaning forward to alleviate symptoms. The onset is sudden and it is rapidly progressive. Dyspnoea, stridor, dysphonia, drooling, tachycardia, lethargy, hypoxia and cough are other symptoms. Croup (viral laryngotracheitis) is the common differential diagnosis. Patients with croup have a distinctive barking cough. Croup has a more gradual onset and such patients do not have dysphagia or drooling. Most are infants and not toddlers or schoolage children.

4. The lateral X-ray of the neck is diagnostic of epiglottitis. A normal epiglottis is seen as a thin, curved flap of soft tissue that is separated from the base of the tongue by air in the valleculae. In epiglottitis, there is diffuse swelling of the epiglottis (thumbprint sign) and thick aryepiglottic folds. The epiglottis is more vertical and has convex anterior and posterior margins. There is ballooning of the hypopharynx (as a result of sucking of air through an open mouth against an obstruction) with normal subglottic structures. Usually an upright lateral view of the neck is obtained using portable equipment in A&E. If there is a clinical suspicion of epiglottis, the patient should not be moved to the radiology department without precautions, because an acute airway obstruction can develop anytime. The patient should not be made to lie supine or sent to the radiology department without skilled, experienced professionals. An enlarged epiglottis can also be seen in other disorders such as burns, foreign body, epiglottic cysts, neoplasms, granulomatous disease (TB, Wegener's granulomatosis, sarcoidosis) and angioneurotic oedema. Direct examination of the pharynx or anxiety caused by diagnostic tests or crying may precipitate acute airway obstruction. X-ray quality can be affected by inability to hyperextend the neck as a result of irritability.

5. Maintenance of airway with endotracheal or nasotracheal intubation/tracheostomy is of paramount importance till the swelling subsides. Intravenous antibiotics (based on culture/broad-spectrum antibiotics till results are obtained) are used. Effective antibiotics include ampicillin with chloramphenicol, ceftriaxone and cefotaxime. Airway obstruction is the life-threatening emergency.

Case 1.37: Answers

1. The chest X-ray shows a normal left lung. The right lung is larger and appears darker than the left lung. There is a mild shift of the trachea to the left side.

2. This appearance is probably secondary to an inhaled foreign body, which is lodged in the right main bronchus. During inspiration, there is less air entering the right lung, so its volume is less and it is lucent. During expiration there is a ball-valve mechanism, causing air trapping on the right side, which makes it larger than the normal left side.

3. Inhaled foreign bodies are common in children aged < 3 years. It is usually diagnosed within a few days, but occasionally it might take weeks to months. Most of the foreign bodies are of vegetable origin and are radiolucent, such as lentils, beans, peas, peanut and barley grass. Teeth are aspirated more commonly in adults.

4. An inhaled foreign body is commonly lodged in the right bronchus, because it is short, straight and narrow. Clinical presentation is with cough, obstructive overinflation and reflex vasoconstriction, atelectasis or infiltrate. Air trapping is seen in expiratory films. If the foreign body is trapped in the distal airways, it might cause lobar or segmental overinflation. A radio-opaque foreign body is seen in 10%. A CT scan can be used to diagnose radiolucent foreign bodies.

5. Bronchiectasis might result from chronic retention of a foreign body.

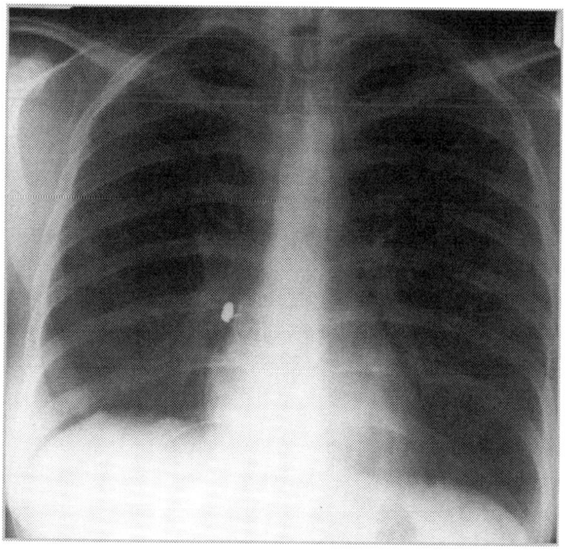

This X-ray in another patient shows a foreign body in the right lower lobe bronchus.

2

GASTROINTESTINAL AND HEPATOBILIARY RADIOLOGY QUESTIONS

Case 2.1

A 3-week-old boy delivered normally at full term presents with recurrent episodes of bilious vomiting and abdominal distension.

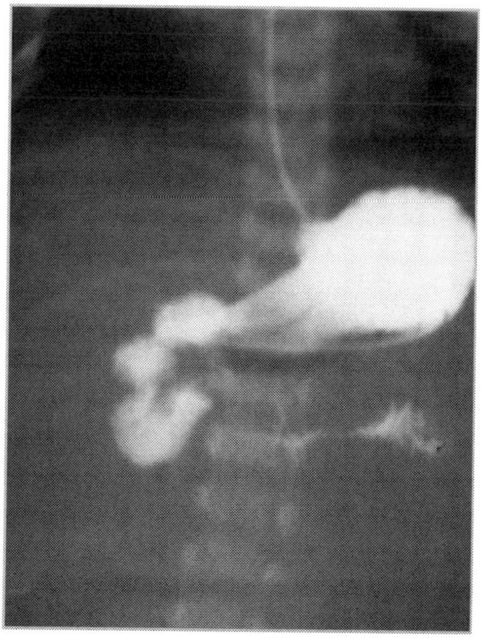

Fig 2.1a

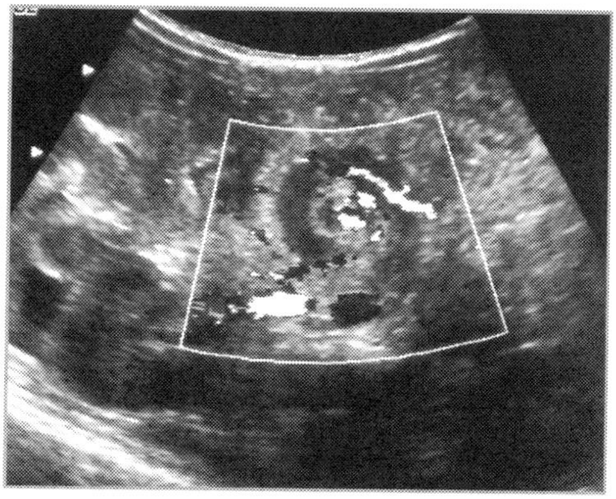

Fig 2.1b

1. What do you see on the plain film of the abdomen?
2. What do you see on Doppler ultrasonography of the abdomen?
3. What are the diagnosis and the development of this condition?
4. What are the radiological features?
5. What are the complications?

Answers *on pages 119–154*

Case 2.2

A 6-week-old boy, delivered at term, presents with projectile vomiting and feeding difficulties. On examination, there is a palpable mass in the upper quadrant of the abdomen.

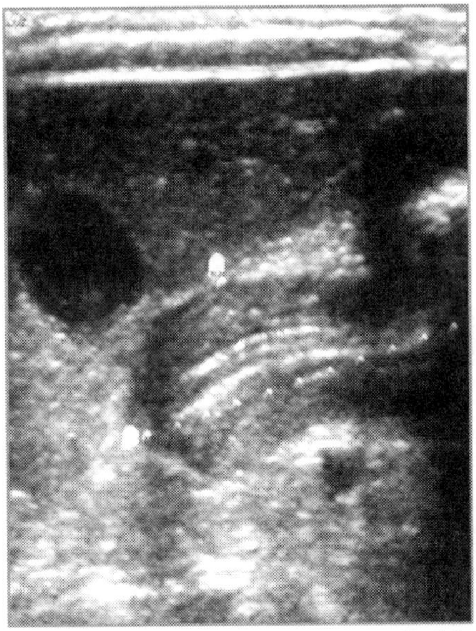

Fig 2.2a

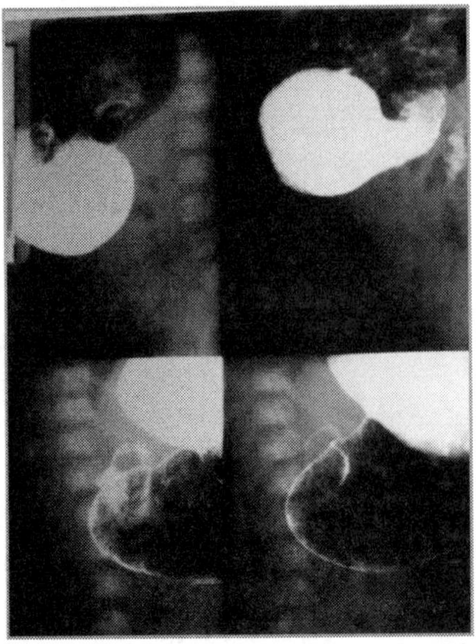

Fig 2.2b

1. What do you observe on this ultrasound examination and contrast study?
2. What is the diagnosis?
3. What are the aetiology and clinical features of this disease?
4. What are the radiological features?
5. What is the differential diagnosis?
6. What is the treatment?

Answers *on pages 119–154*

Case 2.3

A term neonate presents with difficulty feeding and drooling of saliva. Clinical examination revealed bilateral râles and features of respiratory distress.

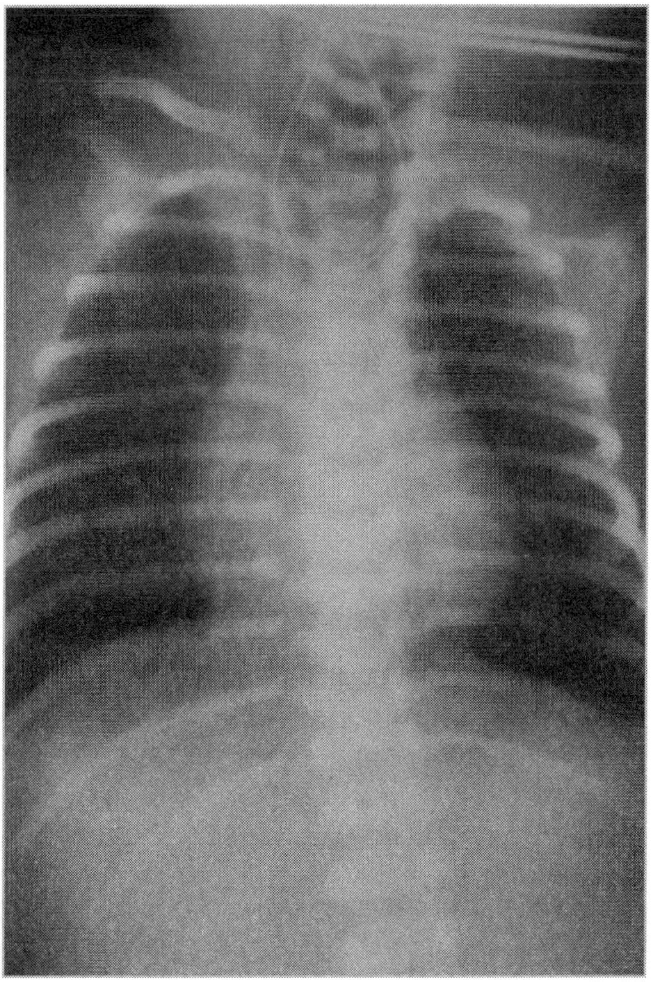

Fig 2.3

1. What are the findings on the plain X-ray of the chest?
2. What is the diagnosis?
3. What is the classification of this disease?
4. What are the clinical features and physiology of this disease?
5. What are the radiological tests and features?
6. What are the associations of this condition?

Answers *on pages 119–154*

Case 2.4

A full-term baby boy delivered naturally develops jaundice, dark urine and light stools in the first week. On examination the liver is enlarged and firm. Lab examination shows conjugated hyperbilirubinaemia

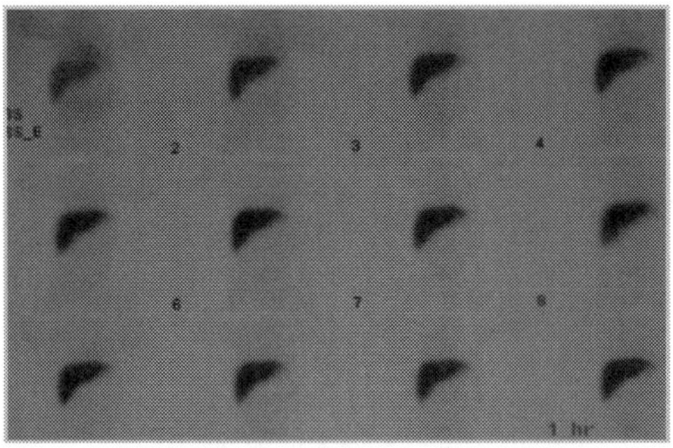

Fig 2.4a

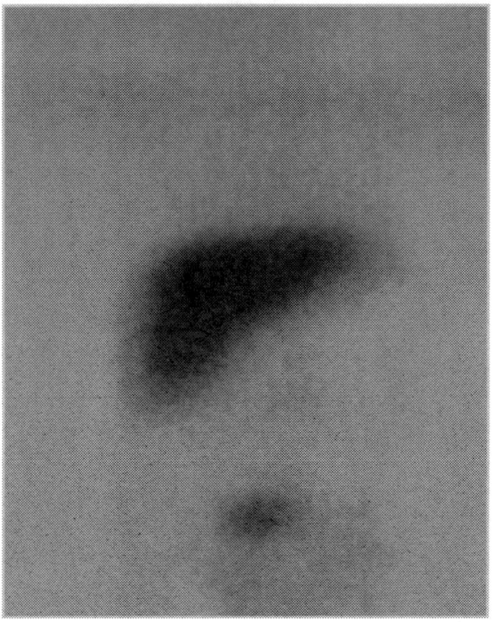

Fig 2.4b

1. What are the findings on the scintiscan? The first film was done immediately and the second film after 6 hours.
2. What is the diagnosis?
3. What are the radiological features?
4. What are the associations?
5. What is the common differential diagnosis?

Answers *on pages 119–154*

Case 2.5

A 12-year-old girl presents with colicky abdominal pain, nausea, vomiting and dyspepsia. On examination she is afebrile. There is no point tenderness in the abdomen. Bowel sounds are normal.

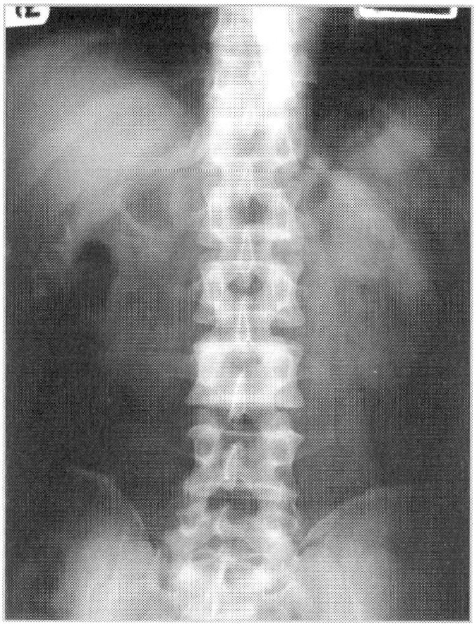

Fig 2.5a

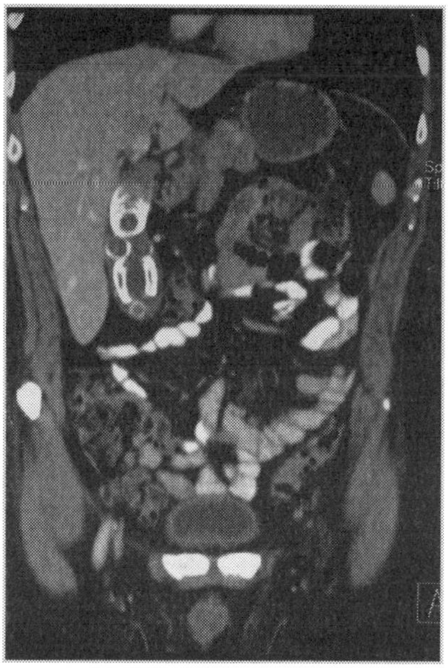

Fig 2.5b

1. What do you observe on the X-ray and CT scan?
2. What is the diagnosis?
3. What is the aetiology of this disease?
4. What are the types of this disease and what is the role of imaging?
5. What are the complications?

Answers *on pages 119–154*

Case 2.6

A 16-month-old baby presents with diarrhoea, rectal bleeding and an incessant cry. An X-ray and ultrasound scan of the abdomen were performed.

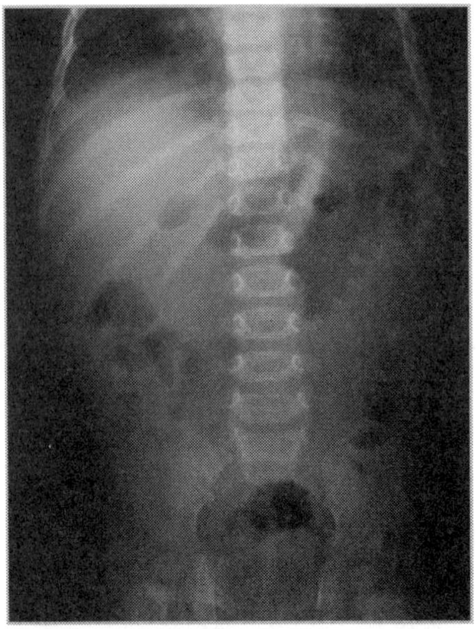

Fig 2.6a

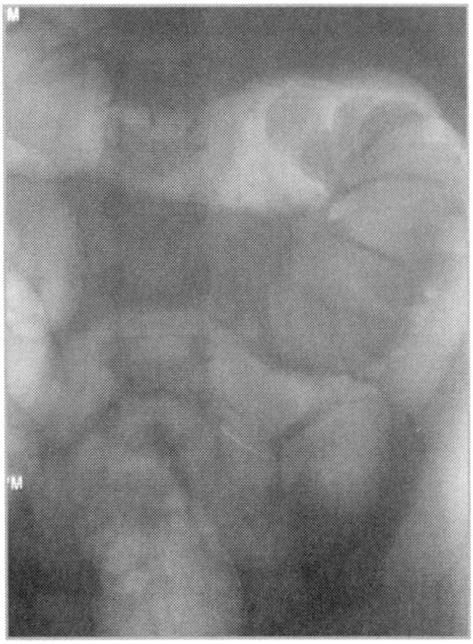

Fig 2.6c

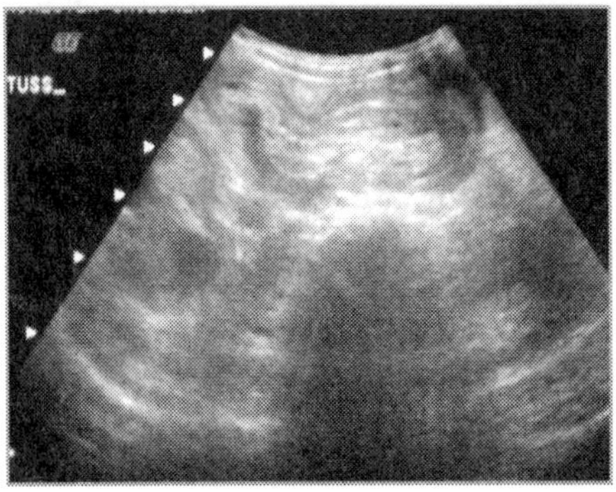

Fig 2.6b

1. What do you observe on the plain X-ray and ultrasound scan?
2. What is the diagnosis?
3. What are the clinical features?
4. What are the radiological features?
5. What do you see on the third picture and what is the management of this patient?

Answers *on pages 119–154*

Case 2.7

A 9-year-old girl presented with severe abdominal pain and rectal bleeding. On examination, she was haemodynamically stable. Tenderness was elicited in the lower abdomen.

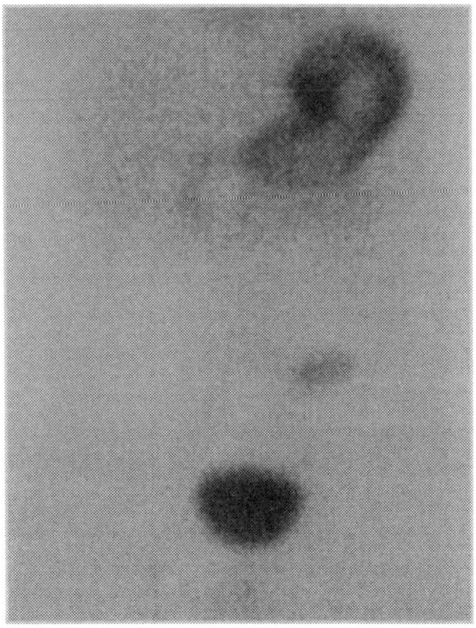

Fig 2.7a

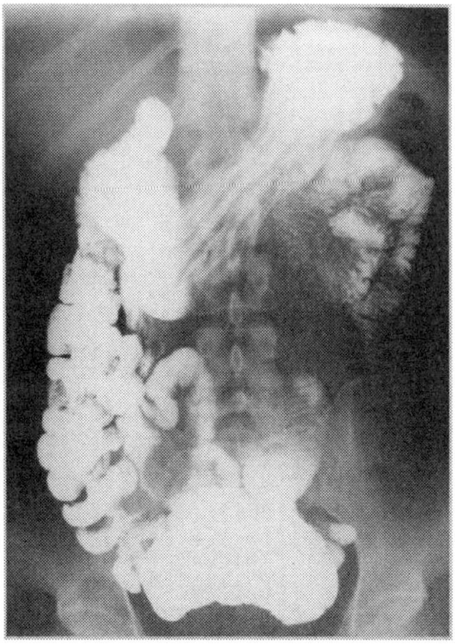

Fig 2.7b

1. What is this test? What are the findings in this patient?
2. What is the diagnosis?
3. How is this scan done?
4. What are the differential diagnosis and radiological features?
5. What are the clinical features?
6. What do you see on the second picture, which was taken after a week? What are the complications?

Answers *on pages 119–154*

Case 2.8

A preterm neonate, born at 30 weeks, with a birthweight of 1000 g, developed severe abdominal distension, bilious vomiting and blood in the stools. Clinically she was febrile, with a distended abdomen and no bowel sounds.

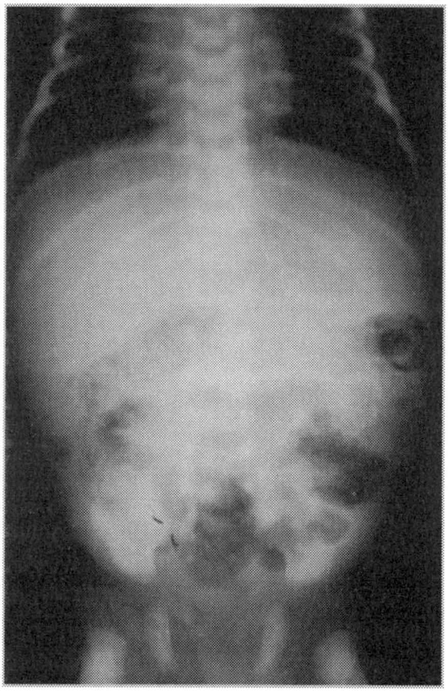

Fig 2.8a

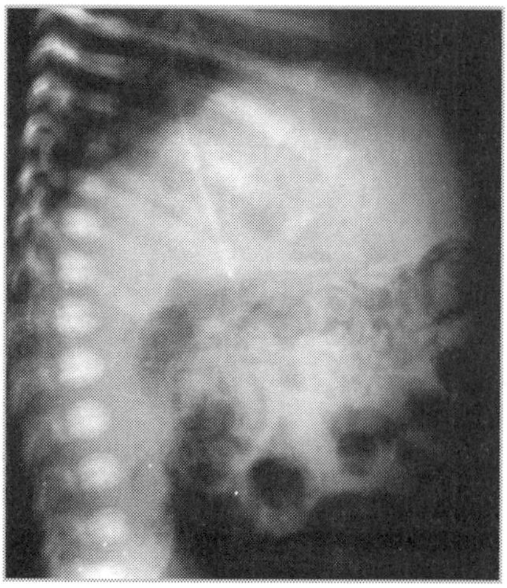

Fig 2.8b

1. What do you observe on the abdominal X-ray?
2. What is the diagnosis?
3. What are the aetiology and predisposing factors for this condition?
4. What are the clinical features?
5. What are the radiological features of this condition?

Answers *on pages 119–154*

Case 2.9

A newborn term infant presents with abdominal distension, vomiting and failure to pass meconium.

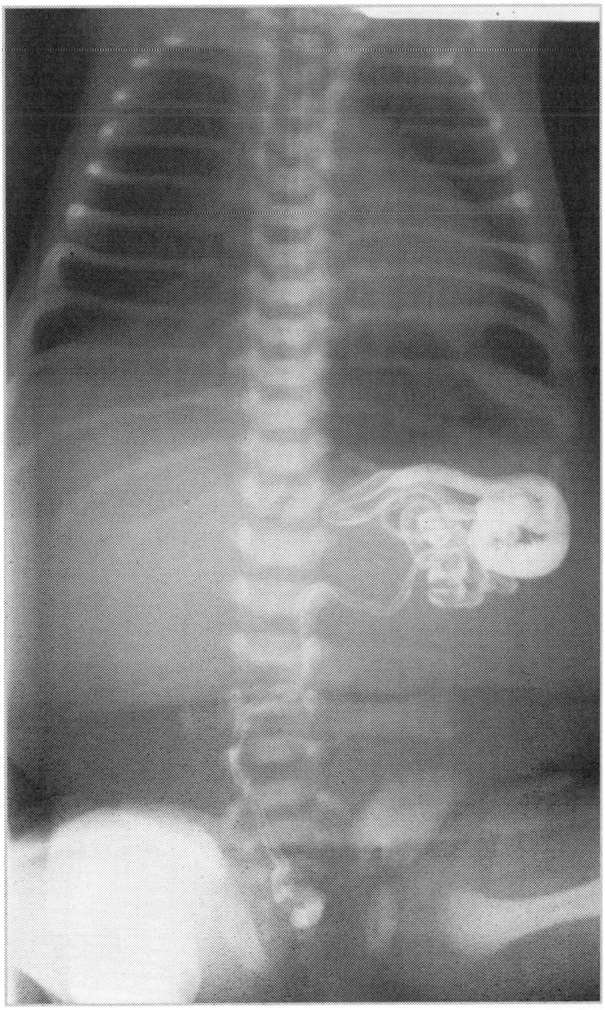

Fig 2.9

1. What do you see on the barium study?
2. What is the diagnosis?
3. What is the aetiology?
4. What are the common differential diagnosis and pathophysiology of this condition?
5. What are the radiological features and differential diagnosis?

Answers *on pages 119–154*

Case 2.10

A 3-year-old boy presents with severe abdominal pain, vomiting, nausea and tenderness. On examination, there is severe rebound tenderness in the abdomen. He is febrile and tachycardic.

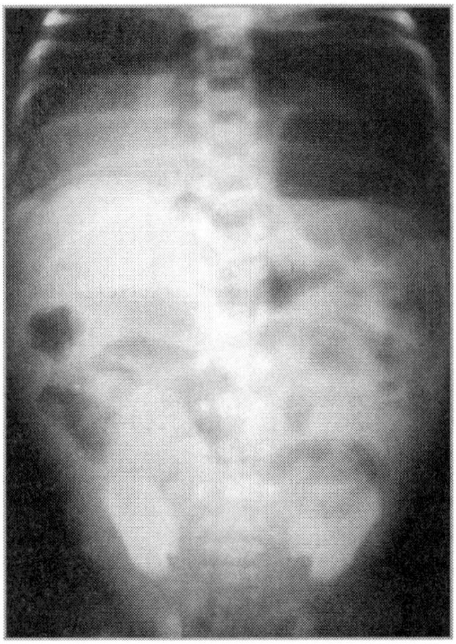

Fig 2.10a

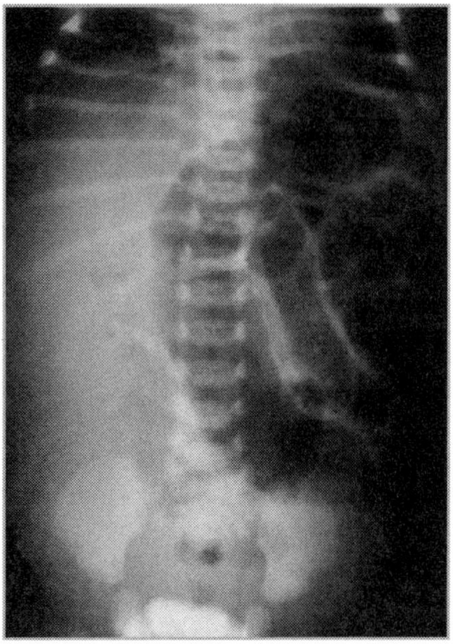

Fig 2.10b

1. What do you observe on the plain abdominal X-rays?
2. What is the diagnosis?
3. What are the radiological signs of this presentation?
4. What are the causes of this appearance?
5. What are the important tips in the radiology of this condition?

Answers *on pages 119–154*

Case 2.11

A 10-year-old boy presents with failure to thrive, poor appetite, drooling, vomiting and coughing. On examination there are mild rhonchi bilaterally.

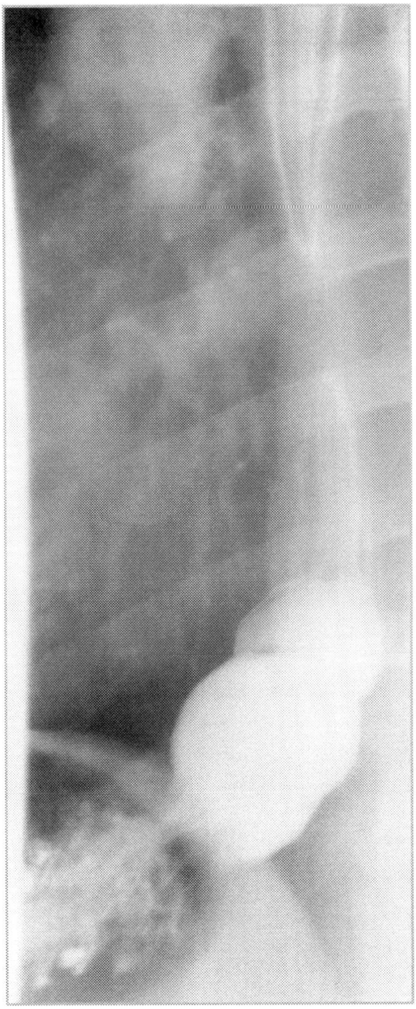

Fig 2.11a

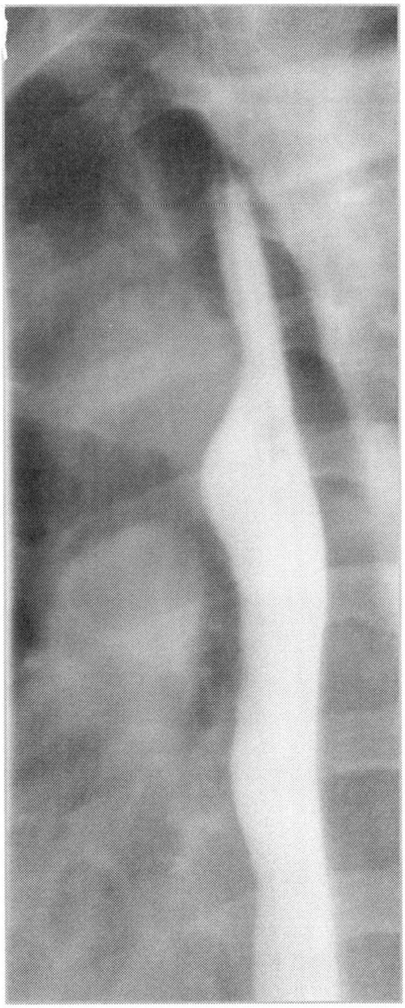

Fig 2.11b

1. What is this test and what do you observe?
2. What is the diagnosis?
3. What other techniques can be used in diagnosis?
4. What are the types and predisposing factors?
5. What are the clinical manifestations?
6. What are the complications and treatment?

Answers *on pages 119–154*

Case 2.12

A 5-day-old newborn boy, delivered normally at full term, presents with bilious vomiting and abdominal distension.

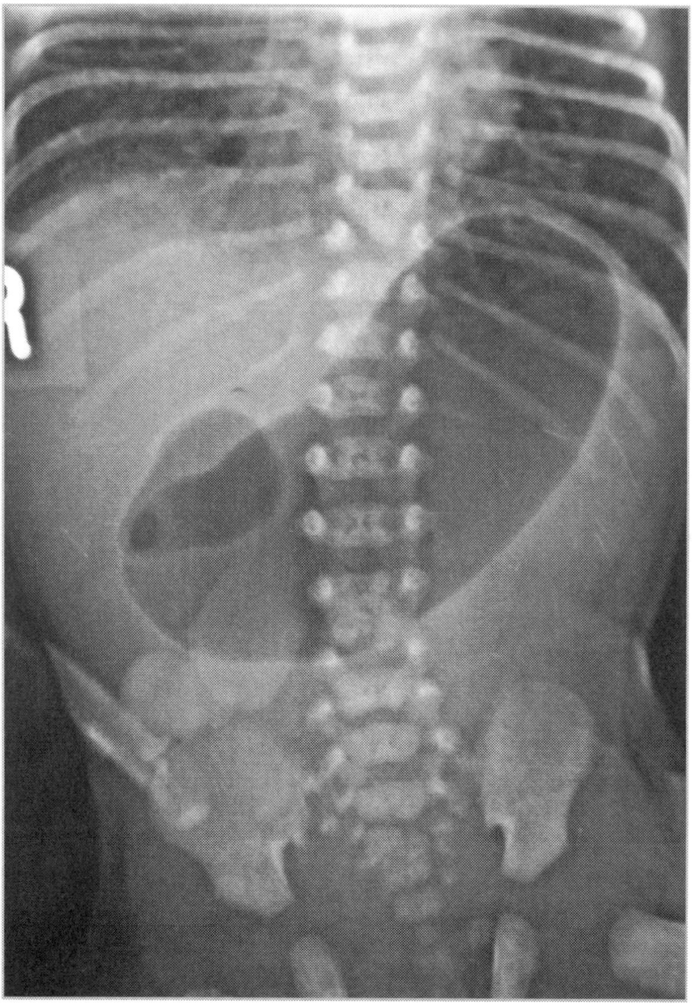

Fig 2.12

1. What do you see on the plain abdominal film?
2. What is the diagnosis?
3. What is the most common association with this condition?
4. What are the development and the clinical features?
5. What are the radiological features?
6. What is the differential diagnosis of this appearance?

Answers *on pages 119–154*

Case 2.13

A newborn term baby fails to pass meconium along with abdominal distension and vomiting. On clinical examination, the abdomen is grossly distended and there are no bowel sounds.

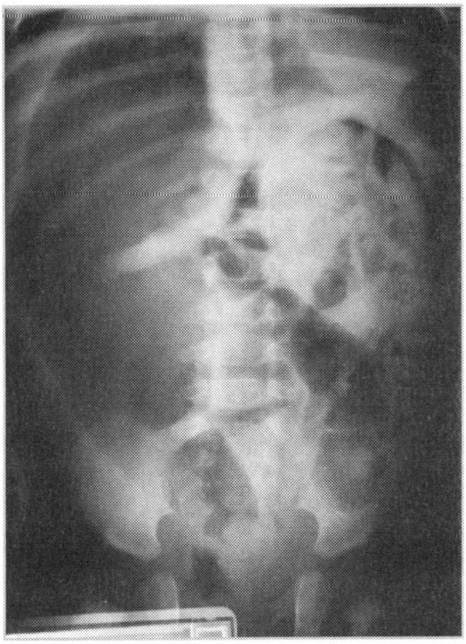

Fig 2.13a

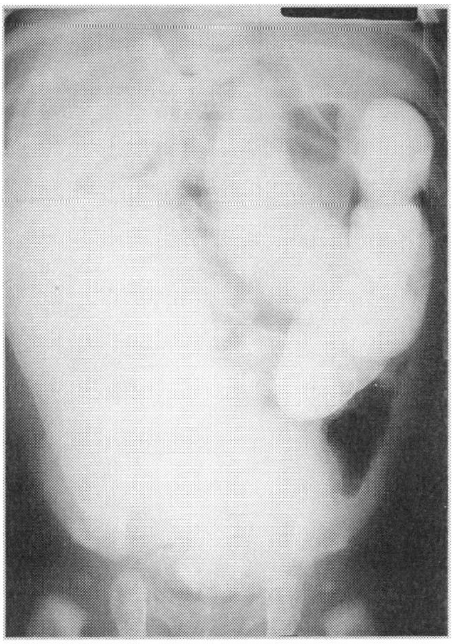

Fig 2.13b

1. What do you see on the plain X-ray?
2. What do you observe on the second examination and what does it show?
3. What is the diagnosis?
4. What are the aetiology and the clinical features?
5. What are the radiological procedures and the findings?

Answers *on pages 119–154*

Case 2.14

A 7-year-old boy presents with severe pain in the lower abdomen, nausea and vomiting. On physical examination there is rebound tenderness in the right lower quadrant. The WBC count is 15 000.

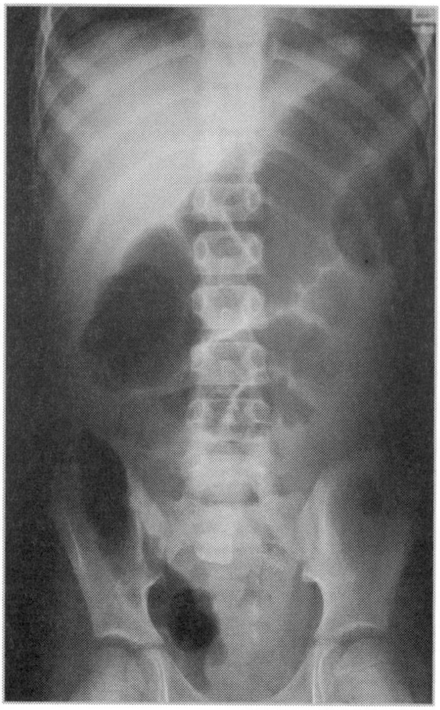

Fig 2.14a

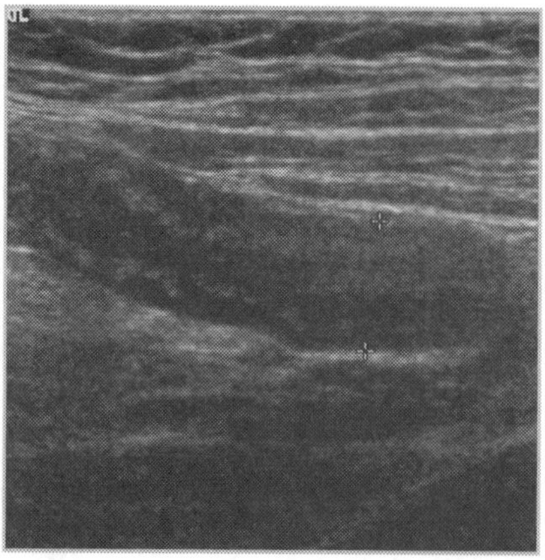

Fig 2.14b

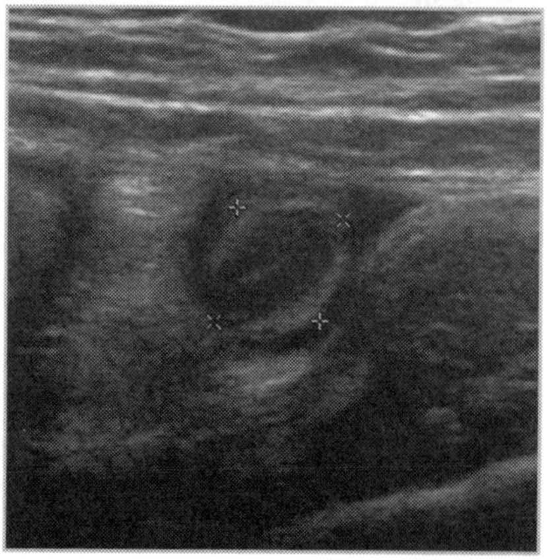

Fig 2.14c

1. What do you see on the X-ray of the abdomen?
2. What do you see on ultrasonography?
3. What is the diagnosis?
4. What are the clinical presentations of this disease?
5. What are the radiological features and treatment of this disease?

Answers *on pages 119–154*

Case 2.15

A 12-year-old girl presents with abdominal pain, nausea, vomiting and weight loss. On examination there is a palpable mass.

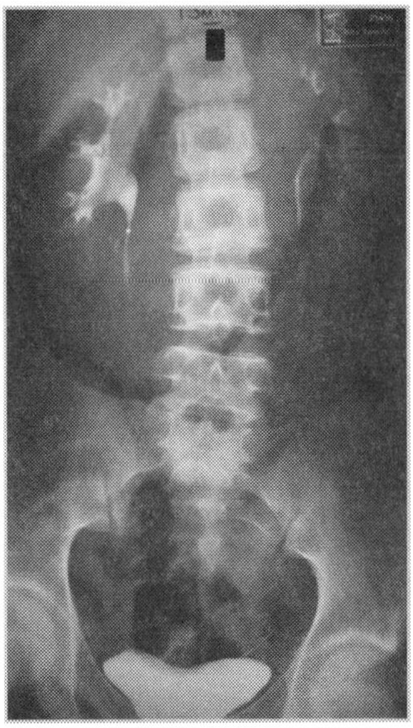

Fig 2.15a

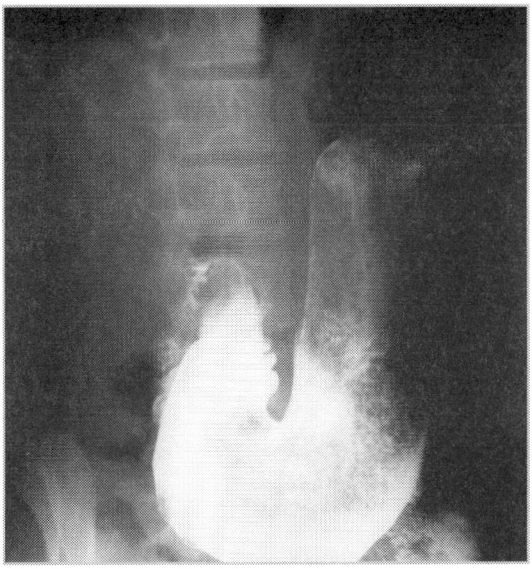

Fig 2.15b

1. What are the findings on the intravenous urogram (IVU) and barium meal?
2. What is the diagnosis?
3. What causes this condition?
4. What are the various subtypes?
5. What are the radiological findings and complications?
6. What are the differential diagnosis and treatment?

Answers *on pages 119–154*

Case 2.16

A 9-year-old boy presents with recurrent abdominal pain and tenderness. On examination he has a mass in the left upper quadrant.

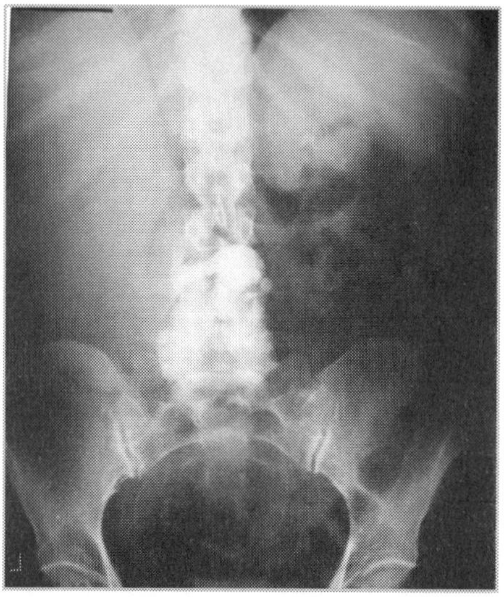

Fig 2.16a

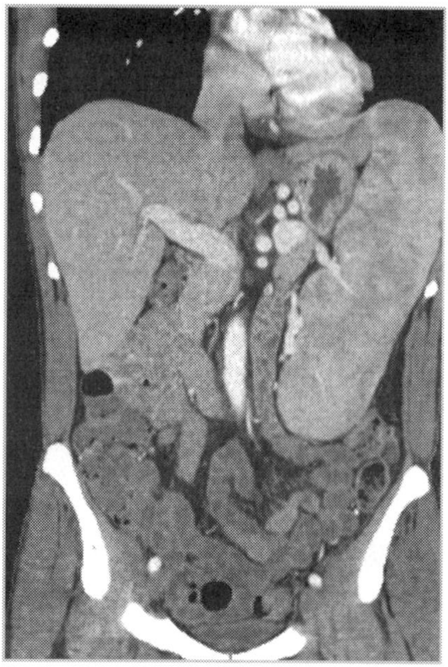

Fig 2.16b

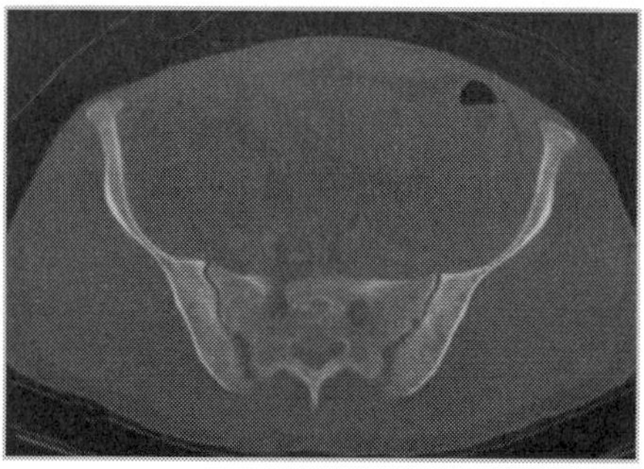

Fig 2.16c

1. What do you observe on the IVU?
2. What do you observe on the CT scan?
3. What are the common causes of this condition?
4. What are the radiological criteria?
5. What are the further investigations?

Answers *on pages 119–154*

Case 2.17

A 15-year-old female pedestrian was hit by a truck and presented to A&E with low BP and upper abdominal pain.

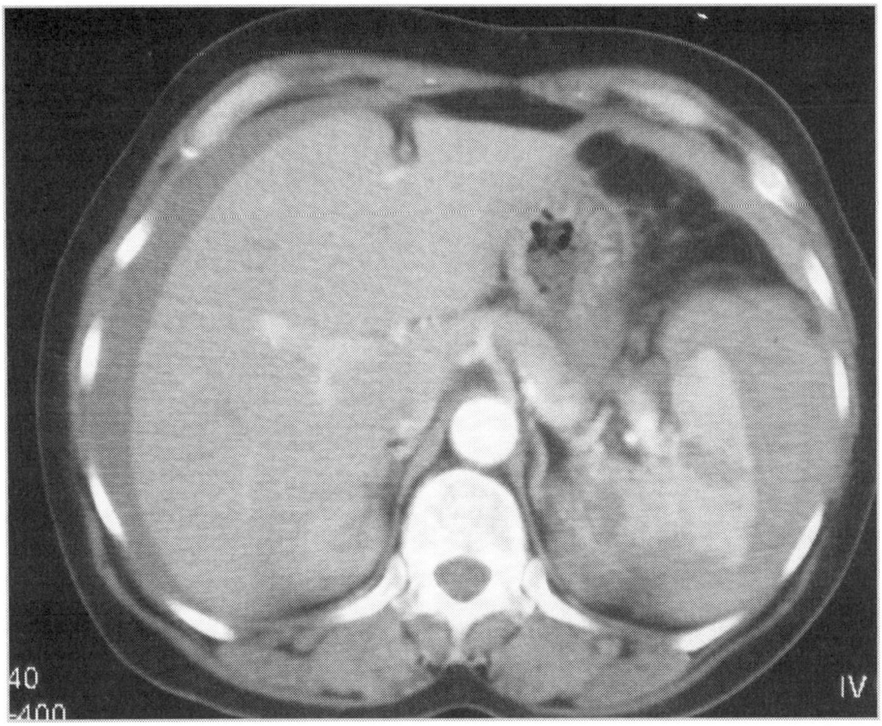

Fig 2.17

1. What do you see on the CT scan of the abdomen?
2. What is the diagnosis?
3. What is the mechanism of injury and what are the clinical features?
4. What are the radiological features and grading?
5. What is the management? What are the indications for surgery and what are the complications?
6. What are the non-traumatic causes of this disorder?

Answers *on pages 119–154*

Case 2.18

A 3-year-old boy presents with jaundice and vomiting. On clinical examination, there is large mass in the right side of the abdomen, which is non-tender.

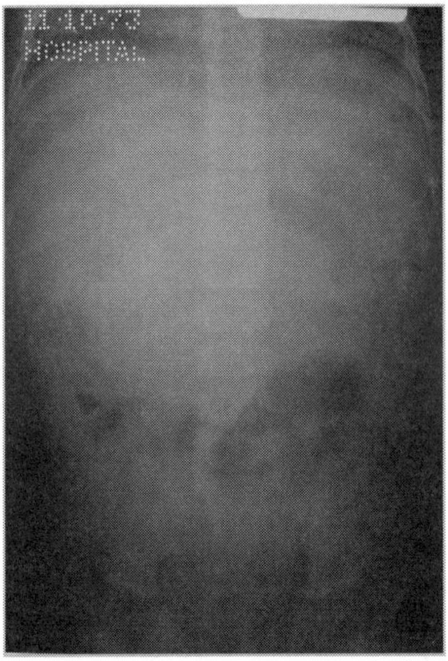

Fig 2.18a

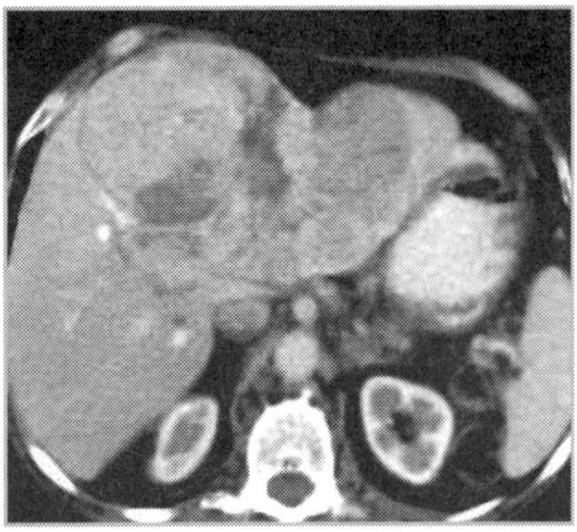
Fig 2.18b

1. What are the findings on the X-ray and CT of the abdomen?
2. What is the diagnosis?
3. What are the aetiology, pathology and presenting features?
4. What are the radiological features?
5. What are the differential diagnosis and the treatment?

Answers *on pages 119–154*

Case 2.19

A 3-year-old girl presents with right upper quadrant colicky pain, fever and jaundice. On examination, she is febrile, tender on the right upper quadrant, with no palpable mass.

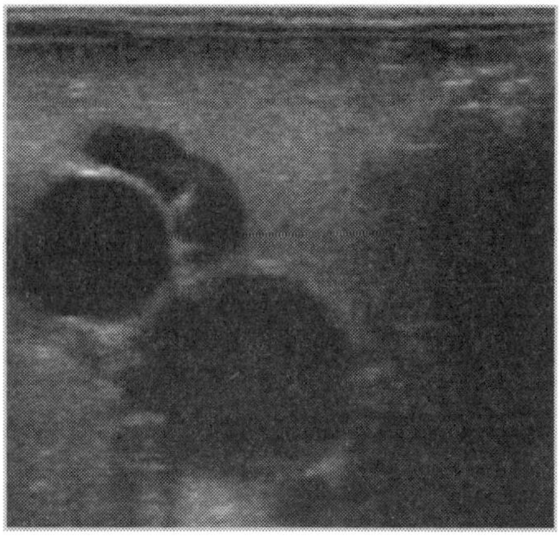
Fig 2.19a

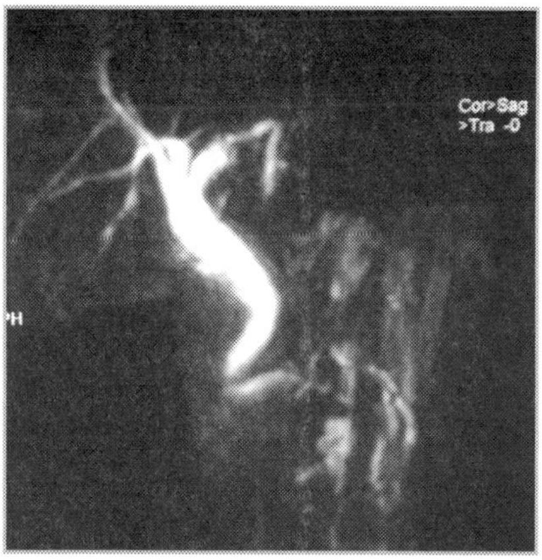

Fig 2.19b

1. What are the findings on abdominal ultrasonography?
2. What are the findings on the MR scan?
3. What is the diagnosis?
4. What are the aetiology and the classification of this disease?
5. What are the clinical features and the complications?
6. What are the radiological features?

Answers *on pages 119–154*

Case 2.20

A 10-year-old boy presents with severe epigastric pain, abdominal distension and retching. On examination, there is severe tenderness in the epigastric region, with no palpable mass.

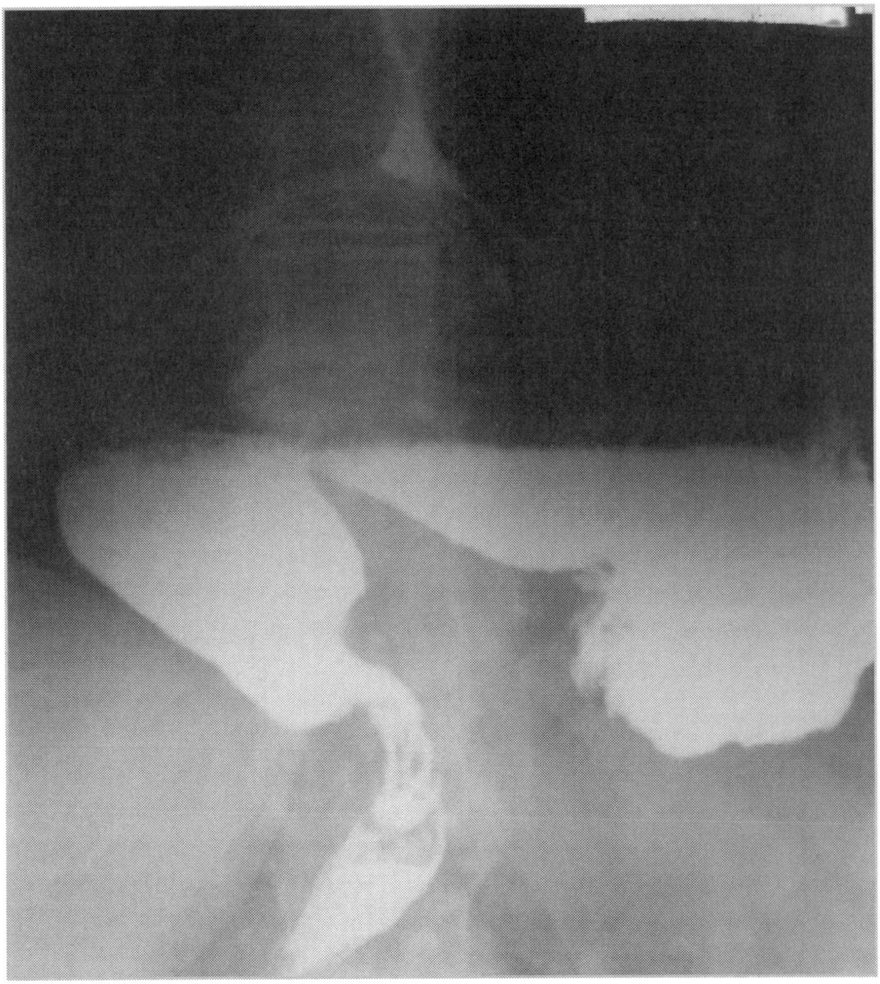

Fig 2.20

1. What are the findings in this barium meal?
2. What is the diagnosis?
3. What causes this condition?
4. What are the types and radiological features?
5. What are the clinical features and complications?

Answers *on pages 119–154*

Case 2.21

A 7-year-old girl presented with acute abdominal pain and fever. On examination there was rebound tenderness in the left upper quadrant. White cell markers were raised.

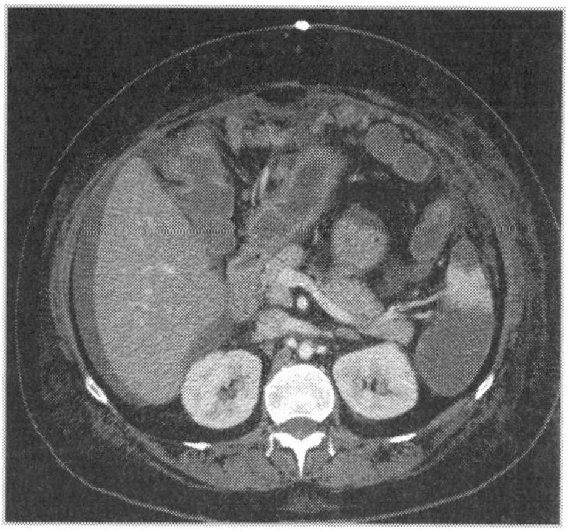

Fig 2.21a

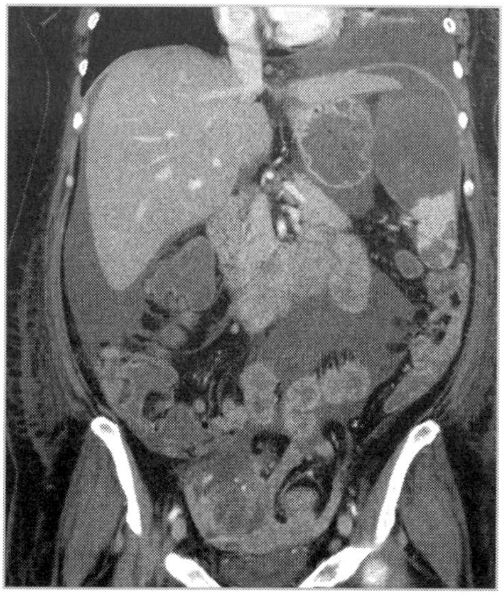

Fig 2.21b

1. What do you observe on the abdominal CT scan?
2. What is the diagnosis?
3. What are the causes of this condition?
4. What are the radiological features?
5. What are the complications and the management?

Answers *on pages 119–154*

Case 2.22

A 7-year-old boy presents with an emergency to the paediatric department. An X-ray of the chest is shown.

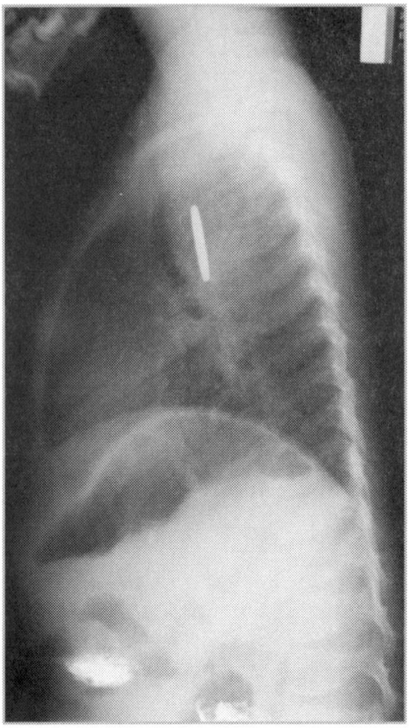

Fig 2.22a

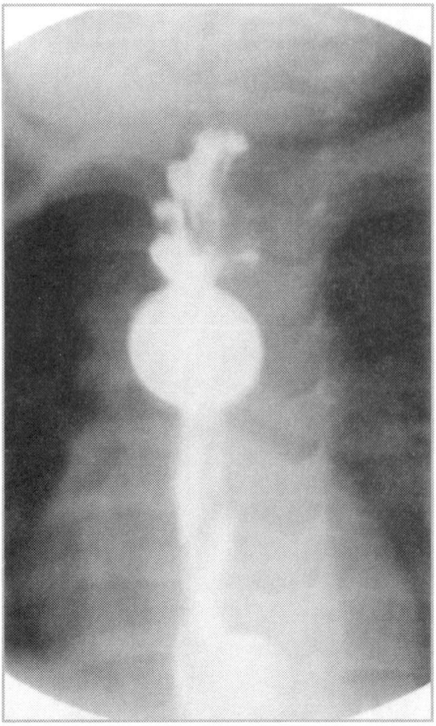

Fig 2.22b

1. What do you see on the X-ray of the abdomen?
2. What do you observe on the second investigation and what is the diagnosis?
3. What are the common sites of this problem?
4. What are the clinical features?
5. What is the treatment?

Answers *on pages 119–154*

Case 2.23

A 17-year-old girl presents with abdominal pain, loss of weight, loose stools with blood and fever. On examination she is febrile. There is tenderness in the right iliac fossa. The bowel sounds were normal.

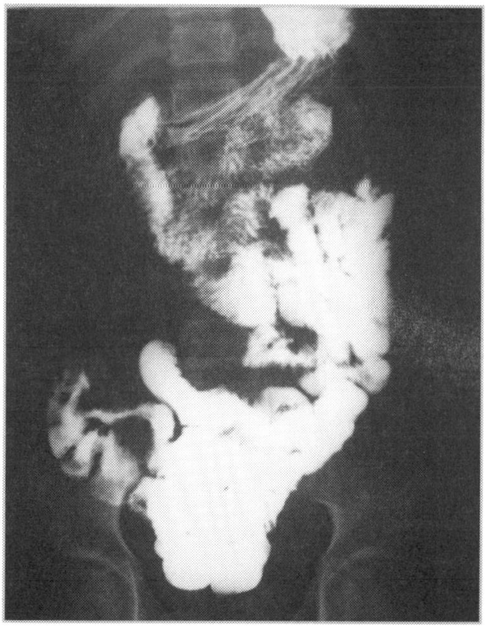

Fig 2.23a

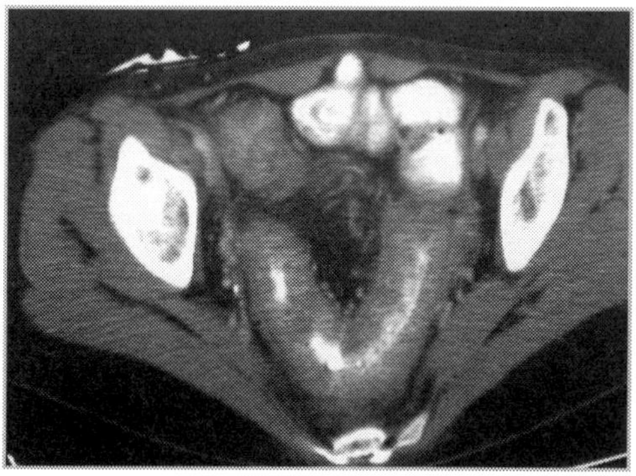

Fig 2.23b

1. What are the findings in the first picture?
2. What do you observe on the CT scan of the abdomen?
3. What is the diagnosis?
4. What are the clinical features, the complications and the treatment?
5. What are the radiological features and the differential diagnosis?

Answers *on pages 119–154*

Case 2.24

A 15-year-old girl presents with severe right upper quadrant pain and vomiting. Clinical examination shows tenderness in the right upper quadrant, without any palpable mass.

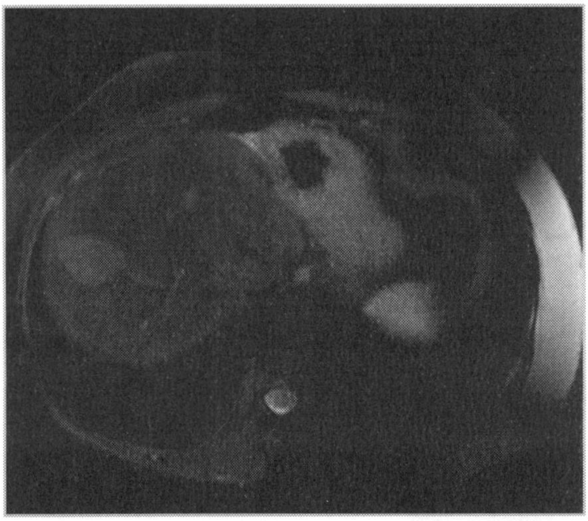

Fig 2.24a

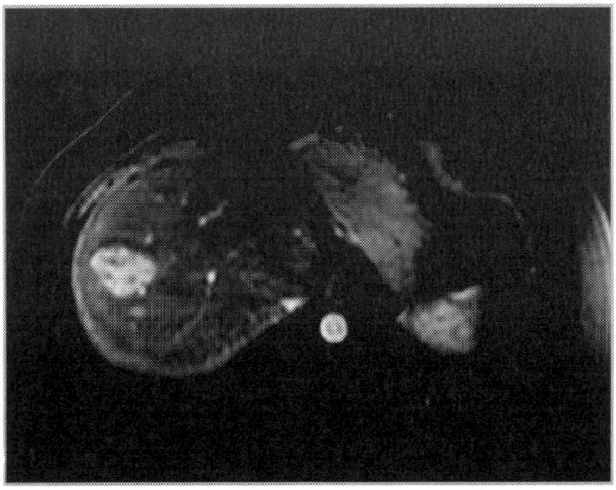

Fig 2.24b

1. What do you see on MRI of the liver?
2. What is the diagnosis?
3. What are the causes?
4. What are the imaging findings?
5. What is the differential diagnosis?
6. What are the complications?

Answers *on pages 119–154*

Case 2.25

A 7-year-old girl presents with right upper quadrant colicky pain, fever and jaundice. On examination, she is febrile and tender in the right upper quadrant, with no palpable mass.

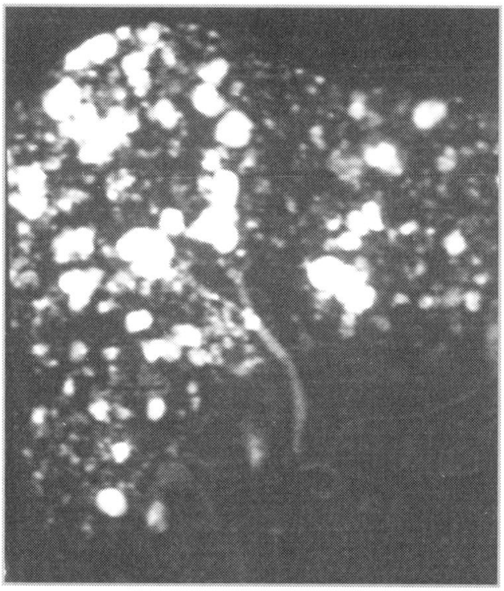

Fig 2.25a

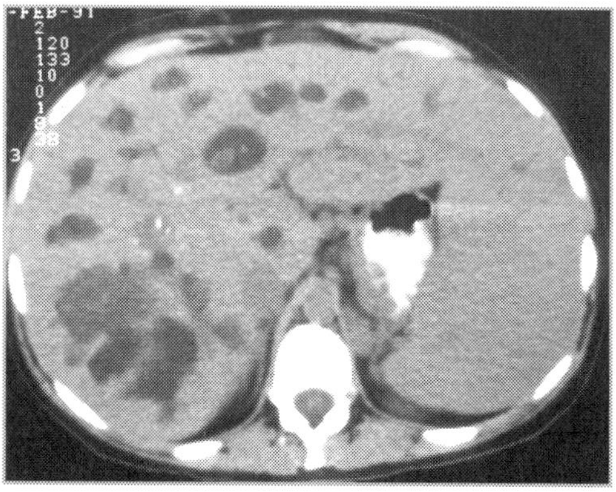

Fig 2.25b

1. What are the findings on MRI and on the CT scan of the liver?
2. What is the diagnosis?
3. What are the aetiology and classification of this disease?
4. What are the clinical features?
5. What are the complications?
6. What are the radiological features and differential diagnosis?

Answers *on pages 119–154*

Case 2.26

A 4-year-old boy presented with pain and lump in the lower abdomen on the right side. Clinical examination revealed a tender lump in the right inguinal region. Bowel sounds were sluggish and the abdomen was distended.

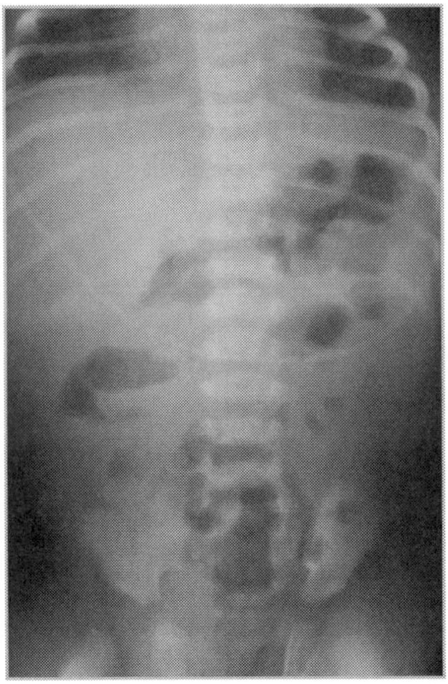

Fig 2.26a

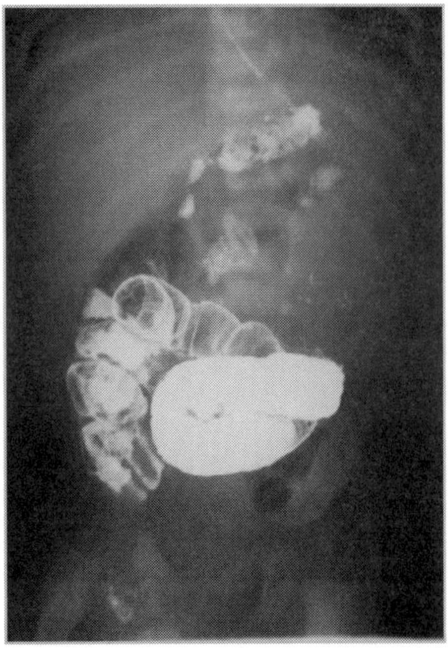

Fig 2.26b

1. What do you see on the plain film?
2. What do you see on the barium study? What is the diagnosis?
3. What is the anatomical location of this lesion?
4. What are the common types? What are the clinical features and complications?
5. What are the salient features in imaging?

Answers *on pages 119–154*

Case 2.27

A 14-year-old girl presented with abdominal pain, fever, weight loss and bloody diarrhoea. On examination she has tenderness in the lower abdomen.

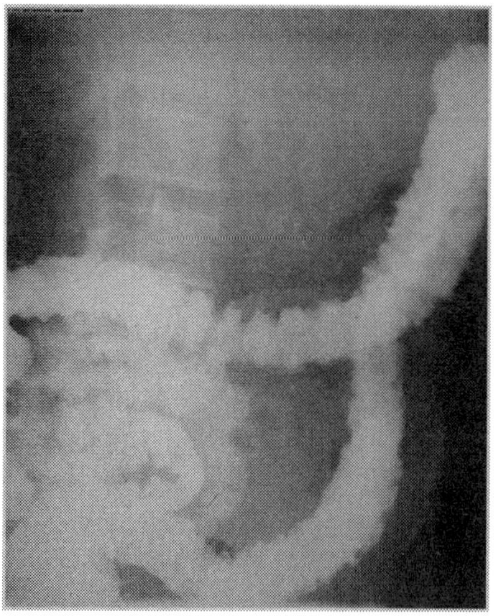

Fig 2.27a

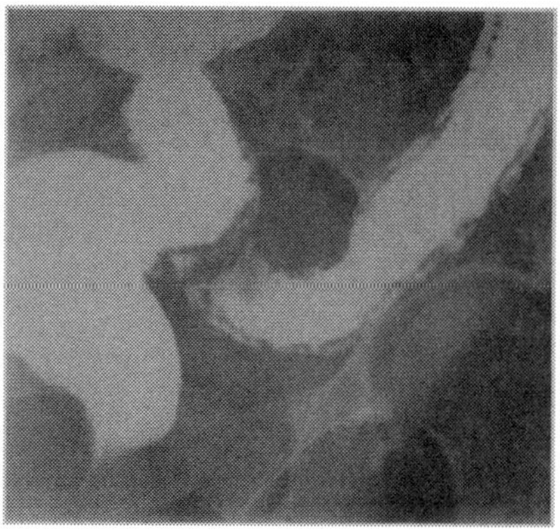

Fig 2.27b

1. What are the findings in the barium enema?
2. What is the diagnosis?
3. What are the clinical features and the characteristic locations?
4. What are the radiological findings?
5. What is the differential diagnosis?
6. What are the complications and the treatment?

Answers *on pages 119–154*

Case 2.28

A 12-year-old boy was involved in a road traffic accident and presents with abdominal pain, tenderness and a high pulse rate.

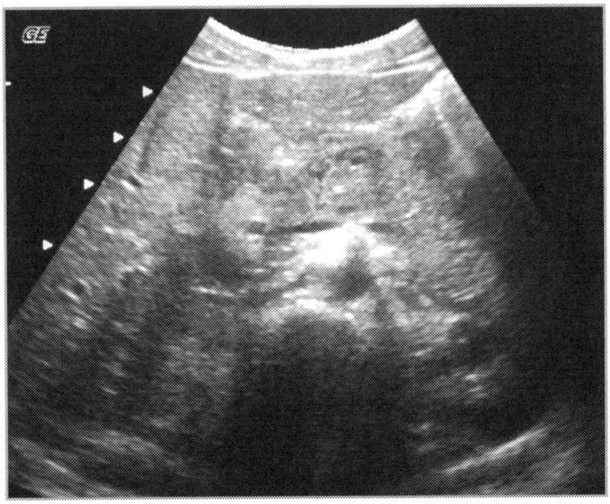

Fig 2.28a

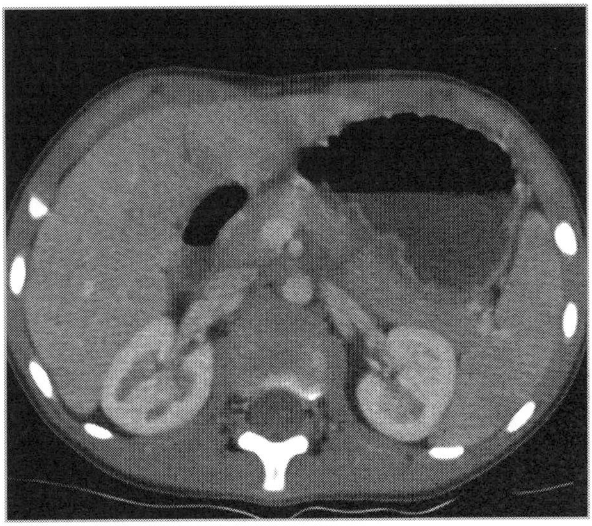

Fig 2.28b

1. What do you see on the ultrasound and CT scans of the abdomen?
2. What is the diagnosis?
3. What is the grading of this lesion? What are the common locations?
4. What are the radiological features and the differential diagnosis?
5. What are the complications and the treatment?

Answers *on pages 119–154*

Case 2.29

A neonate presented with vomiting and failure to pass meconium.

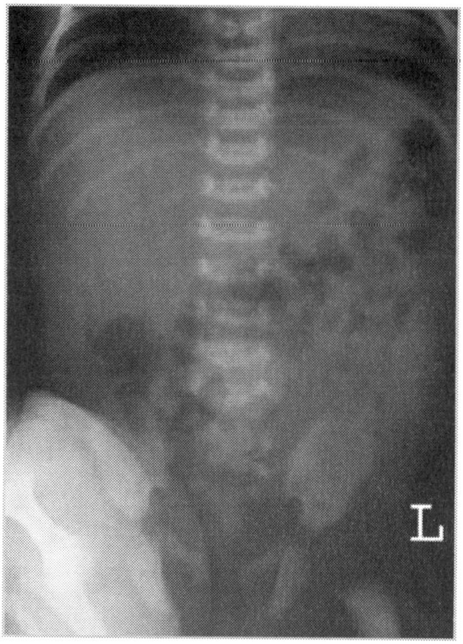

Fig 2.29a

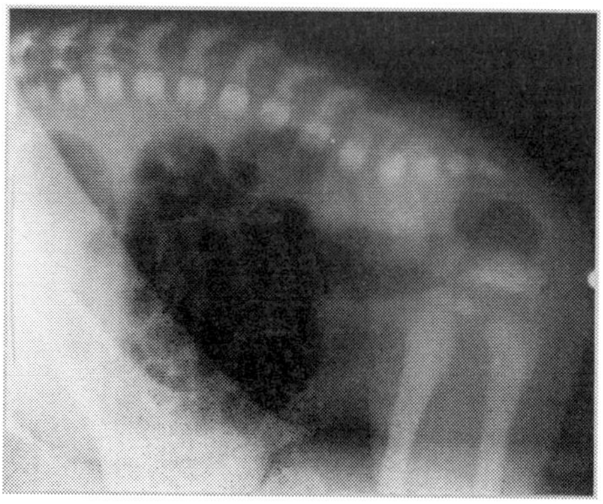

Fig 2.29b

1. What do you observe on the plain X-ray?
2. What is the diagnosis?
3. What is the development of this disease?
4. What are the classification and the radiological features?
5. What is the treatment?
6. What syndrome is associated?

Answers *on pages 119–154*

Case 2.1: Answers

1. The barium meal shows a distended stomach. The duodenojejunal flexure is situated in the right side of the lumbar vertebrae and there is some contrast flowing into the proximal jejunum.

2. Doppler ultrasonography of the abdomen shows a whirlpool appearance of twisted mesentery. The superior mesenteric artery (SMA) is situated to the right of the superior mesenteric vein (SMV).

3. Intestinal malrotation. Normal rotation takes place around the SMA as axis. The proximal duodenojejunal loops and distal colic loops make a total 270° in rotation during normal development. Both loops start in vertical plane parallel to the SMA and end in a horizontal plane.

Stage **I** (5–10 weeks): the bowel herniates into the base of the umbilical cord. The duodenojejunal loop begins superior to the SMA at 90° and rotates 180° in a counterclockwise direction. At 180° the loop is to the right of the SMA and by 270° it is beneath it. The caecal loop begins beneath the SMA at 270°, rotates 90° counterclockwise and ends at the left of the SMA at 0°. Both loops maintain these positions until bowel returns to the abdominal cavity. The midgut lengthens along the SMA and a broad pedicle is formed at the base of mesentery.

Stage **II** (week 10): bowel returns to the abdominal cavity. The duodenojejunal loop rotates 90° to end at the left of the SMA. The caecal loop turns 180° more to place it to the right of the SMA at 180°.

Stage **III** (11 weeks till term): the descent of the caecum to the right lower quadrant and mesentery fixation. Arrest in development of stage I causes **non-rotation** (duodenojejunal junction not inferior and left of the SMA, caecum not in right lower quadrant, narrow base of mesentery, midgut volvulus). **Incomplete rotation** is stage II arrest – peritoneal bands, midgut volvulus depending on rotation before arrest, internal herniations; **incomplete fixation** is no mesenteric fixation, resulting in hernial pouch formation, and volvulus if the caecum remains unfixed.

4. A plain X-ray shows a double-bubble appearance. A barium meal is the mainstay in the diagnosis of malrotation. Small volumes of barium are fed and rapid fluoroscopic images acquired. The duodenum and jejunum are located to the right of the spine. The duodenojejunal junction (ligament of Trietz), which is normally located to the left of the spine at the level of T12, is located on the right side. Colonic loops are seen on the left side of the abdomen. A corkscrew appearance indicates midgut volvulus. Doppler ultrasonography is used to confirm the diagnosis of malrotation. In normal Doppler ultrasonography, the SMV is located to the right of the SMA, but this is reversed in malrotation. Another sign is the whirlpool sign, which is caused by twisted mesentery at the base of the bowel.

5. Complications: volvulus (resulting from clockwise rotation of the midgut), obstruction, ischaemia, perforation, Ladds' bands and internal herniation. Surgery is done when there is malrotation associated with volvulus or obstruction

Case 2.2: Answers

1. This is an ultrasound scan of the upper abdomen. The pylorus is visualised here and is very thick, measuring 14 mm. A target sign is seen with a central bright area surrounded by dark areas. The length of the pyloric channel, which is the hyperechoic area in the centre of the pylorus, measures 20 mm. The redundant pyloric channel is protruding into the gastric antrum. A contrast study shows narrow, tapered pylorus and proximally a distended stomach filled with contrast.

2. Congenital hypertrophic pyloric stenosis.

3. Hypertrophic pyloric stenosis is idiopathic hypertrophy of the circular muscle fibres of pylorus, extending into the gastric antrum. It is seen between 2 and 8 weeks and is common in boys with a family history. It is seen in first-born boys and inherited in an autosomal dominant fashion. The baby has projectile vomiting and there might be a palpable olive-shaped mass in the epigastric region.

4. Ultrasonography is the mainstay in the diagnosis of pyloric stenosis. It is done after feeding:

(a) target sign: refers to thickened hypoechoic pylorus with central hyperechoic band

(b) pyloric wall thickness > 3 mm; pyloric transverse diameter > 13 mm

(c) elongated pyloric channel > 17 mm

(d) pyloric volume > 1.4 cm^3

(e) pyloric length + 3.64 × muscle thickness > 25

(f) cervix sign: indentation of muscle mass on a fluid-filled antrum.

(g) antral nipple sign: redundant pyloric channel protruding into the antrum

(h) increased peristaltic waves

(i) delayed gastric emptying of fluid into the duodenum.

Contrast study is also useful. It shows the following:

String sign: contrast flowing via a small streak through the pyloric channel

Double-track sign: crowding of mucosal folds into the pyloric channel

Diamond sign: irregular tent-like clefts in the midportion of the pyloric canal

Teat sign: outpouching along the lesser curvature

Beaking: mass impression on the antrum

Mushroom sign: indentation of the base of the bulb.

5. Infantile pylorospasm has similar features to pyloric stenosis, with thick muscle, antral narrowing and elongation of the pylorus. However, it undergoes spontaneous resolution or responds to metoclopramide. Gastritis/milk allergy (circumferential thickening of antral mucosa), gastric diaphragm and duodenal obstruction from a midgut volvulus (whirlpool sign – twisted mesentery, reversal of SMA and SMV) are other differential diagnoses.

6. Once the diagnosis has been confirmed, the metabolic abnormality such as hypochloraemic metabolic alkalosis is corrected. Treatment is with Heller's myotomy, where the pylorus is split longitudinally.

Case 2.3: Answers

1. The plain X-ray shows a nasogastric tube coiling in a blind-ending oesophagus indicating absence of distal oesophagus. In the abdomen, there is no gas in the stomach.

2. Oesophageal atresia.

3. **Type A**: oesophageal atresia without fistula (pure oesophageal atresia) (10%); **type B**: oesophageal atresia with proximal tracheo-oesophageal fistula (<1%); **type C**: oesophageal atresia with distal tracheo-oesophageal fistula (85%); **type D**: oesophageal atresia with proximal and distal tracheo-oesophageal fistulae (<1%); **type E**: tracheo-oesophageal fistula without oesophageal atresia or so-called H-type fistula (4%); and **type F**: congenital oesophageal stenosis (< 1%).

4. Oesophageal atresia is one of the tracheo-oesophageal fistula subtypes. Absence of distal oesophagus prevents swallowing of food. The pouch gets filled with saliva, which then overflows. There is a high risk of aspiration, which might be saliva or gastric secretions depending on the type of fistula. Air from the trachea flows into the stomach whenever the child cries and this causes abdominal distension and possible perforation. Oesophageal atresia is caused by faulty development of the early trachea and oesophagus in which a dorsal fold lies too ventrally, resulting in incomplete division of an early tracheo-oesophagus. Oesophageal vascular or ischaemic events are predicted to be predisposing factors. The trachea is also weak and D shaped, rather than the usual C shape, and this results in cough and pneumonias.

5. A replogle tube can be placed through the oral cavity and 5–10 ml air is injected, after which an X-ray of the chest is taken. The X-ray shows coiling of the tube and a gas-distended pouch. The second important thing to look for is the gastric bubble. If there is no gas, it indicates an absence of distal tracheo-oesophageal fistula (unless there is a fistula occluded by mucus plugs). The lungs may show features of aspiration pneumonitis. To demonstrate the presence of a fistula a contrast study is done with injection of 1 ml isotonic water-soluble contrast, to prevent airway spillage. A catheter with an end-hole is used. If there is an upper pouch fistula, contrast flows freely into the airway. Oesophageal atresia can be diagnosed on prenatal ultrasonography, which shows polyhydramnios (as the fetus cannot swallow amniotic fluid). A gastric bubble is absent or present depending on the presence of fistula and VACTERL malformations (**v**ertebral defects, **a**norectal malformation, **c**ardiovascular defects, **t**racheo-o**e**sophageal defects, **r**enal anomalies and **l**imb deformities). If associated syndromes are suspected, renal ultrasonography, spinal and limb ultrasonography, and echocardiography should be done. If there is no gas in the distal oesophagus, it is assumed that there is a long gap between the atretic proximal and the distal oesophagus. This can be confirmed by doing a gap-o-gram. A replogle tube is placed proximally and a dilator is placed through a distal gastrostomy; both these tubes are pushed towards each other and find the least distance between them, which is the gap between the atretic ends. A gap of two to three vertebral bodies is good for anastomosis.

6. Oesophageal atresia is associated with the VACTERL malformation. It is also associated with the CHARGE syndrome (**c**oloboma, **h**eart, **a**t**r**etic choanae, **g**enital hyoplasia and **e**ye defects).

Case 2.4: Answers

1. This is a scintiscan (hydoxyiminodiacetic acid or HIDA scan) augmented with phenobarbital administration. An HIDA scan is used for assessing the function of the liver. Phenobarbital is given at the rate of 5 mg/kg per day for 5 days to induce hepatic enzymes, which results in increased conjugation and excretion of bilirubin; this in turn increases the sensitivity of the scan. In normal patients the isotope is taken up by the liver and gallbladder and excreted into the bile ducts and then the duodenum. In this patient, there is good uptake into the liver, but the gallbladder and biliary ducts are not seen. The bowel is not visualised, even in delayed films.

2. Congenital biliary atresia. This characterised by obliteration or discontinuity of the extrahepatic biliary system. It is believed to be caused by the same process as neonatal hepatitis, but with additional vascular injury/sclerosis of the bile ducts. It is more common in boys. There are many types: focal/intrahepatic biliary atresia (common), extrahepatic biliary atresia with patient intrahepatic bile ducts (subtype 1 – bile duct remnant in porta hepatis; subtype 2 – no bile duct remnant in porta hepatis) The various types are:

Type 1: obliteration of common duct with normal proximal ducts

Type 2: atresia of hepatic duct with cystic structures in porta hepatis

Type 3: atresia of the right and left hepatic ducts to the level of the porta hepatis (most common).

Intrahepatic biliary hypoplasia is a distinct entity.

3. Ultrasonography: the gallbladder is not seen (occasionally it is seen and can be small or large (if the obstruction is distal to a cystic duct). Liver is normal or large.

Triangle cord sign: hyperechoic tubular opacities in the porta hepatis as a result of fibrous tissue. Bile ducts are not dilated. Bile duct remnant and choledochal cyst can be seen.

HIDA scan: normal uptake in the liver within 5 min, but no biliary excretion or bowel activity even in 6- and 24-hour delayed films. Increased renal excretion and delayed cardiac clearance are seen.

MR cholangiography can be used for proper evaluation. Liver biopsy is used for confirmation and differentiation from other lesions.

4. Of cases of this condition 10–35% are associated with polysplenia, situs inversus, trisomy 18, malrotation, azygos continuation of IVC, bilobed liver, situs inversus, preduodenal portal vein, anomalous hepatic arteries, bilobed right lung and complex heart disease.

5. The most common differential diagnoses are: **neonatal hepatitis** (common in preterm neonates, slow and decreased hepatic uptake, bowel activity seen in 24 hours, associated with TORCH syndrome **T**oxoplasmosis, **O**ther agents, **R**ubella, **C**ytomegalovirus, **H**erpes simplex); **sclerosing cholangitis**; and **Alagille syndrome** (arteriohepatic dysplasia – abnormal facies, butterfly vertebra, pulmonary stenosis). Complications include sclerosing cholangitis and secondary biliary cirrhosis.

Case 2.5: Answers

1. The X-ray of the abdomen shows multiple, laminated opacities in the right upper quadrant. The CT scan shows multiple, dense calculi inside the gallbladder. The wall of the gallbladder is not thickened and there is no fluid collection around the gallbladder.

2. Cholelithiasis.

3. Causes of cholelithiasis in children: sickle cell disease, hereditary spherocytosis, other haemolytic anaemias, cystic fibrosis, malabsorption, Crohn's disease, total parenteral nutrition, intestinal resection and choledochal cyst. Causes of calculi in neonates: haemolytic anaemia, infection, parenteral nutrition, dehydration, starvation, phototherapy, biliary atresia, short gut syndrome and furosemide.

4. Calculi can be cholesterol or pigment stones. Pure cholesterol stones are radiolucent and not seen on an X-ray. On CT, they are hypodense and float in contrast-enhanced bile. A mixture of cholesterol and calcium carbonate stones is laminated and opaque on plain films (20%). Pigment stones (30%) are denser than bile. On an X-ray, 85% of stones are lucent and 15% opaque; of the lucent stones 85% are cholesterol and 15% pigment; of the opaque stones, 67% are pigment and 33% cholesterol. Calcium phosphate is deposited centrally in cholesterol stones. Calcium carbonate is deposited peripherally around cholesterol. On ultrasonography, the gallstones might appear to float. This is caused by pure cholesterol or gas-containing stones, and a rise in specific gravity. Gas-containing stones result from dehydration of older stones and internal shrinkage and nitrogen gas filling (Mercedes Benz sign). Ultrasonography and CT can confirm the presence of calculi, and are also useful in evaluating the complications of gallstones such as cholecystitis.

5. Complications of gallstones are acute cholecystitis, chronic cholecystitis, perforation, abscess, porcelain gallbladder and carcinoma. Acute cholecystitis will be seen as thick-walled, oedematous gallbladder with pericholecystic fluid collection. Chronic cholecystitis has thick walls. In perforation, the gallbladder wall is irregular, stones might be seen outside the gallbladder and there is gas in the peritoneum. Focal fluid collections can be seen outside the gallbladder.

Case 2.6: Answers

1. The plain film shows a claw (meniscus) sign in the middle of the abdomen at the level of the L2 vertebra, with a soft-tissue opacity protruding into a gas shadow of the colon. Ultrasonography shows pseudokidney sign, with central hyperechogenicity and surrounding hypoechogenicity.

2. Intussusception.

3. Intussusception is a common cause of acute abdomen in infancy, and occurs when a segment of bowel, the intussusceptum, telescopes into the bowel distally, the intussuscipiens. It is usually seen between age 6 months and 2 years. Most are ileoileal or ileo-ileocolic; most cases are idiopathic and do not have any lead point other than lymphoid hypertrophy. About 2% have lead points, which include Meckel's diverticulum, duplication cyst, lymphoma, polyps, Henoch–Schönlein purpura and inspissated mucus in cystic fibrosis. Characteristic features include intermittent colicky abdominal pain with drawing up of legs, vomiting, red-currant jelly stools and palpable abdominal mass. Drowsiness and lethargy can be seen. Mechanical small bowel obstruction and ischaemia are the complications if untreated.

4. A plain X-ray demonstrates a soft-tissue mass in the right upper quadrant, dilated loops or the classic claw sign, in which the apex of the intussusceptum is outlined by gas in the colon. Bowel obstruction, perforation and sparse amount of bowel gas are other features. A plain X-ray can be normal. Ultrasonography is the most sensitive method in diagnosis. Multiple concentric rings, or a pseudokidney or doughnut sign, can be seen, resulting from varying appearances of the telescoping bowel loops. Enlarged Peyer's patches can be seen. Fluid in the intussusceptum indicates vascular compromise.

5. This picture demonstrates air reduction of intussusception. The bowel loops are distended with gas, which has entered the small bowel, indicating successful reduction. The standard treatment is air reduction using oxygen or carbon dioxide. A Foley catheter is inserted into the rectum and a tight seal maintained. Air is delivered inside the bowel, with a maximum pressure of 120 mmHg. Successful reduction is indicated by air entering the small bowel. Three attempts can be made with 3-min intervals. Reduction is less likely to be successful if the symptoms have lasted more than 48 hours, or if there is rectal bleeding or small bowel obstruction. Perforation and tension pneumoperitoneum are complications of air reduction. Surgery is performed for failed reductions, but 5–10% recur after surgical or non-surgical reduction.

Case 2.7: Answers

1. This is a pertechnate scan (Meckel scan). There is a high focus of activity in the left side of the lower abdomen. This area of uptake has the same intensity as that of the stomach uptake.

2. Meckel's diverticulum

3. A pertechnate scan is the gold standard in the diagnosis of Meckel's diverticulum. As Meckel's diverticulum has ectopic gastric mucosa with its mucoid cells, it excretes [^{99m}Tc]pertechnate. The patient is prepared for the test by avoiding any irritative procedure for 48 hours and fasting for 3–6 hours, which decreases gastric secretion and intestinal motility. The bowel and bladder are evacuated before the study, and 5–20 mCi [^{99m}Tc]pertechnate injected and scans are acquired for 30–45 min. Cimetidine (decreased gastric secretion), pentagastrin (stimulates uptake) and glucagon (decreases intestinal peristalsis) can be used to improve the scans. The scan shows a focal collection of tracer in the right lower quadrant, appearing at the same time or shortly after the gastric activity, and the tracer activity increases in intensity with time parallel to that of the stomach. Meckel's diverticulum should bleed at a rate of at least 0.1 ml/min to be picked up by the scan. The sensitivity of this scan is 75–100% and specificity up to 80%. A false-positive scan can be seen if there are other lesions with ectopic gastric mucosa, such as a duplication cyst with gastric wall, normal small bowel or Barrett's oesophagus, or lesions with an increased blood pool – haemangioma, aneurysm, AVM (arteriovenous malformation), hypervascular tumour, duodenal ulcer, appendicitis, ulcerative colitis, Crohn's disease, laxative abuse, intestinal obstruction, intussusception, volvulus, urinary obstruction and meningomyelocele. The test will not be useful after adolescence, because these patients are unlikely to have ectopic gastric mucosa without symptoms. False-negative tests are also seen when there is insufficient gastric mucosa or dilution of activity as a result of peristalsis or hypersecretion. Other tests that would be useful are a contrast study of the small bowel (enteroclysis), where Meckel's diverticulum would be seen as a smooth, club-like intraluminal mass parallel to the long axis of the distal ileum. An angiogram shows persistent vitelline artery and is useful when the bleeding is more than 1 ml/min.

4. Meckel's diverticulum is the most common congenital abnormality of the gastrointestinal tract. It results from the persistence of the omphalomesenteric duct (which connects the midgut to the yolk sac) and normally obliterates by week 5. It is seen in 2% of the population, located within 0.6 m of the ileocaecal valve in the antimesenteric border, symptomatic before age 2 years, and usually is 6 cm long. It contains ectopic mucosa, which can be gastric (80%), colonic, jejunal or pancreatic. It is supplied by the right vitelline artery.

5. Most patients are asymptomatic and detected incidentally in a barium study. Development of symptoms indicates a complication, the most common being bleeding from peptic ulceration of gastric mucosa. Definitive treatment of the condition is excision of the diverticulum along with the adjacent ileal segment.

6. This is a barium study of the small bowel. There is a well-defined, smooth, filling defect in the distal ileum, parallel to the long axis of the ileum. Complications are acute diverticulitis, acute gastrointestinal bleeding, intussusception, volvulus, bands, internal hernia leading to obstruction and associated malignant tumours (carcinoid, sarcoma and carcinoma).

Case 2.8: Answers

1. The X-ray of the abdomen shows distended loops of small and large bowel. There are subtle areas of gas collection in the wall of the large bowel. Gas is also seen in the peritoneum, and is best seen in the lateral view. There is no gas in the portal veins.

2. Necrotising enterocolitis

3. Necrotising enterocolitis is the most common gastrointestinal emergency in neonates. It is an ischaemic bowel disease secondary to hypoxia, perinatal stress, infection (no single causative organism) and congenital heart disease. It is common in preterm infants (abnormal intestinal flora, ischaemia and mucosal immaturity), those with Hirschsprung's disease, and bowel obstruction resulting from small bowel atresia, pyloric stenosis, meconium ileus and meconium plug syndrome. It is most commonly seen in the terminal ileum, followed by the caecum and right colon. It develops in the first 2–3 days after birth. Pathologically there is widespread transmural necrosis and acute inflammation with mucosal ulceration.

4. Clinically, the neonates present with gross abdominal distension, bilious emesis, delayed gastric emptying, feeding intolerance, decreased bowel sounds, explosive diarrhoea, blood-streaked stools, apnoea, lethargy, shock and generalised sepsis. Elevated WBC count, anaemia, thrombocytosis, metabolic acidosis and hyponatraemia are worrisome features. Complications are inflammatory stricture and bowel perforation, which are seen in 30% of patients. Short gut syndrome results from the removal of long segments of bowel, causing malabsorption. Some 75% of patients survive, of whom 50% develop complications. Treatment of necrotising enterocolitis depends on the degree of bowel involvement and severity of its presentation. Parenteral nutrition and fluid support are initiated. Broad-spectrum antibiotics are given after blood culture. Surgery is indicated when there is bowel perforation.

5. The X-ray shows dilated small and large bowel loops, with or without air–fluid levels, especially in the right lower quadrant. The bowel gas pattern is disarrayed rather than the normal polygonal pattern. Bowel wall thickening with thumbprinting is also seen. The bowel loops are fixed and do not show any change in sequential films. Pneumatosis intestinalis is a characteristic finding and is characterised by curvilinear (serosal) or bubbly (mucosal) gas collection (hydrogen bubbles produced by bacterial fermentation of intestinal contents). The bowel appears bubbly as a result of gas in the wall and faecal matter, which is a mix of blood, sloughed colonic mucosa, intraluminal gas and faecal material. Gas is seen in the branches of the mesenteric vessels and portal vein. Gas in the portal vein does not necessarily imply a grave outcome. Pneumoperitoneum is seen as a result of bowel perforation and warrants surgery. Barium enema is contraindicated in these patients. Absence of bowel gas indicates distension with fluid and is also worrisome. When ascites develops as a result of perforation, the bowel loops float in the centre of the abdomen Ultrasonography can find the portal gas, any local abscess formation and other abnormalities.

Case 2.9: Answers

1. The barium enema shows the very small calibre of the descending and transverse colon.

2. Small left colon syndrome.

3. Small left colon syndrome is caused by transient functional obstruction resulting from immaturity of the mesenteric plexus. It is seen in maternal diabetes and substance abuse. The appearance is the same as that of meconium ileus syndrome, but here the meconium plug is seen as a sequela of functional obstruction rather than the cause, and it undergoes spontaneous resolution within weeks.

4. Meconium ileus syndrome is seen in cystic fibrosis, Hirschsprung's disease, prematurity and maternal magnesium sulphate treatment. There is local inspissation of meconium in the large bowel. Clinical features are abdominal distension, vomiting and failure to pass meconium. An X-ray shows dilated small bowel and proximal large bowel loops up to the splenic flexure, with a bubbly appearance of colon caused by meconium inspissation. The distal large bowel is small and collapsed and there is no air in the rectum. A barium enema has a double-contrast effect with barium between the meconium plug and the colonic wall. Treatment is by water-soluble enema.

5. In small left colon syndrome, the large bowel is small. An X-ray may show dilated loops of proximal bowel. A barium enema demonstrates the small calibre of the bowel lumen.

Case 2.10: Answers

1. There is air under the dome of the diaphragms, and also air outlining the falciform ligament. The X-ray done in the supine position shows clear visualisation of the bowel wall, as a result of the air outlining it on either side.

2. Pneumoperitoneum resulting from hollow viscus perforation.

3. The radiological findings: on an erect film, air collects under the diaphragm. In supine views, diagnosis may depend on subtle findings:

   Rigler's sign: air on both sides of the bowel (indicates > 1000 ml gas)

   Football sign: large pneumoperitoneum outlining the entire abdomen

   Tell's triangle sign: air among three loops of bowel

Inverted V sign: outlining of both lateral umbilical ligaments

Outlining of medial umbilical ligaments: falciform ligament

Urachus sign: outlining middle umbilical ligament

Doges' cap sign: triangular collection in Morrison's pouch

Falciform ligament sign: linear lucency

Ligamentum teres sign: vertical, slit/oval area between ribs 10 and 12

Ligamentum teres notch: V shaped and inverted, under the liver

Cupola sign: gas below central tendon of the diaphragm

Diaphragmatic muscle misses visualisation.

---

4. Causes of pneumoperitoneum:

Trauma: blunt/penetrating

Iatrogenic: postoperative (absorbed in 1–24 days; air after 3 days is suspicious), laparoscopy, endoscopy, enema tip injury, intussusception reduction

Gastrointestinal tract diseases: hollow viscus perforation, perforated appendix, foreign body, inflammatory bowel disease, obstruction, tumours, imperforate anus, Hirschsprung's disease, meconium ileus

Ruptured pneumatosis

Idiopathic perforation in preterm infants

Extension from chest

Gas-forming peritonitis

Introduction through female genital tract.

---

5. **False positive**: other gas-filled structures such as a diverticulum, Chiladiti syndrome (hepatic flexure interposition between liver and diaphragm), diaphragmatic hernia, abscess, subdiaphragmatic fat, omental fat between liver and diaphragm, basal atelectasis, irregular diaphragm, pneumothorax.

False negative: erect X-ray should be taken 5 min after keeping the patient in erect position, otherwise it will be negative. Lateral decubitus films may be acquired for confirmation. Ultrasonography is useful in skilful hands to identify air.

Case 2.11: Answers

1. This is a barium swallow under videofluoroscopic observation. There is lot of dense contrast in the stomach, which is seen extending back to the lower and midoesophagus in the films.

2. Gastro-oesophageal reflux disease. A barium study is useful in evaluating the upper gastrointestinal tract. On videofluoroscopy studies, the contrast can be seen passing through the oesophagus into the stomach. In those with gastro-oesophageal reflux, the contrast will reflux back into the oesophagus from the stomach. The barium meal is not a very sensitive test. Provocative manoeuvres might be required for eliciting the reflux, such as a prone oblique position, coughing or Valsalva manoeuvre. Hiatus hernia can be observed. Gastro-oesophageal reflux is episodic and might be missed. It is graded according to the extent of reflux. Reflux just into lower oesophagus is graded as **mild**, to midoesophagus is **moderate** and into cervical oesophagus is **severe.**

3. Other studies are:

Gastric **scintiscan**: ^{99m}Tc-labelled sulphur colloid in orange juice is administered and reflux is assessed by oesophageal counts. Late postprandial reflux cannot be evaluated.

A **24-hour pH probe measurement** in distal oesophagus (gold standard).

Manometry and **endoscopy** are other procedures.

4. Gastro-oesophageal reflux is caused by an incompetent lower oesophageal sphincter. It is the most common oesophageal disorder in children. Chalasia refers to reflux across a dilated sphincter. All children have a functional gastro-oesophageal reflux that is minor and development is normal. Pathogenic gastro-oesophageal reflux disease occurs in 1/300–1/1000 and can result in strictures, malnutrition, respiratory disorders, oesophagitis, bleeding and dysplasia. Secondary gastro-oesophageal reflux is caused by underlying conditions such as hiatus hernia and gastric obstruction. The pathogenesis is transient lower oesophageal sphincter relaxation, which promotes reflux, especially in supine or slumped-seated position. A fluid diet in infants increases the risk. Delayed gastric emptying is seen in preterm infants. Decreased gastric compliance and rapid filling, with abdominal wall contraction, propel refluxate into the oesophagus and regurgitation. Cerebral palsy, Down syndrome, developmental delay and head injury increase the risk. Medications, poor dietary habits, allergies, greasy food, antral dysmotility, small reservoir capacity of infant's oesophagus, obesity and supine position (smoking, alcohol in adolescents) are other predisposing factors.

5. Symptoms of gastro-oesophageal reflux can start in neonates: 85% vomit in the first week and symptoms stop without treatment in 60% by 2 years, as a result of the upright position. Some have persistent reflux till 4 years. Pathogenic gastro-oesophageal reflux disease is seen in 2–10%. Crying, irritability, apnoea, poor appetite, failure to thrive, vomiting, wheezing, chest pain, stridor, weight loss, pneumonitis, sore throat, chronic cough, waterbrash and hoarseness are symptoms.

6. Strictures, malnutrition, asthma, sudden infant death syndrome (SIDS), chronic blood loss, oesophagitis, failure to thrive and recurrent respiratory infections are the complications. Functional gastro-oesophageal reflux requires only reassurance. Upright positioning after feeding, elevating the head, prone positioning and small frequent feeds help in controlling reflux. In older children, prone position, thick feeds with cereal and burping after feeds are enough. Medications can be given to reduce gastric secretion and increase gastric emptying. Antireflux surgery is indicated when complications develop.

Case 2.12: Answers

1. The X-ray of the abdomen shows no gas in the small or large bowel. There is a double-bubble appearance with a gas-filled, distended stomach and proximal duodenum.

2. Duodenal atresia.

3. Down syndrome is the most common association with duodenal atresia (associated with 11 pairs of ribs). Other associated conditions are congenital heart disease, urinary tract anomalies, vertebral and rib anomalies, biliary atresia, duodenal duplication, annular pancreas, Meckel's diverticulum, malrotation, preduodenal portal vein, transposed liver, oesophageal atresia and imperforate anus.

4. Duodenal atresia is caused by defective vacuolation of the duodenum, between 6 and 11 weeks of gestation. It is the second most common site

of bowel atresia and the most common cause of duodenal obstruction. In 80%, the obstruction is distal to the ampulla of Vater, but in 20% it is seen in the proximal duodenum. Newborns present with persistent bilious vomiting and electrolyte imbalance.

5. An X-ray shows the characteristic double-bubble sign, which is caused by the air–fluid levels in a distended stomach and proximal duodenum. There is no gas in the distal small and large bowel. Colon is of normal calibre. The double-bubble appearance can also be detected on antenatal ultrasonography, which is associated with polyhydramnios. The diagnosis can be confirmed by a contrast study, which will demonstrate obstruction at the level of the duodenum.

6. Differential diagnoses of duodenal obstruction are annular pancreas, duodenal diaphragm, bands, choledochal cyst and duplication anomalies.

Case 2.13: Answers

1. The plain X-ray shows dilated loops of small bowel and large bowel, indicating distal obstruction in the large bowel. There is no gas in the rectum and no pneumoperitoneum.

2. This is a contrast study of the large bowel. A rectal tube is inserted and a radio-opaque contrast is introduced to distend the rectum. The study shows a transition point from a normal calibre bowel to grossly dilated proximal bowel.

3. Hirschsprung's disease.

4. Hirschsprung's disease is characterised by the absence of myenteric (Auerbach) and submucosal (Meissner) ganglion cells in the distal alimentary tract as a result of failure of neural crest cells to populate the embryonic colon at around 5–12 weeks of gestation. Hirschsprung's disease can be classified as classic (75%), where the rectosigmoid is involved, or long segment (20%) or total colonic (3–12%). Neonates present with failure to pass meconium, abdominal distension and vomiting. Older children present with constipation, abdominal distension, vomiting and failure to thrive. Associated conditions are Down syndrome, multiple endocrine neoplasia and Waardenburg syndrome. Treatment depends on the age of the patient and extent of involvement. The aganglionic bowel is removed or bypassed, with anastomosis of normally innervated intestine to the distal rectum. This can be performed by means of a preliminary colostomy followed by a definitive pull-through procedure or an immediate definitive procedure

5. The X-ray shows features of bowel obstruction with no gas in the rectum, implying a low large bowel obstruction. Another feature is the presence of mixed barium stool pattern on delayed X-rays. Hirschsprung's disease is diagnosed by the presence of a transition zone that marks the junction between aganglionic narrow distal bowel and proximal, dilated, normally innervated bowel. This sign is highly reliable, but not always seen. Other findings are irregular bowel contractions in the aganglionic segment, thick nodular mucosa proximal to the transition point and delayed evacuation of contrast. The false-negative rate is 24%. Rectal manometry shows an absence of normal relaxation of the internal sphincter, with a reduction in the intraluminal pressure in the anal canal when the rectum is distended with a balloon. Rectal biopsy (suction or full thickness) has a 100% negative predictive value. If ganglion cells are present, then Hirschsprung's disease is excluded. Other findings are hypertrophy and hyperplasia of nerve fibres, and an increase in acetylcholinesterase-positive nerve fibres in the lamina propria and muscularis mucosa.

Case 2.14: Answers

1. The X-ray shows a dense calcification in the right iliac fossa, which is likely to be an appendicolith. There is also an abnormal collection of gas in the right lower quadrant, which is situated outside the bowel loops.

2. Ultrasonography done over the right iliac fossa shows a distended tubular structure, measuring 7 mm, which could not be compressed by the ultrasonic probe.

3. Acute appendicitis.

4. Appendicitis begins when the appendiceal lumen is blocked by food/stool/parasites/barium or hyperplastic lymphoid tissue, resulting in oedematous mucosa, and leading to increased intraluminal pressure, inflammation and exudates. Growth of bacteria within the lumen enhances the inflammatory response. Perforation ensues if the diagnosis is not made early and obstruction continues, resulting in peritonitis. Unlike in adults or adolescents where the omentum walls off perforated appendix, causing a focal abscess, in young children the omentum is not well developed, resulting in peritonitis. It is usually seen in children aged 6–10 years. The younger the age, the higher the risk of perforation. Clinically the symptoms start with ill-defined pain in the periumbilical region, with anorexia, nausea and vomiting. Subsequently the pain moves to the right lower quadrant, and is more intense. Children are usually afebrile or have a low fever. On examination the child lies still with maximal tenderness seen in McBurney's point in the right lower quadrant. Cough, Rovsing's, psoas and obturator signs are other signs of peritoneal irritation. Rectal examination may show impacted stool, mass or right-sided tenderness. The WBC count is elevated, but can be normal in 10%. A WBC count > 15 000 cells/cm^2 indicates perforation. Urinalysis can show WBCs as a result of bladder wall irritation. A WBC count > 20/Hpf indicates urinary infection. Positive triple test: CRP (C-reactive protein) values > 8 μg/ml, total WBC count > 11 000/ml, and neutrophil percentage > 75.

5. On X-rays, an appendicolith is seen in 10% of cases. Other features that are suggestive of, but not specific for, appendicitis are scoliosis concave to the right side, obliteration of the right psoas shadow, gas–fluid level on the right side, air in the appendix and localised ileus. Ultrasonography is the most useful modality used in diagnosis of appendicitis. The presence of a dilated (> 6 mm), non-compressible appendix has a high sensitivity and specificity in diagnosis. Other features are fluid in the appendix, appendicolith, transverse diameter > 6 mm and focal rebound tenderness. Appendiceal abscess and phlegmon are diagnosed by the presence of loculated fluid collections. An ultrasound scan excludes other causes of right-sided pain including ovarian cysts, pyelonephritis, renal stones and cholecystitis. A CT scan can be used in obese children, in whom ultrasonography is difficult. The appendix is enlarged, with an appendicolith with surrounding soft-tissue stranding. No contrast enters the appendix from the caecum. Children with appendicitis can undergo laparoscopic appendectomy without incurring a greater risk for complications. Of appendectomies 15–20% are performed in cases for which test results are later determined to be falsely positive, because appendicitis is difficult to diagnose in infants and toddlers. Non-toxic patients with a localised, walled-off abscess may be candidates for initial medical management with antibiotics, followed by an elective appendectomy.

Case 2.15: Answers

1. On the IVU, there is normal appearance of the urinary collecting system. However, the stomach is grossly distended. There is a large soft-tissue density within the stomach and a crescenteric rim of air between the soft tissue and the gastric wall. In the barium meal, the stomach is distended and there is a large heterogeneous filling defect with interstices of air within it.

2. Gastric bezoar.

3. Gastric bezoar is concretion in the stomach that increases in size by accumulation of non-absorbable food or fibres. (Bezoar comes from the Arabic word *Badzahr* which means antidote.) It is more common in those with previous surgery, altered gastrointestinal anatomy (inflammation, obstruction, malrotation, strictures), gastric motility disorders (gastroparesis, hypothyroidism, Guillain–Barré syndrome, myotonic dystrophy, medication), psychiatric complications, elderly people, hepatitis, cholestasis, cystic fibrosis, dehydration and dialysis, and those on drugs such as opiates, anticholinergics, ganglion blockers and antihistamines.

4. The various subtypes are **trichobezoar** (hair, mucus, undigested fat), **phytobezoar** (plant and vegetable matter), **diospyrobezoars** (persimmons) and **lactobezoar** (milk). Trichobezoars are caused by swallowing hair, which gets trapped in the gastric folds, resists peristalsis and forms hair balls. In **Rapunzel syndrome**, the trichobezoar extends continuously from the stomach along the entire length of the small intestine. Lactobezoars are seen in neonates as a result of poor motility, concentrated formulas and dehydration. Other compositions are medications including the shells of medications such as bulk-forming laxatives, extended-release products, ion exchange resins, vitamins and other natural products. Clinical features are nausea, vomiting, bloating, swelling, weight loss, anorexia, intolerance of solid food and gastric outlet obstruction. Examination might show tenderness, palpable mass or foul breath.

5. A plain X-ray shows a filling defect outlined by gas, which is amorphous, calcified granular or bubbly. A barium meal shows heterogeneous intraluminal filling defects with interstices of air within them, and not attached to any wall. A CT scan is better for evaluating the bezoar, because it shows the composition of the bezoar and air entrapped

within the mass. Ultrasonography shows an acoustic shadow surrounded by an echogenic arc of air. Complications are bleeding, obstruction, malabsorption and perforation.

6. Differential diagnoses include other intraluminal lesions such as tumours and polyps. Endoscopy is required for confirmation. Diet modification, pharmacotherapy (metoclopramide, erythromycin), gastric lavage, enzymatic disruption (*N*-acetylcysteine, papain, cellulase), endoscopic therapy and surgical therapy are done.

Case 2.16: Answers

1. The IVU shows a large soft-tissue opacity in the left upper quadrant of the abdomen, which displaces the bowel loops inferiorly and to the right side. The left renal collecting system is also displaced inferiorly and to the right side.

2. The CT scan shows a large spleen, which extends almost to the pelvic brim. Note that there are no lesions within the spleen. The second CT scan shows dense bones. This was a case of myelofibrosis.

3. The causes of splenomegaly in children are:

Infections:

– viral: Epstein–Barr virus, CMV, hepatitis

– bacterial: TB, endocarditis, typhoid, syphilis, brucellosis

– protozoal: malaria, schistosomiasis, kala-azar, hydatid

Inflammation: collagen vascular disease, juvenile rheumatoid arthritis, haemolytic anaemias – spherocytosis, thrombotic thrombocytopenic purpura, primary neutropenia

Neoplasia: acute lymphoblastic leukaemia (ALL), non-Hodgkin's lymphoma, acute/chronic myeloid leukaemia (AML/CML), metastatic neuroblastoma, histiocytosis

Congestive: portal vein thrombosis, cirrhosis, congestive cardiac failure, cystic fibrosis, acute splenic sequestration crisis of sickle cell anaemia

Storage disorders: Gaucher's disease, Niemann–Pick disease, mucopolysaccharidoses, haemochromatosis, diabetes

Trauma: haematoma, pseudocysts

Congenital: cysts

Miscellaneous: extramedullary haematopoiesis, thalassaemia major, osteopetrosis, idiopathic myelofibrosis.

4. Splenomegaly is diagnosed by clinical examination. Ultrasonography, CT and MRI can diagnose splenomegaly easily. Normalised curves exist for splenic sizes and volumes in children and splenomegaly is confirmed by comparing with these measurements. In older children and adults, a craniocaudal length > 13 cm is considered splenomegaly. As a rule of thumb, if the inferior tip of the spleen extends below the right lobe of liver or if the AP diameter of the spleen is more than two-thirds of the abdominal diameter, it is called splenomegaly. Focal lesions in the spleen can be identified in these imaging modalities. Extrasplenic lesions can also be evaluated. Myelofibrosis is an idiopathic, chronic disease, characterised by bone marrow fibrosis, splenomegaly and anaemia with immature and tear drop-shaped red blood cells (RBCs). Diagnosis is established by excluding other conditions that cause secondary myelofibrosis such as tumours (leukaemia, polycythaemia, myeloma, lymphoma, marrow metastasis), infections (TB, osteomyelitis), toxins (radiation, benzene, thorium) and autoimmune (SLE). Treatment is usually supportive.

5. The investigations used in the evaluation of splenomegaly are full blood count (FBC), liver function tests, antinuclear antibodies (ANAs) for SLE, immunoglobulin levels, neutrophil function, T-cell subclasses, viral antibody titres for Epstein–Barr virus, CMV, *Toxoplasma* spp., HIV, blood cultures, bone marrow examination and biopsy.

Case 2.17: Answers

1. The CT scan shows the completely irregular and disrupted architecture of the spleen, with hypodense areas indicating laceration and perisplenic collection, suggestive of haematoma.

2. Splenic rupture secondary to trauma.

3. Blunt abdominal trauma is the most common cause of splenic rupture. The spleen is the most common organ in the abdomen to be involved in blunt trauma. It is often associated with other visceral or bowel injuries, rib fractures, left kidney injury and diaphragm injuries. Twenty per cent of those with left rib fractures have splenic injuries, and 25% of those with left kidney injury have splenic injury. Left upper quadrant pain/tenderness, shoulder pain, abdominal distension and circulatory collapse are features of splenic injury.

4. Grading is done using a CT scan, which is the main investigation in a stable patient. There are many classification systems. There are various grading systems for splenic trauma.

Grade I: tear < 1 cm, subcapsular < 25%

Grade II: tear 1–3 cm, subcapsular 25–50%, parenchymal < 5 cm

Grade III: tear > 3 cm, trabecular vessels involved, subcapsular > 50%, parenchymal > 10 cm

Grade IV: segmental/bilobar vessels with devascularisation

Grade V: shattered spleen or total devascularisation.

CT is the procedure of choice for the diagnosis of splenic injuries. Splenic injuries can be haematomas, lacerations, vascular injuries or perisplenic haematoma. Haematoma is a round, hypodense, inhomogeneous region with or without hyperdense clot. Subcapsular haematoma is a crescentic region of hypodensity along the splenic margin. Contusion is mottled enhancement and laceration a linear, hypodense, parenchymal defect connecting the opposing visceral surfaces. Fracture is hypodense haematoma with separation of splenic fragments, a laceration extending across two capsular surfaces; shattered spleen is multiple lacerations and perisplenic haematoma a sentinel clot adjacent to spleen. **Active extravasation** of high-density contrast indicates vascular injury/pseudoaneurysm. **Haemoperitoneum** indicates splenic capsular disruption. Differential diagnoses of splenic injury include patchy enhancement in arterial phase of scan, normal lobulations, unopacified jejunum mimicking spleen and ascites/bile leak mimicking haemoperitoneum. Complications are scar, fibrosis, pseudocyst, pseudoaneurysm and delayed rupture.

5. Management is conservative in the earlier stages. If the injury is severe and the patient unstable, a splenectomy is performed. A haemodynamically unstable patient, higher grades of injury, haemoperitoneum, associated injuries and comorbid factors are all taken into consideration when surgery is planned. Bleeding, injury to adjacent structures, infection, thrombocytosis and splenosis are some of the complications of splenectomy. Immunisation against capsulated organisms such as *Haemophilus* spp., pneumococci and meningococci is indicated because normal spleen phagocytoses capsulated organisms.

6. Infections, congestive splenomegaly, infiltrative disorders and tumours are other causes of non-traumatic splenic rupture.

Case 2.18: Answers

1. The X-ray of the abdomen shows a large mass arising in the right upper quadrant, which is causing inferior displacement of the bowel loops. A CT scan of the abdomen with intravenous contrast shows a large, well-defined, round, contrast-enhancing mass in the left lobe of the liver.

2. Hepatoblastoma.

3. Hepatoblastoma is the most common liver cancer in children and the third most common abdominal malignancy after neuroblastoma and Wilms' tumour. It is seen at age < 3 years and peak age is 18–24 months, with a male preponderance. It can present as an incidental finding or with anorexia, nausea, vomiting, jaundice, pain or precocious puberty (as a result of ectopic hormone production). Elevated liver function tests and α-fetoprotein are noted. Pathologically, it can be a epithelial type or mixed type. It can be associated with hemihypertrophy and Beckwith–Weidemann syndrome.

4. An X-ray may show a large mass in the right side of the abdomen, which displaces the bowel loops inferiorly and medially. Calcification is very rarely seen (6%). Ultrasonography is often the first imaging modality. The tumour usually shows a heterogeneous echogenicity, with areas of calcification and necrosis, and is predominantly hyperechoic (bright). Of these tumours 80% are solitary and are more common in the right lobe. CT shows a hypodense tumour with peripheral rim or inhomogeneous enhancement. It is also useful for assessing the involvement of adjacent structures. An MR scan shows the lesion of heterogeneous signal intensity, with a low signal in T1 and a high signal in T2. Haemorrhagic areas are high signal in T1 and T2. Fibrous septa can be seen within the tumour, which are of low signal in T1 and T2 with slow delayed enhancement. Sulphur colloid scan shows a photopenic defect. An angiogram shows a hypervascular mass. A CT scan of the chest is useful for pulmonary metastasis and a bone scan for bone metastasis.

5. Common differential diagnoses of abdominal tumours in this age group are **Wilms' tumour** and **neuroblastoma**, both of which can be clearly identified on CT scans. Other liver tumours in children are **haemangioendothelioma** (granular calcifications), haemangioma (hypodense, bright in T2 on MRI, rim enhancement with slow centripetal filling of contrast), **juvenile embryonal sarcoma** (more cystic components), hepatocellular carcinoma (> 5 years, no calcification), **mesenchymal hamartoma** (cystic with septations), **metastatic neuroblastoma**, **lymphoma** and **leukaemia.** Of these tumours 60% are resectable. An epithelial tumour has a better prognosis. A combination of chemotherapy (cisplatin/5-fluorouracil [5FU]/vincristine or cisplatin/doxorubicin regimen) and surgery is used. Preoperative chemotherapy can eradicate pulmonary metastasis and make the tumour more resectable. Postoperative chemotherapy is also useful.

Case 2.19: Answers

1. Ultrasonography shows a dark hypoechoic lesion in the liver. This is a prominent bile duct and not an intrahepatic cyst.

2. MRI shows cystic dilatation of the common bile duct. There is no dilatation of the intrahepatic biliary radicles.

3. Choledochal cyst, type IA

4. Choledochal cysts are congenital anomalies with cystic dilatation of the biliary tree. The La Todani classification of choledochal cysts:

Type I (80–90%): saccular or fusiform dilatations of the common bile duct

- **IA**: saccular, entire extrahepatic bile duct or most of it
- **IB**: saccular, limited segment of the bile duct,
- **IC**: fusiform, most or all of the extrahepatic bile duct

Type II: diverticulum arising from the common bile duct

Type III: choledochocele arising from the intraduodenal portion of the common bile duct

Type IVA: multiple dilatations of the intrahepatic and extrahepatic bile ducts

Type IVB: multiple dilatations involving only the extrahepatic bile ducts

Type V (Caroli's disease) consists of multiple dilatations limited to the intrahepatic bile ducts.

5. Choledochal cyst is seen in childhood or older age groups. It presents with recurrent cramps, fever, jaundice and cirrhosis, with portal hypertension in late cases. Complications include bile stasis with cholelithiasis, cholangitis, liver abscess, septicaemia and cholangiocarcinomas.

6. Ultrasonography shows cystic dilatation of the bile duct. The location depends on the type of choledochal cyst. Demonstration of communication with the biliary tree is essential to make a diagnosis. Doppler ultrasonography is used to evaluate the liver and portal hypertension. A CT scan shows a dilated duct and coronal and sagittal reconstructions show continuation with the bile duct. Sludge or calculi are seen in dilated ducts. MRCP can be done and it shows dilatation of the bile ducts. Hepatobiliary nuclear scans can demonstrate communication between the cysts and the bile ducts. Ultrasound-guided aspiration of cysts will confirm the presence of bile and the diagnosis of cholangitis. Differential diagnoses include other causes of cysts such as simple liver cyst, abscess, hydatid and cystic tumours.

Case 2.20: Answers

1. The barium meal shows a twisted stomach with abnormal configuration. The stomach is rotated around the long axis of the stomach.

2. Gastric volvulus.

3. Gastric volvulus is twisting of one part of stomach around another part. It is caused by unusually long gastrohepatic and gastrocolic mesenteries or by abnormality of the suspensory ligaments (hepatic, splenic, phrenic or colic).

4. There are two types: **organoaxial** (the stomach is rotated around a line extending from the cardia to the pylorus along the long axis of the stomach) and **mesenteroaxial** (rotation around an axis extending from

the lesser to the greater curvature). A barium meal is used to diagnose the volvulus and find the type. It demonstrates the area of twist. There might be a delay in the entry of barium into the stomach. A CT scan can be used for further characterisation.

5. The characteristic **Borchardt's triad** is epigastric pain, retching and inability to pass the nasogastric tube into the stomach. Complications are ischaemia, gastric empyema and perforation. Differential diagnoses are gastric atony, acute gastric dilatation and pyloric obstruction. It is associated with paraoesophageal hiatus hernia and eventration.

Case 2.21: Answers

1. The axial and coronal post-contrast CT scans of the abdomen show an enlarged spleen, which has non-enhancing hypodense areas within it and only a thin rim of normal enhancing splenic parenchyma.

2. Splenic infarct in a patient with sickle cell disease.

3. Causes of splenic infarct are:

   Embolic: endocarditis (50%), vasculitis, cardiac thrombosis, atrial fibrillation, infarcted graft, metastasis, HIV

   Thrombosis: sickle cell disease, CML, lymphoma, polycythaemia, myelofibrosis, Gaucher's disease, SLE, portal hypertension

   Vasculitis: periarteritis nodosa

   Vascular compromise: thrombus from splenic artery aneurysm, splenic torsion

   Iatrogenic: hepatic embolisation, pancreatectomy

   Trauma: blunt, torsion, vasopressin injection

   Miscellaneous: pancreatitis, amyloidosis, pancreatic tumours, ARDS, toxic shock syndrome

   Wandering spleen, where the spleen is attached by a long stalk, is a predisposing factor for splenic infarction.

4. The infarct can be focal or global. Global infarcts are uncommon. The spleen is hypodense and does not show any contrast enhancement. Focal infarcts are seen as wedge-shaped hypodensities in the periphery of the spleen. There are three phases depending on the evolution of the infarct. In the **hyperacute phase** (day 1), a mottled area or a large focal area of hyperdensity is seen on the CT. In the **acute** (2–4 days) and **subacute phase** (days 4–9), the lesions get more demarcated with hypodense areas, showing no enhancement. In the **chronic phase** (2–4 weeks) the size decreases and the density returns to normal. Usually the resolution is complete with just a residual contour defect and areas of calcification. Ultrasonography can also show ill-defined hypoechoic lesions in the early stages, which become more organised and smaller and wedge shaped in the later phases.

5. Most of the splenic infarcts are occult and caused by outstripping of the splenic vascular supply. They can present with left upper quadrant pain, fever, chills, nausea, vomiting, left pleuritic pain and left shoulder pain. The WBC count, ESR and LDH are elevated. Complications of splenic infarct are acute febrile illness, abscess formation, pseudocyst, splenic rupture or haemorrhage. Complications warrant surgical intervention, otherwise the infarcted spleen is left *in situ* and the patient observed.

Case 2.22: Answers

1. The X-ray shows a radio-opaque foreign body in the upper chest.

2. Contrast swallow outlines the oesophagus and demonstrates that the foreign body is within the oesophagus. The child has swallowed a coin.

3. The most common sites of lodgement of a foreign body are: **in the oesophagus** 70% are at the level of upper oesophageal sphincter, which is the cricopharyngeus, at the level of C6; 15% are lodged in the mid-oesophagus and 15% in the lower oesophageal sphincter. Congenital or acquired oesophageal abnormalities are often frequent sites of lodgement of a foreign body. **In the bowel** foreign bodies usually pass freely, unless they are too long or too wide or sharp to pass the pyloric sphincter. The ileocaecal valve is a common site of lodgement of foreign bodies. Congenital anomalies and surgeries are frequent sites of lodgement of foreign bodies in the gastrointestinal tract (eg Meckel's diverticulum).

Repeated cases of foreign body ingestion suggest neglect or abuse or gastrointestinal abnormalities or attention-seeking behaviour or bulimia.

4. Unlike adults, children often do not present with any complications of foreign body ingestion. Foreign bodies in the stomach and bowel often do not produce any symptoms. An oesophageal foreign body can produce dysphagia, food refusal, drooling, vomiting, foreign body sensation, chest pain, sore throat, stridor and cough. Stomach/lower gastrointestinal tract foreign bodies produce abdominal distension, haematochalazia and unexplained fever. When foreign bodies are impacted or inflamed, they can cause pain, bleeding, scarring, obstruction or perforation. Foreign bodies migrating through the oesophagus can cause mediastinitis or aortoenteric fistula. Pneumothorax, pneumomediastinum and peritonitis can be manifestations. Drooling or pooling of secretions suggests an oesophageal foreign body. Streaks of blood or oedema in hypopharynx suggests a proximal swallowing-related trauma.

5. Most of the foreign bodies ingested by children are radio-opaque, unlike in adults where most are radiolucent. In small children a single X-ray that includes the whole body will localise the foreign body. If the object is below the diaphragm, further imaging is not required, unless there are gastrointestinal disorders such as previous surgery or congenital anomalies. If the object is in oesophagus, a frontal and lateral view of the chest are done to find whether the object is in the oesophagus or airway, and to be sure that there are not two adherent objects. Coins can be localised to the airway or oesophagus by their position in frontal views. If they are oriented en face (coronal) on a frontal film, they are unlikely to be in the airway. Coins in trachea are oriented sagittally in the frontal view. Although the coins have a smooth border, button batteries have a distinct two-step border. If the object is radiolucent, it can be localised only if there are secondary changes such as airway compression. An alternative is to use a dilute contrast or CT scan. Other tests include endoscopy or metal detectors (useful in coins or aluminium cans). Coins in the oesophagus may require endoscopy for location and removal. Coins in the abdomen usually pass out without complications.

Case 2.23: Answers

1. The first study is a small bowel study with barium. There is a long abnormal segment of terminal ileum, which is narrowed with focal areas of ulcerations. There are proximally dilated small bowel loops.

2. The CT scan shows diffuse circumferential wall thickening of the terminal ileal loops. There is increased density of fat in the adjacent mesentery and retroperitoneum, with fat creeping. There are few dilated loops of bowel proximally.

3. Crohn's disease of the small bowel.

4. Crohn's disease is a chronic inflammatory disease of bowel with discontinuous, asymmetrical involvement of the gastrointestinal tract. Complications are fistula, sinus, abscess, perforation, toxic megacolon, hydronephrosis and adenocarcinoma in the ileum. Fatty liver, liver abscess, gallstones, cholecystitis, sclerosing cholangitis, urolithiasis, hydronephrosis, amyloidosis, cystitis, clubbing, ankylosing spondylitis, erosive arthritis, avascular necrosis, osteomyelitis, septic arthritis and abscesses are other complications. Treatment consists of 5-aminosalicylic acid preparations, antibiotics such as metronidazole, corticosteroids, immunosuppressants (methotrexate, 6-mercaptopurine, azathioprine, antibodies to tumour necrosis factor [TNF]-α). Surgery is performed when medical therapy fails and complications develop.

5. A barium meal shows involvement of the terminal ileum in the form of thickened and nodular folds, aphthous ulcers, cobblestone mucosa or a medial caecal defect. There is rigidity of the small bowel loops with wide separation. Postinflammatory polyps, mucosal granularity and pseudodiverticula can be seen. There can be diarrhoea, rectal bleeding and abdominal pain, weight loss, anaemia, joint pain, growth failure and delayed puberty. The small intestine disease usually manifests with evidence of malabsorption, including diarrhoea, abdominal pain, growth deceleration, weight loss and anorexia. Pathologically Crohn's disease is characterised by transmural involvement and granulomas. A CT scan shows homogeneous thickened walls or a double-halo configuration (lumen surrounded by oedematous, hypodense mucosa and soft-tissue density). There are skip lesions of asymmetrical bowel wall thickening. A characteristic feature on CT is the creeping fat sign, where there is massive proliferation of mesenteric fat that separates the bowel loops. Dilated bowel loops, sinus, fistula, adenopathy and abscesses are other features. Radiological differential diagnoses are TB (involvement of caecum, pulmonary TB), *Yersinia* spp. (resolution in 3–4 months), radiation enteritis, lymphoma (no spasm, nodular/aneurysmal), actinomycosis, carcinoid and eosinophilic gastroenteritis.

Case 2.24: Answers

1. MRI of the liver shows two bright lesions in the right lobe. Other lesions were seen in the left lobe (not shown here).

2. Hepatic adenomas.

3. Hepatic adenoma is the most frequent liver tumour in young women as a result of the use of oral contraceptives. It is a benign tumour composed of sheets of hepatocytes without portal veins or central veins. Causes are oral contraceptives, steroids, pregnancy, diabetes mellitus, glycogen storage disease type 1a (von Gierke's) and Fanconi's anaemia. The tumour increases and may rupture during pregnancy. In those with diabetes, the tumour regresses after restoration of serum glucose levels.

4. The most common location of adenoma is the right lobe in a subcapsular location. It is a round, well-circumscribed, pseudoencapsulated mass. It can be pedunculated in 10%. On ultrasonography, it is seen as a well-defined solid mass and can be bright, dark or complex. On CT it is hypodense, but can be hyperdense if there is haemorrhage. It enhances during the arterial phase and is isodense in delayed images. On MRI it is inhomogeneous in all sequences. It is hypointense in T1 and isointense in T2, showing early arterial enhancement, and isointense in delayed images. In angiography it is very vascular.

5. Differential diagnoses are: **focal nodular hyperplasia** (central scar that is hypointense in T1 and hyperintense in T2 and may have calcifications), **haemangioma** (nodular enhancement, centripetal slow persistent filling), **hepatocellular** carcinoma (early enhancement and early washout, seen in cirrhotic liver).

6. Complications are spontaneous rupture and haemorrhage with haemoperitoneum, malignant transformation and recurrence after resection. Treatment is with surgical resection. Biopsy has a high risk of bleeding.

Case 2.25: Answers

1. MRI (T2-weighted sequence) shows multiple cystic lesions, which are bright (hyperintense) as a result of their fluid content. The CT scan shows multiple hypodense (less dense than adjacent liver) lesions in the liver. Some of these cysts have small dense nodules within them.

2. Caroli's disease.

3. Caroli's disease is segmental saccular dilatation of intrahepatic bile ducts, probably secondary to perinatal hepatic artery occlusion or hypoplasia of fibromuscular wall components. The La Todani classification of choledochal cysts is as given for the answer to question 2.19 on page 146.

4. Caroli's disease is seen in childhood or older age group. It presents with recurrent cramps, fever, jaundice, cirrhosis with portal hypertension in late cases. It is associated with renal tubular ectasia, medullary sponge kidney, choledochal cyst and congenital hepatic fibrosis.

5. Complications include bile stasis with cholelithiasis, cholangitis, liver abscess, septicaemia and cholangiocarcinomas. In patients without hepatic fibrosis, the frequency and severity of cholangitis determine the prognosis. In those with hepatic fibrosis, cholangitis and portal hypertension are the complications.

6. Ultrasonography shows multiple cystic structures that are dilated biliary radicles, converging towards porta hepatis. These are more prominent in the superior aspect of the liver. Portal branches protrude into the cysts. Extrahepatic ductal dilatation is seen only if there is another cause such as a stone. Doppler ultrasonography is used for evaluating the liver and portal hypertension. CT has the characteristic central dot sign, where the portal radicles are completely surrounded by dilated bile ducts. Sludge or calculi are seen in dilated ducts. MRCP can be done and shows segmental saccular dilatation of the bile ducts. Hepatobiliary nuclear scans can demonstrate communication between the cysts and bile ducts. Ultrasound-guided aspiration of cysts will confirm the presence of bile and the diagnosis of cholangitis. A common differential diagnosis is polycystic liver disease, which is usually associated with multiple, renal cysts.

Case 2.26: Answers

1. The plain X-ray shows dilated loops of small bowel. There is a subtle area of soft-tissue density in the right inguinal region.

2. The barium study demonstrates dilated loops of small bowel. One of the contrast-filled small bowel loops is seen herniating inferiorly in the right inguinal region. This patient has incarcerated right inguinal hernia with proximal small bowel obstruction.

3. The inguinal region has muscle and fascial layers. The inguinal ligament is the lower border of an external oblique aponeurosis, attached between the anterosuperior iliac spine and the pubic tubercle; it forms the floor of the inguinal canal. The deep inguinal ring is a defect in the transversalis fascia. A superficial inguinal ring is a defect in the external oblique aponeurosis, above and lateral to the pubic tubercle. The inferior epigastric artery is situated medial to the deep inguinal ring. Hasselbach's triangle is bounded inferiorly by the inguinal ligament, medially by the lateral margin of rectus abdominis and superiorly by the inferior epigastric artery. The inguinal canal extends from the deep to the superficial ring. The roof is formed by fibres of internal oblique and transverse abdominis muscles, the floor by inguinal ligament, augmented by the lacunar ligament medially, anterior wall by the external oblique aponeurosis, augmented by the internal oblique aponeurosis laterally and the posterior wall by transversalis fascia, augmented by conjoint tendon medially.

4. Inguinal hernias can be direct or indirect. An indirect inguinal hernia occurs through the deep inguinal ring, which is lateral to the inferior epigastric artery and superior to the inguinal ligament, and extends for a variable distance into the inguinal canal. It can pass through the canal, emerge via the superficial ring and extend into the scrotum (complete hernia). Contents may be small bowel loops, mobile colon segments (caecum, sigmoid, appendix), mesenteric fat or urinary bladder. Direct hernia occurs through the inferior aspect of Hesselbach's triangle, which is medial to the inferior epigastric artery. Patients with inguinal hernia present with dull aching pain and a lump, worsened on exercise or straining. On examination, a soft or firm lump that is more prominent with provocative manoeuvres is seen. A cough impulse is noted. In an inguinal hernia, the neck of the sac is situated above and medial to the ligament. Complications are incarceration, obstruction and strangulation. When the hernia is strangulated, there is pain, tenderness, swelling and redness, with a toxic

appearance. Obstruction presents with nausea, vomiting, constipation and distension. Hernias are more common in boys and bowel incarceration is more common in girls. In children hernias are caused by idiopathic failure of closure of processus vaginalis.

5. On ultrasonography, an indirect inguinal hernia is seen lateral to the inferior epigastric artery. A direct inguinal hernia arises medial to the inferior epigastric artery in Hesselbach's triangle. Ultrasonography differentiates a groin swelling from an abscess, lymph node or aneurysm. On a CT scan, the sac is situated medial to the pubic tubercle. Complications such as obstruction and strangulation are diagnosed. In obstruction, bowel loops are dilated. In strangulation, the bowel loops are thickened, with poor contrast enhancement, and gas may be seen in the bowel wall. Herniogram is useful in indeterminate cases. Elective repair is herniotomy or herniorrhaphy. Emergent surgery is required for complications.

Case 2.27: Answers

1. The barium enema shows absence of haustrations in the colon. Multiple ulcers are seen, scattered throughout the colon. There are mucosal islands noted in the transverse colon.

2. Ulcerative colitis.

3. Ulcerative colitis is an idiopathic inflammatory bowel disease, with symmetrical continuous involvement of the colon. It presents with bloody diarrhoea, fever and cramps. Extracolonic features are iritis, pyoderma gangrenosum, erythema nodosum, pericholangitis, sclerosing cholangitis, chronic active hepatitis, rheumatoid arthritis, spondylitis and thrombotic complications. Twenty per cent start in childhood or adolescence. Usually, ulcerative colitis begins in the rectum and spreads proximally and symmetrically. Rectosigmoid is involved in 95%. When the colitis extends proximal to the splenic flexure, it is called universal colitis and, when it extends to the terminal ileum, it is called backwash ileitis.

4. The findings on a barium enema depend on the stage. In the acute stage there is fine mucosal granularity and tiny superficial ulcers. Collar-button ulcers, double-tracking and thumbprinting are other findings.

Pseudopolyps are seen as a result of scattered areas of oedematous mucosa and re-epithelialised granulation tissue within an area of denuded mucosa. Presacral space is widened as a result of inflammation. Rectal folds are obliterated. In later stages, the haustra are lost. Inflammatory polyps are seen and the colon is short and rigid. The term 'burnt-out colon' is used when there is distensible colon with no haustral markings and no mucosal pattern. Postinflammatory polyps are small sessile nodules (filiform polyps).

5. **Familial polyposis**: haustrations are seen. No inflammation in polyps.

Cathartic colon: more extensive changes are seen in the right colon.

Crohn's disease is the most important clinical differential diagnosis.

Crohn's disease is more common in the small bowel with deep ulcers, thick ileocaeal valve, eccentric location and transmural skip lesions. Megacolon is uncommon, but fistulae may be seen. There is a slight increase in the risk of carcinoma. In ulcerative colitis, the colon is involved and the rectum is always involved. There are shallow ulcers with loss of haustrations and a gaping ileocaecal valve. There is symmetrical involvement with no skip lesions. Megacolon is common and there is a high risk of carcinoma.

6. Complications are toxic megacolon (most common cause of death, transverse colon > 5.5 cm), strictures, obstruction and perforation. There is a 5% risk of malignancy, and the risk starts after 10 years. Risk is 0.5% per year for colitis, higher if the onset < 15 years and when it is in the rectosigmoid. The lesion is usually annular or polypoid. Treatment is with ASA derivatives, steroids and immunosuppressants. Surgery is done when complications develop.

Case 2.28: Answers

1. Ultrasonography of the abdomen shows a linear, vertical discontinuity in the pancreatic body. There is disruption of the pancreatic duct. The CT scan shows a vertical split in the body of the pancreas.

2. Pancreatic laceration. Pancreatic injuries are uncommon (0.4/100 000). Injury may follow blunt or penetrating trauma. Most blunt injuries are caused by direct contact with a steering wheel or secondary to seat belt injury or handlebar injury in cyclists/motorcyclists.

3. Classification of pancreatic trauma:

I: simple superficial contusion, minimal parenchymal damage without ductal injury (most common)

II: deep laceration/perforation/transection of body/tail; pancreatic duct may be damaged

III: severe crushing, perforation/transaction of pancreatic head, with or without duct injury, but intact duodenum

IV: combined pancreaticoduodenal injuries – with mild pancreatic injury and with severe pancreatic injury and duct disruption.

The most common location of pancreatic trauma is the junction of the body and tail. Transection is more common to the left of the superior mesenteric vessels and occurs when there is compression over the spine. Injuries to the right of the midline cause serious crushing injuries to the pancreas and duodenum.

4. Ultrasonography and CT are used for diagnosing pancreatic trauma. Contusion is seen as an area of focal hypodensity in the pancreas. Acute haematoma is seen as a high-density area. Laceration is seen as a focal area of linear disruption in the pancreas. Fluid collection can be seen around the SMA, transverse mesocolon and lesser sac, and between the pancreas and splenic vein. There is thickening of pararenal fascia. Other features are pancreatic enlargement, fluid separating the splenic vein and pancreas, high-density fat around the pancreas and intra-/extraperitoneal fluid. Endoscopic retrograde cholangiopancreatography (ERCP) is useful for assessing ductal injuries. MRCP is a non-invasive way of assessing the pancreatic duct. Pancreatitis and tumours are the common differential diagnosis. In pancreatitis, the gland is enlarged with inflammatory fluid seen in the pancreas and around it. Tumours are seen as focal discrete masses.

5. Pancreatitis, pseudocyst formation, pseudoaneurysm, portal vein thrombosis, abscess and fistula are the complications. Many patients have delayed presentations with recurrent pancreatitis and pseudocysts. A patient with a post-traumatic pseudocyst should be considered to have a duct leak unless proved otherwise. Grade I injuries do not require surgery, unless there are serious associated injuries to other organs. Grade II injuries require only drainage, if the main duct is intact. For distal ductal injury, distal pancreatic resection and drainage of pancreatic bed with or without splenectomy are done. Surgery for grade III injuries depends on ductal injury status. Grade IV injuries always require surgery, which is usually pancreaticoduodenectomy.

Case 2.29: Answers

1. the plain X-ray shows dilated bowel loops. There is no gas in the rectum or anus. In the second lateral film, a skin marker has been placed at the location of the anus.

2. Anal atresia.

3. Failure of development of the cloacal membrane.

4. Imperforate anus can be classified into low, intermediate and high anomalies. In **low anomaly** (55%), the bowel has passed through the levator sling and there is a fistula to the perineum/vulva. In **intermediate type**, the bowel ends within the levator muscle and there is a fistula opening low in the vagina/vestibule. In **high anomaly**, the bowel ends above the levator sling and there is a fistulous connection to the perineum/vagina/posterior urethra. X-rays show absence of gas in the anus. A crude method of estimating the size of the atretic segment is to measure the distance between the rectal air and skin. This size varies with crying, increase in abdominal pressure and contraction of levator ani. Transperineal ultrasonography can be done and, if the distance between the anal dimple and the rectal pouch is < 15 mm, it indicates a low anomaly.

5. Low anomalies are easily corrected. Intermediate anomalies are corrected by a two- or three-stage operation. High anomalies require multistage procedures.

6. VACTERL is a well-known congenital malformation association including **v**ertebral, **a**nal, **c**ardiac, **t**racheo-o**e**sophageal, **r**enal and **l**imb anomalies.

3

GENITOURINARY RADIOLOGY QUESTIONS

Case 3.1

A 4-year-old girl presents with recurrent urinary infections, right-sided abdominal pain and oliguria. On examination there is a large, tender mass on the right side of the abdomen in the renal angle.

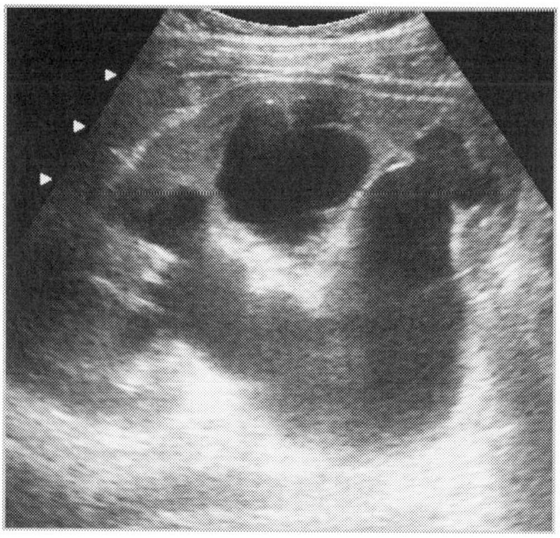

Fig 3.1a

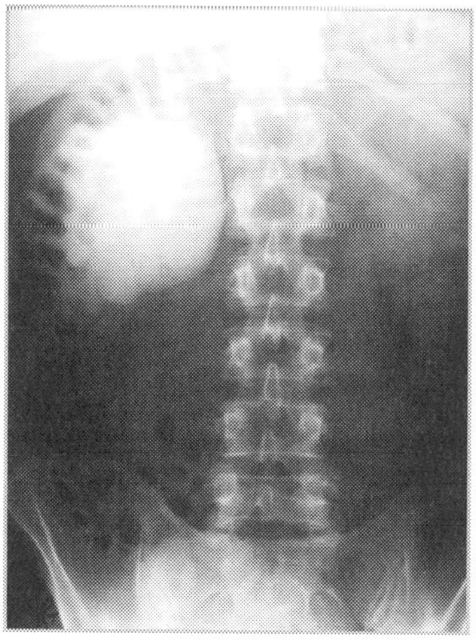

Fig 3.1b

1. What do you note on ultrasonography of kidneys?
2. What do you note on the IVU?
3. What is the diagnosis?
4. What are the aetiology and the clinical features?
5. What are the earliest test to diagnose this condition and the treatment?

Answers *on pages 183–211*

Case 3.2

A 3-year-old boy presents with abdominal pain and failure to thrive. On examination, a tender mass is felt in the right upper quadrant.

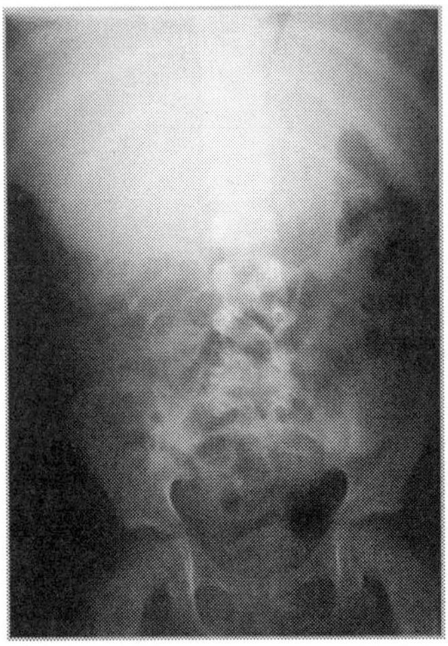

Fig 3.2a

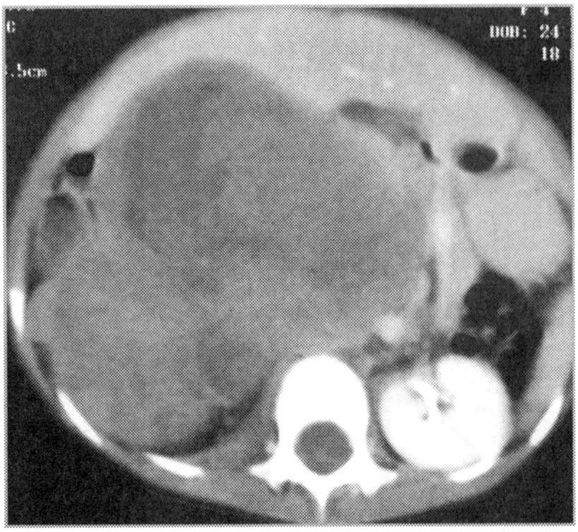

Fig 3.2b

1. What do you see on the plain X-ray and the CT scan?
2. What is the diagnosis?
3. What are the clinical features and associations?
4. What are the radiological features?
5. What is the differential diagnosis in this age group?
6. How will you manage this patient?

Answers *on pages 183–211*

Case 3.3

A 12-year-old boy was involved in a road traffic accident. He presented to the accident and emergency department (A&E) with severe pain in the right side of his abdomen and haematuria. On examination, his pulse was 120 and BP 106/82 mmHg. There was severe tenderness and swelling on the right side of the abdomen.

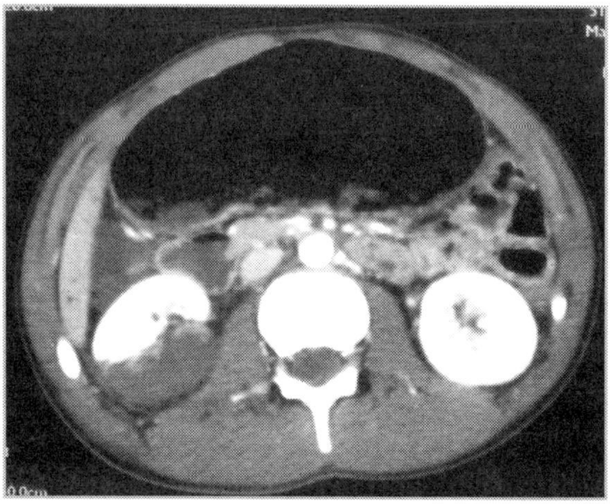

Fig 3.3a

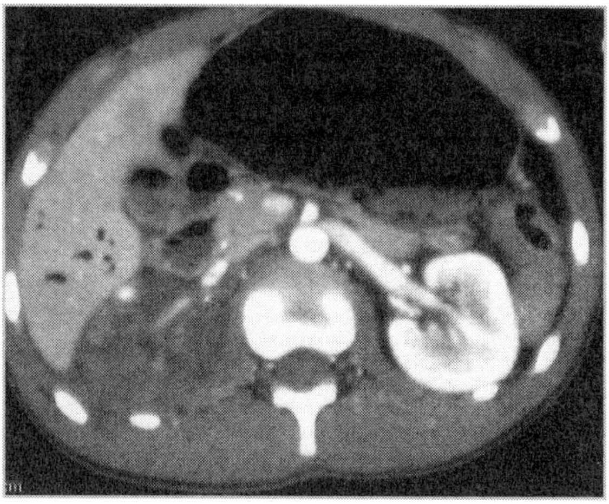

Fig 3.3b

1. What do you observe on the CT scan?
2. What is the diagnosis?
3. How is this categorised?
4. What are the radiological features and the imaging protocol?
5. What are the complications and treatment?

Answers *on pages 183–211*

Case 3.4

A 4-year-old girl presents with abdominal pain, fever and pain on micturition. On examination, there is mild bilateral renal angle tenderness.

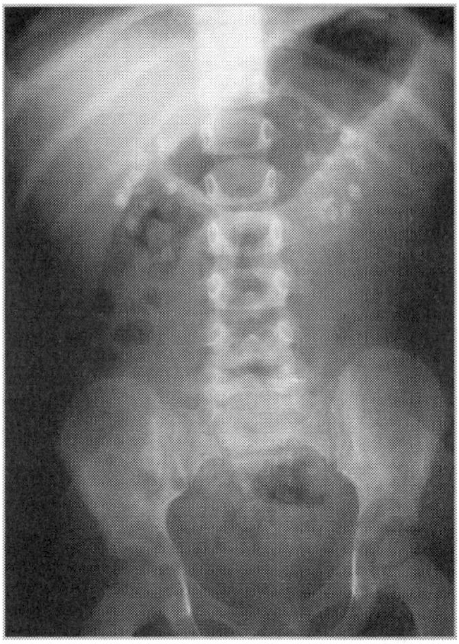
Fig 3.4a

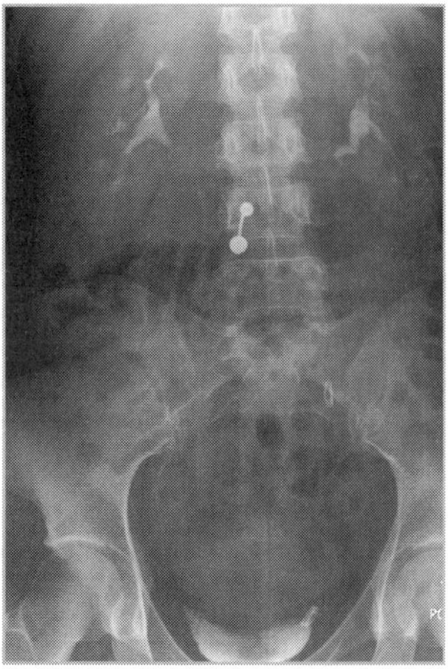

Fig 3.4b

1. What do you see in the plain abdominal X-ray? What do you see in the IVU (follow up IVU done at 13 years of age)?
2. What is the diagnosis?
3. What are the causes of this appearance?
4. What disease does this boy have and what are its clinical features?
5. What are the radiological features?

Answers *on pages 183–211*

Case 3.5

A 1-year-old boy presents with persistent abdominal pain. Clinical examination does not show any focal areas of rebound tenderness.

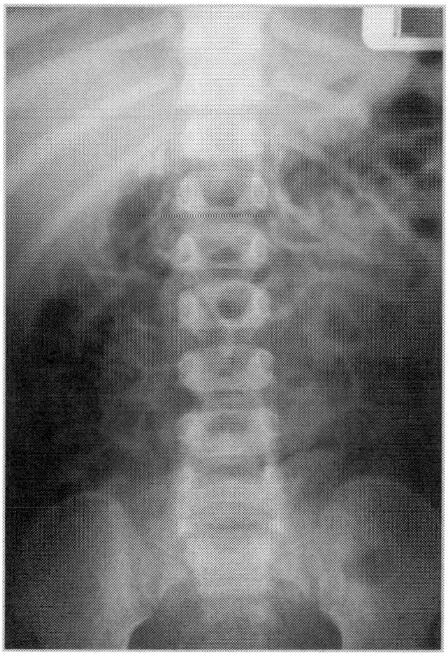

Fig 3.5a

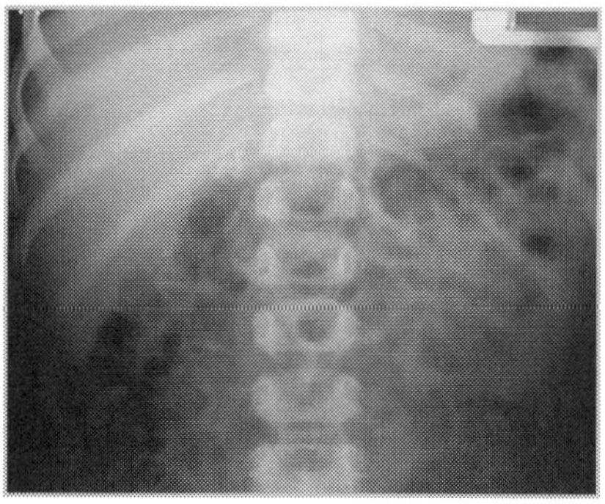

Fig 3.5b

1. What do you see on the X-ray of the abdomen?
2. What is the diagnosis?
3. What are the causes of these findings?
4. What are the clinical and radiological features?
5. What is the differential diagnosis?
6. What is the management of this condition?

Answers *on pages 183–211*

Case 3.6

A 7-year-old boy presents with urinary infections and abdominal pain.

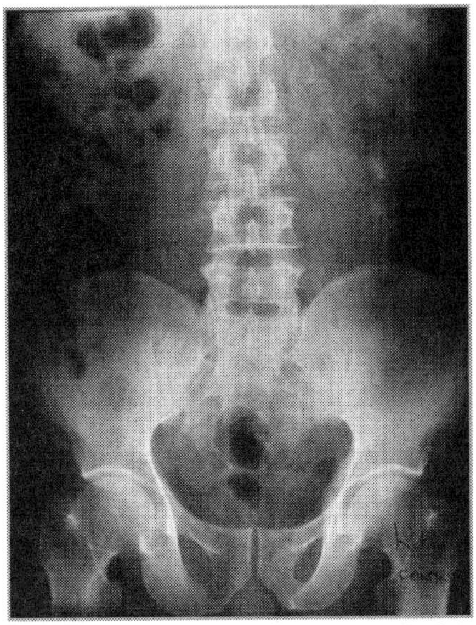

Fig 3.6a

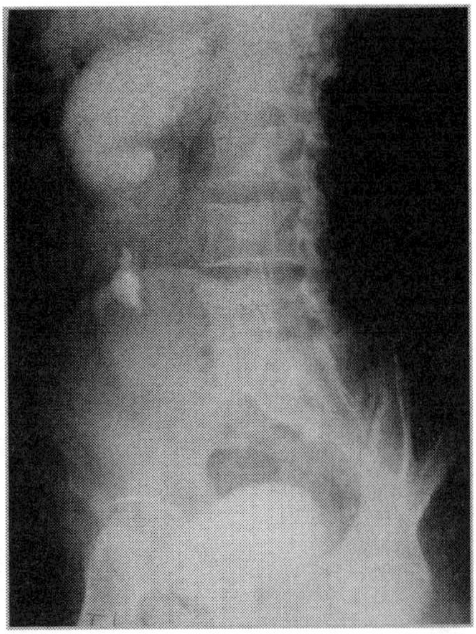

Fig 3.6b

1. What do you observe on the X-ray and the IVU?
2. What is the diagnosis?
3. What is the development of this condition?
4. What are the clinical features?
5. What are the associated features?

Answers *on pages 183–211*

Case 3.7

A 1-year-old boy was brought to the hospital with abdominal distension, urinary infections and abnormal renal function tests.

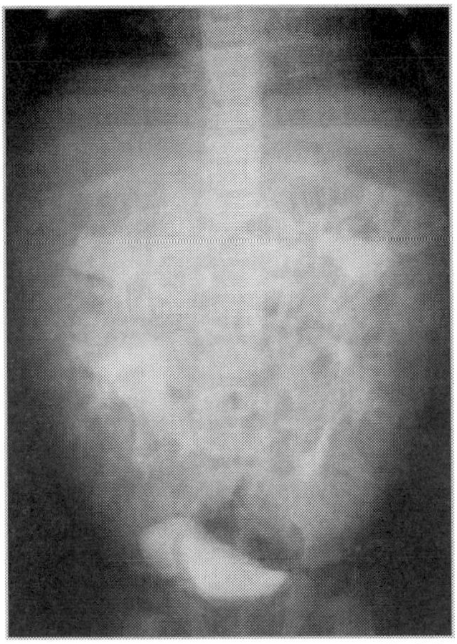

Fig 3.7a

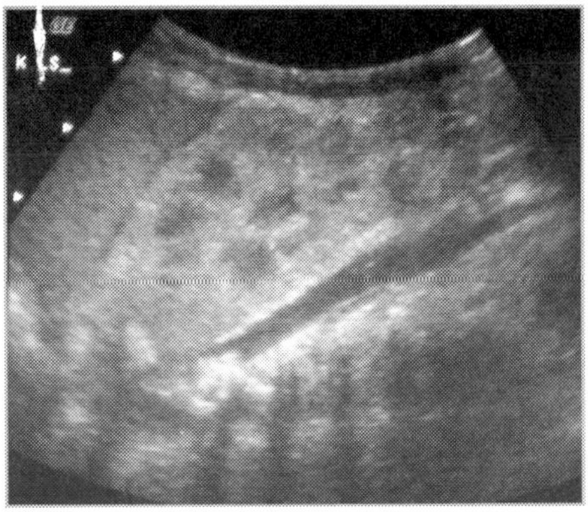

Fig 3.7b

1. What are the findings on the IVU and the ultrasound scan?
2. What is the diagnosis?
3. What are the pathophysiology and classification of this disorder?
4. What are the radiological features?
5. What are the prognosis and the important complications of this condition?

Answers *on pages 183–211*

Case 3.8

A 3-year-old girl presents with recurrent UTIs. Investigations were ordered.

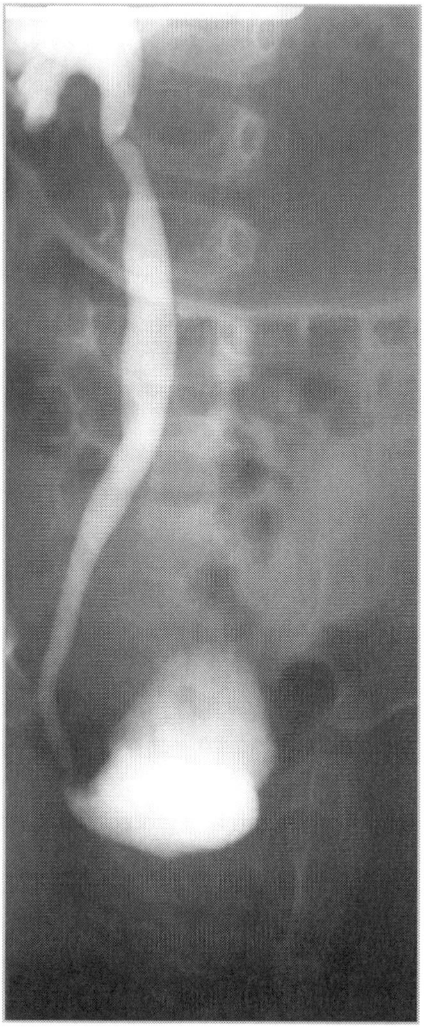

Fig 3.8a

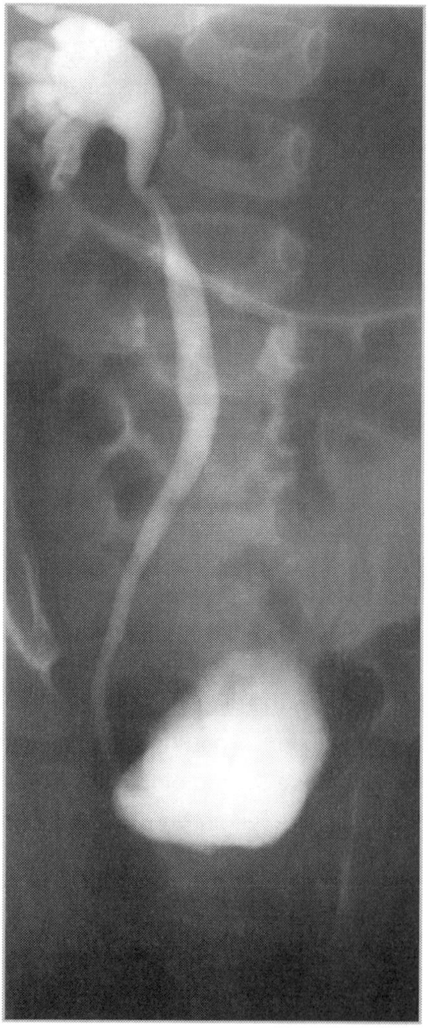

Fig 3.8b

1. What is this investigation? How is it done?
2. What are the findings and the diagnosis?
3. What are the causes of this condition and the complications?
4. What other imaging modalities can be used and how are they graded?
5. What is the imaging protocol for recurrent UTIs?

Answers *on pages 183–211*

Case 3.9

A 5-year-old boy presents with abdominal pain and headache. Clinical examination reveals a large mass in the right side of the abdomen.

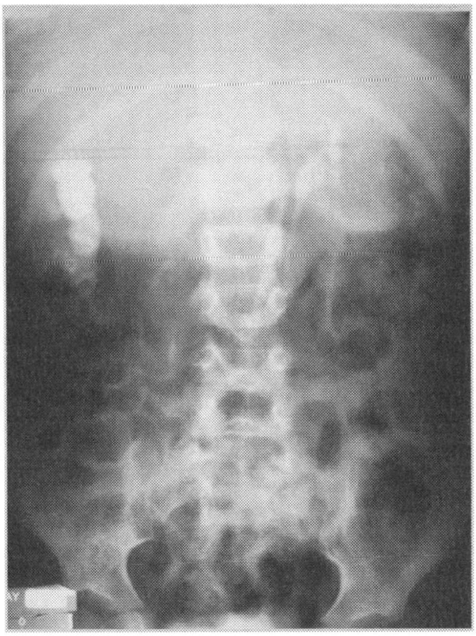

Fig 3.9a

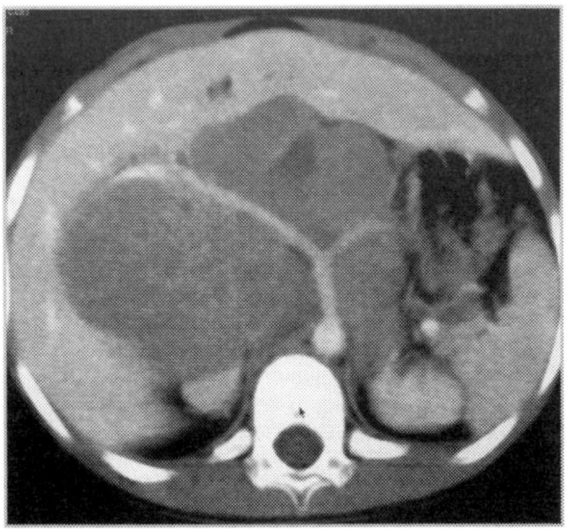

Fig 3.9b

1. What do you see on the IVU and CT scan of the abdomen?
2. What is the diagnosis?
3. What are the clinical features?
4. What are the radiological features and differential diagnosis?
5. What is the further management of this patient?

Answers *on pages 183–211*

Case 3.10

A 14-year-old girl presents with left loin pain. On examination, there is tenderness in the left costovertebral angle.

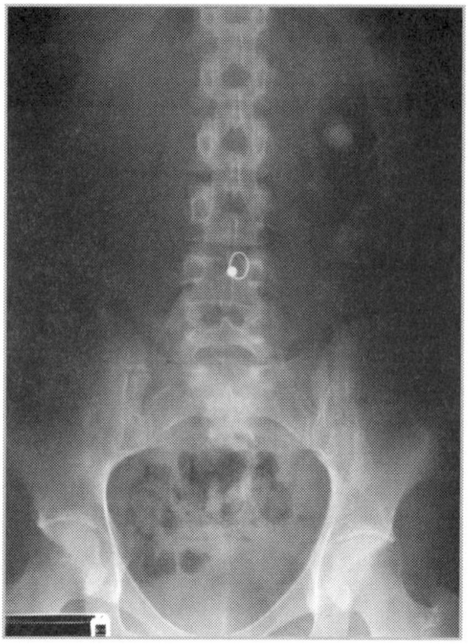

Fig 3.10a

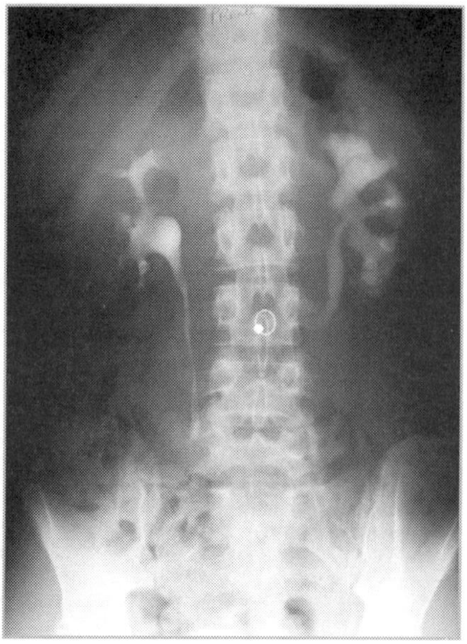

Fig 3.10b

1. What do you see on the X-ray and the IVU?
2. What is the diagnosis?
3. What are the types and causes of this disease?
4. What are the clinical and radiological features?
5. What are the complications and treatment?

Answers *on pages 183–211*

Case 3.11

A 16-year-old girl presents with pain in the right lower quadrant. Clinical examination revealed no rebound tenderness, but mild tenderness in the right lower quadrant and pelvis.

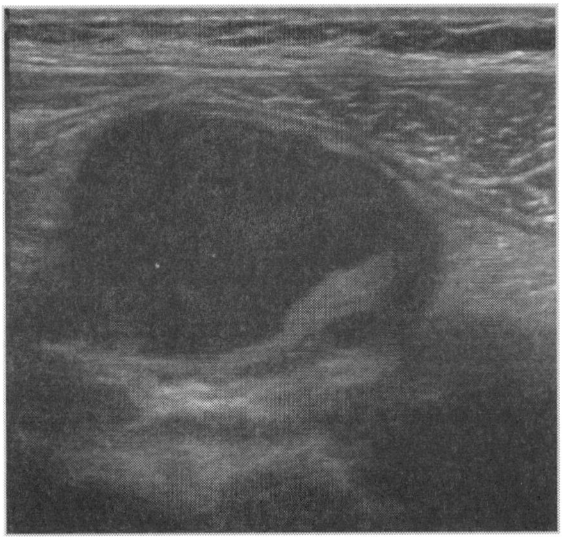

Fig 3.11a

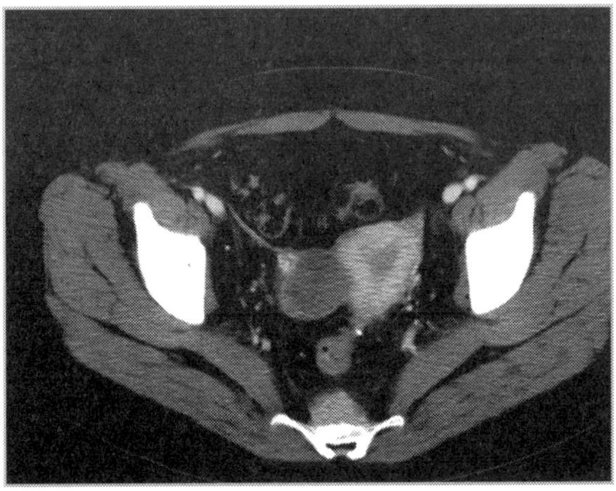

Fig 3.11b

1. What do you see on the ultrasound and CT scans of the pelvis?
2. What is the diagnosis?
3. What are the pathological types and clinical features?
4. What are the radiological features?
5. What are the differential diagnosis and the management protocol?

Answers *on pages 183–211*

Case 3.12

A 13-year-old girl presents with recurrent lower abdominal pain, constipation and dribbling of urine. She has not reached menarche yet. Abdominal examination showed a non-tender mass in the lower abdomen, extending to the pelvis.

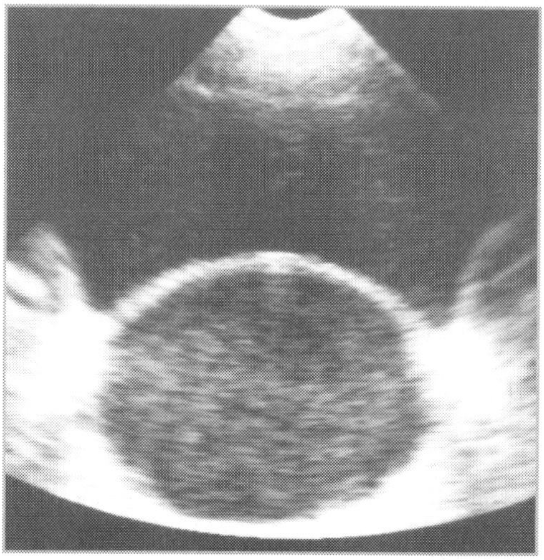

Fig 3.12a

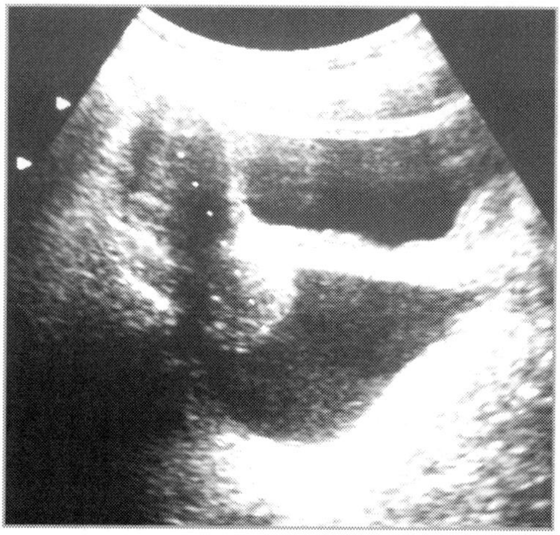

Fig 3.12b

1. What do you observe on the ultrasound examination?
2. What is the diagnosis?
3. What are the types of this disease?
4. What are the clinical and radiological features?
5. What is the differential diagnosis?

Answers *on pages 183–211*

Case 3.13

A 15-year-old girl presents with a history of recurrent UTIs and abdominal pain. Clinical examination is unremarkable.

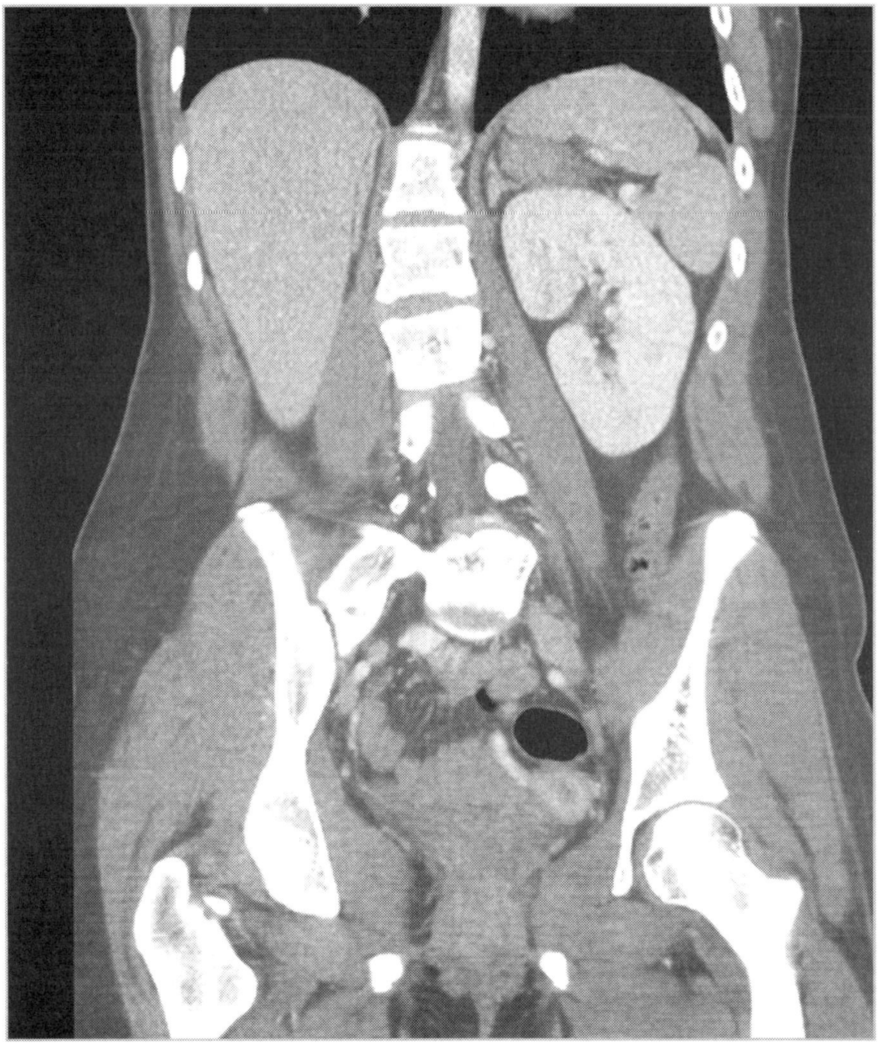

Fig 3.13

1. What are the findings on the CT scan?
2. What is the diagnosis?
3. What are the development and associations?
4. What are the radiological findings?
5. What is the differential diagnosis?

Answers *on pages 183–211*

Case 3.14

A 6-year-old girl was investigated for recurrent renal infections. Ultrasonography done as a part of the work-up showed a normal right kidney, but the left kidney was not visualised. Further investigations were done.

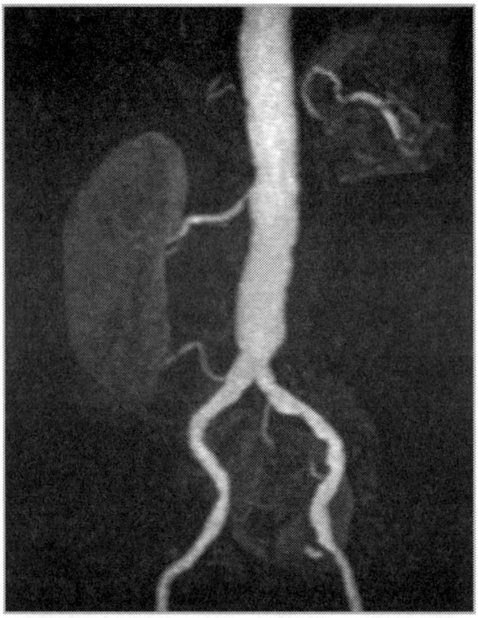

Fig 3.14a

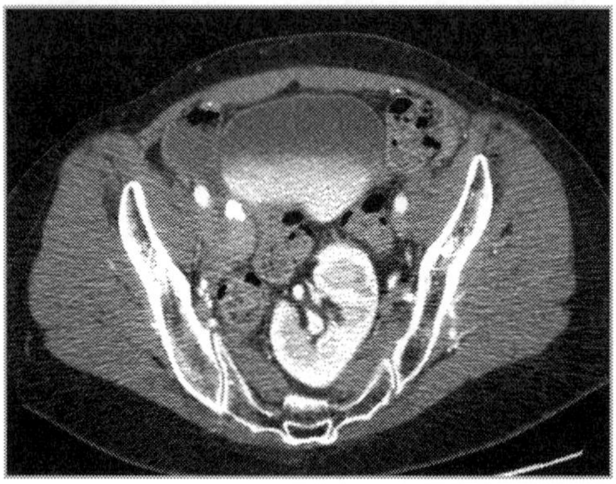

Fig 3.14b

1. What do you observe in these investigations?
2. What is the diagnosis?
3. What is the development of this condition?
4. What are the associated features?
5. What are the complications?

Answers *on pages 183–211*

Case 3.15

A 12-year-old boy presents with recurrent urinary infections and abdominal pain. On clinical examination, there is no mass or tenderness in the abdomen.

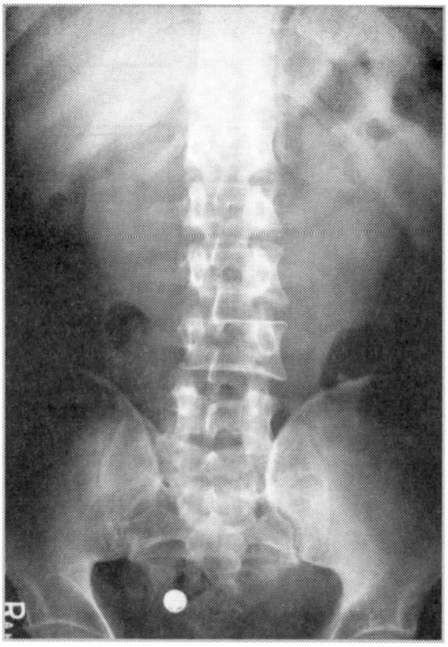

Fig 3.15a

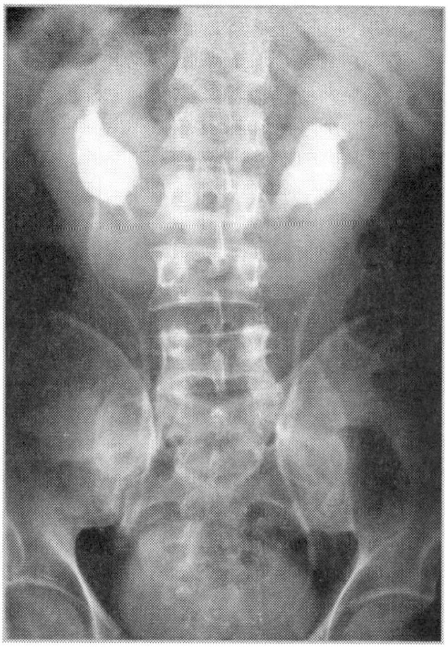

Fig 3.15b

1. What do you observe on the plain X-ray?
2. What do you observe on the IVU and what is the diagnosis?
3. What is the development of this condition?
4. What are the anatomical and radiological features?
5. Is there an increased risk of tumour in this condition? What other conditions are associated?

Answers *on pages 183–211*

Case 3.16

A 4-year-old girl presents with recurrent UTIs, abdominal pain and vomiting. On examination, she has left renal angle tenderness.

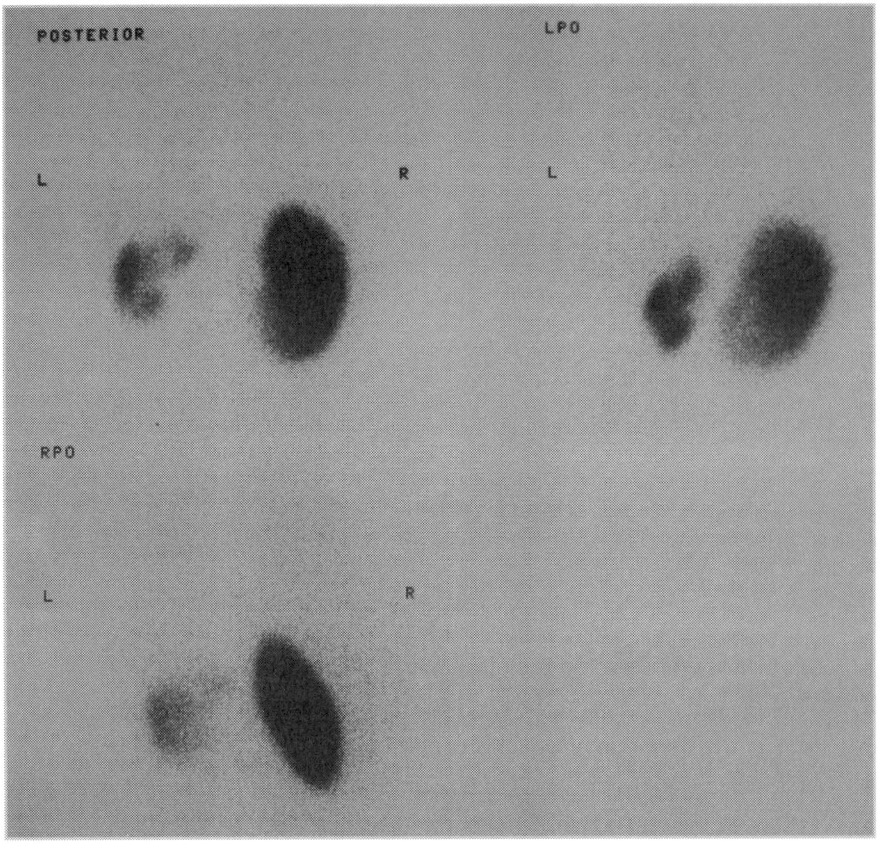

Fig 3.16

1. What is this test and what are the findings?
2. What is the diagnosis?
3. How is this test performed?
4. What are the cause and pathophysiology of this disease?
5. What is the further management of this disease?

Answers *on pages 183–211*

Case 3.17

A 5-year-old girl presents with severe abdominal pain, vomiting, fever, nausea and burning micturition. On examination, she is febrile and tachypnoeic, and has bilateral renal angle tenderness.

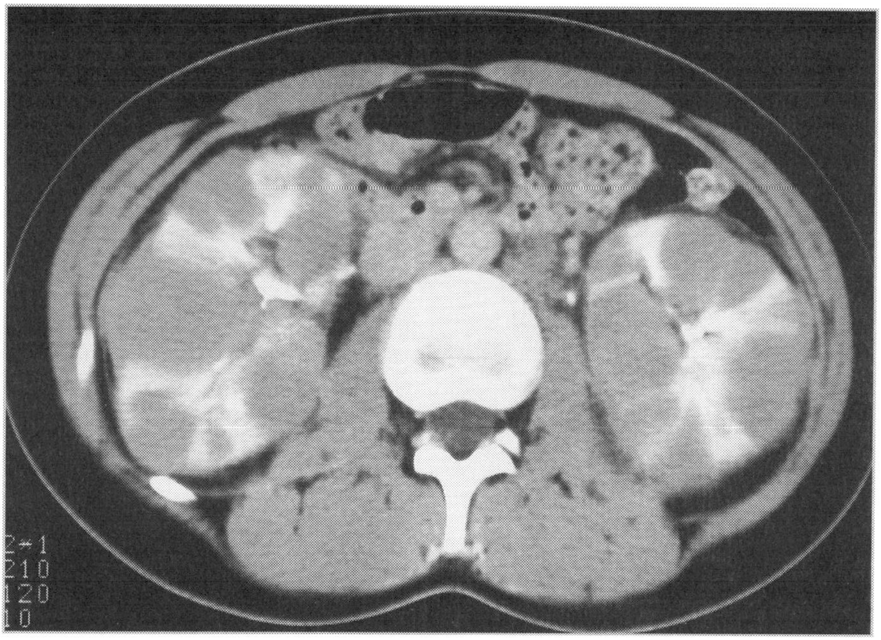

Fig 3.17

1. What do you see on the abdominal CT scan?
2. What is the diagnosis?
3. What are the causative organisms?
4. What are the clinical and radiological features?
5. What are the complications?

Answers *on pages 183–211*

Case 3.18

A 10-year-old boy presents with tenderness in the right side of his abdomen, fever, bloating and oliguria. On examination he has rebound tenderness on the right side of the abdomen and is febrile. He received a renal transplant for Alport syndrome 2 months ago. His serum creatinine is increased and urinary sodium decreased.

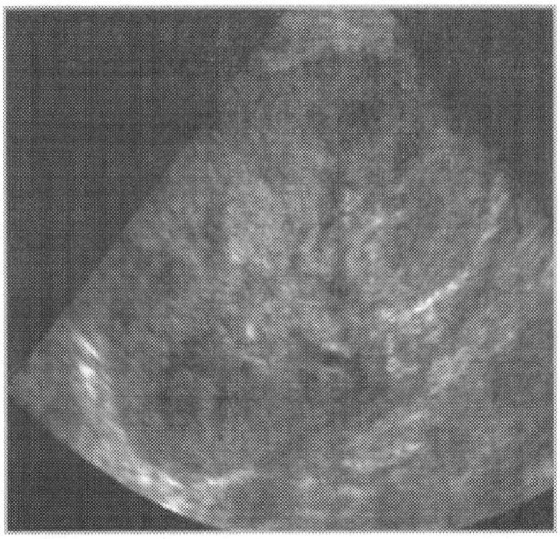

Fig 3.18a

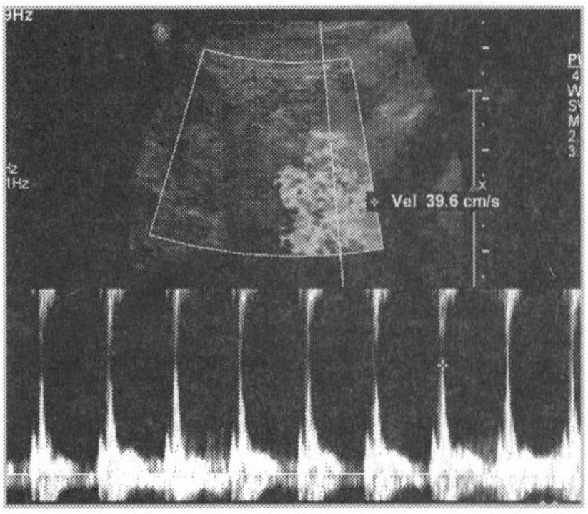

For colour version , see *Colour Images* section from page 411.

Fig 3.18b

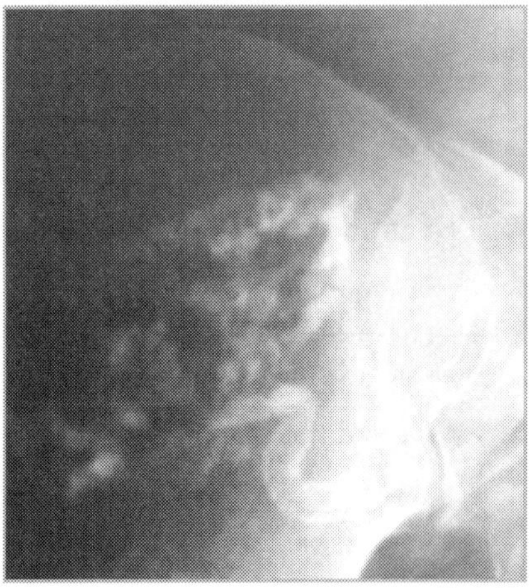

Fig 3.18c

1. What are the findings on the ultrasound scan?
2. What does the X-ray show?
3. What is the diagnosis?
4. What are the radiological features?
5. What are the other conditions that mimic this disease?

Answers *on pages 183–211*

Case 3.19

An 18-month-old boy presents with a history of recurrent UTIs, failure to thrive and dribbling of urine. On examination the abdomen is distended and the bladder palpable.

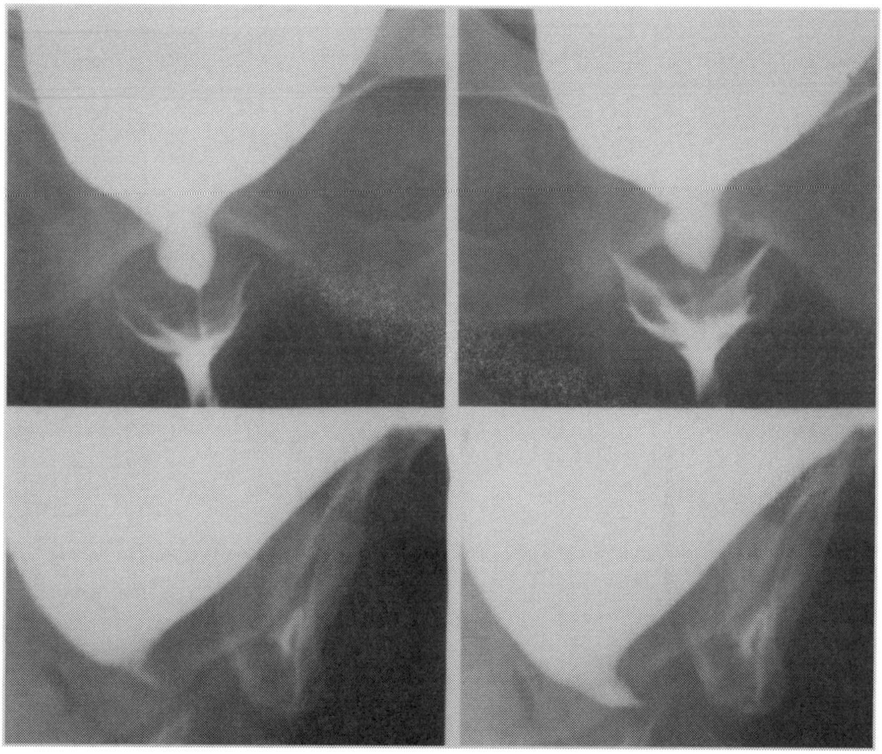

Fig 3.19

1. What is this investigation and what are the findings?
2. What is the diagnosis?
3. What are the radiological findings and types of this disorder?
4. What are the complications?
5. What is the differential diagnosis?

Answers *on pages 183–211*

Case 3.20

A 1-year-old girl is brought to the urology department with abdominal swelling, recurrent UTIs, vomiting and failure to thrive. On clinical examination, she is febrile and tachypnoeic. There is large cystic lump in the left renal fossa.

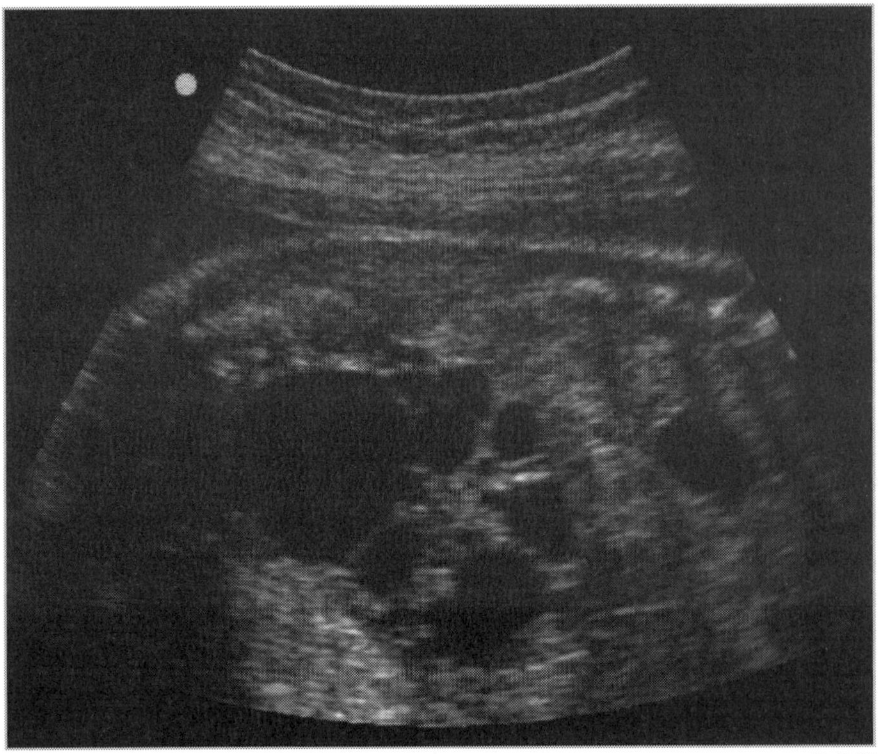

Fig 3.20

1. What do you observe on the abdominal ultrasound scan?
2. What is the diagnosis?
3. What are the development and clinical features of this disease?
4. What are the radiological findings?
5. What is the differential diagnosis?

Answers *on pages 183–211*

Case 3.21

A 9-year-old girl presents with persistent bedwetting and recurrent UTIs. Clinical examination was unremarkable.

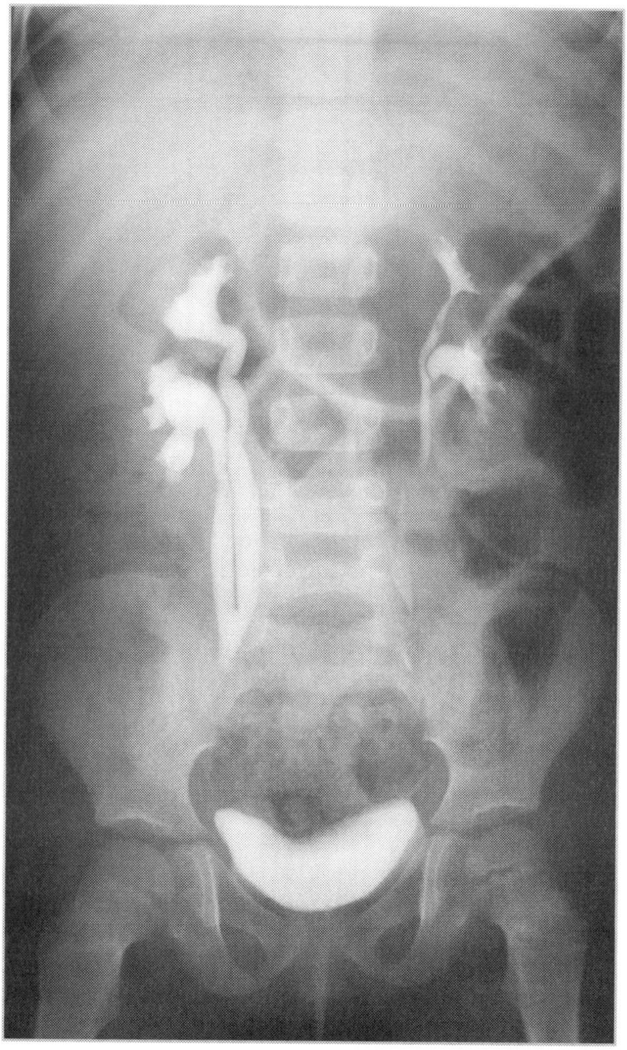

Fig 3.21

1. What do you observe on the IVU?
2. What is the diagnosis and what are the causes of the patient's symptoms?
3. What is the development and clinical features?
4. What is the Weigert–Meyer rule?
5. What are the complications?

Answers *on pages 183–211*

Case 3.22

A 9-year-old boy presents with pain in the lower abdomen and testis, and a testicular lump. On examination there is a tender lump in the right testis that does not reduce or transilluminate.

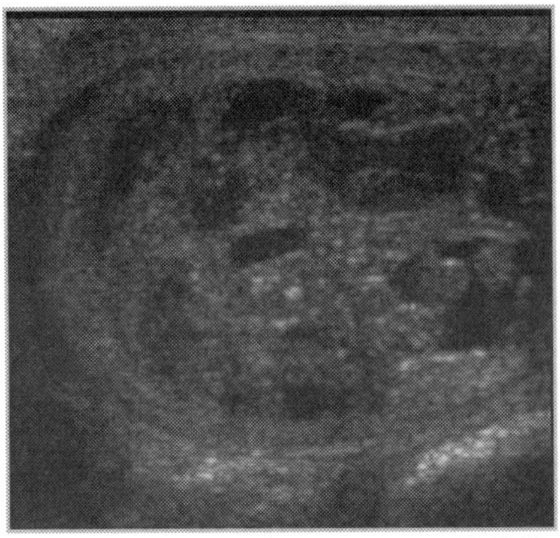

Fig 3.22a

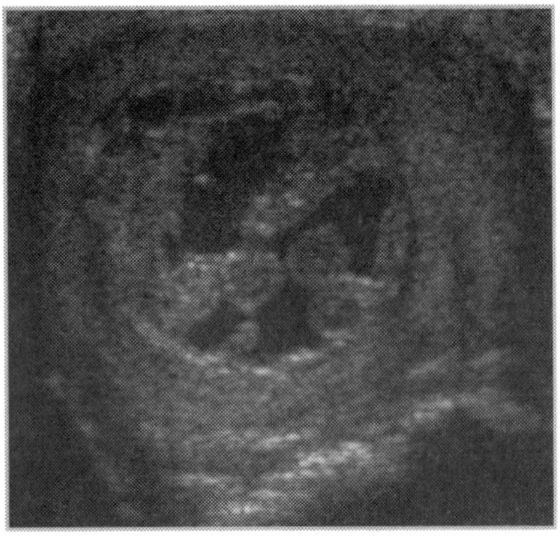

Fig 3.22b

1. What do you observe on the testicular ultrasound scan?
2. What is the diagnosis?
3. What are the different types and the clinical presentations?
4. What are the radiological features?
5. What are the imaging approach and the treatment?

Answers *on pages 183–211*

Case 3.23

A 13-year-old boy presents with fever, severe pain and swelling in his scrotum, and burning micturition. On examination, he has a tender, swollen and red scrotum.

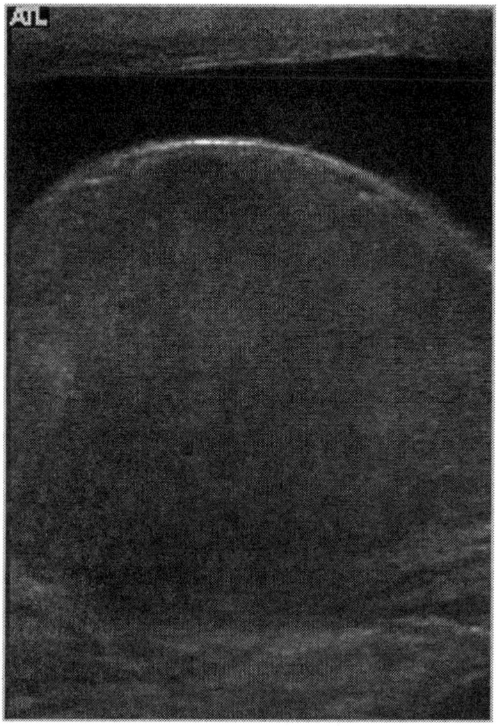

Fig 3.23a

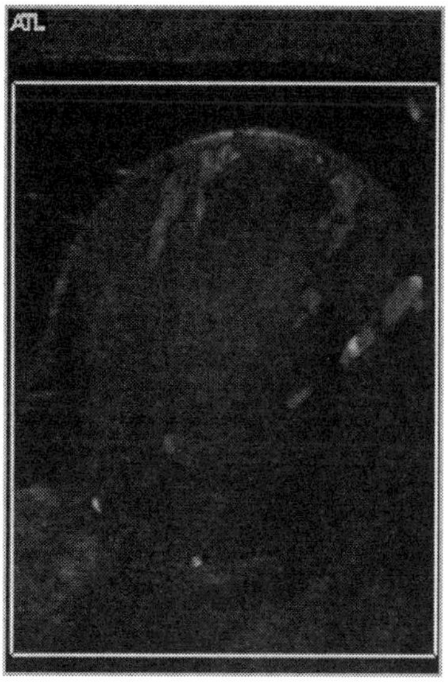

For colour version , see *Colour Images* section from page 411. Fig 3.23b

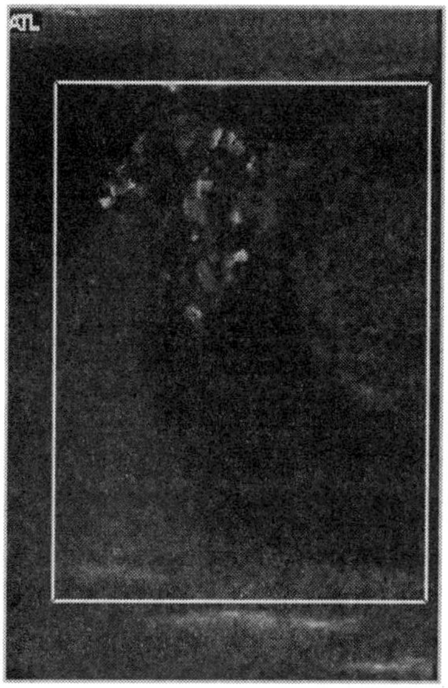

For colour version , see *Colour Images* section from page 411. Fig 3.23c

1. What do you see on ultrasonography of the scrotum?
2. What is the second scan and what do you see?
3. What is the diagnosis?
4. What is the cause?
5. What are the role of radiology and the differential diagnosis?
6. What are the complications?

Answers *on pages 183–211*

Case 3.24

A 14-year-old boy presents with severe pain and swelling of the testis, fever, nausea and vomiting. On examination, the testis is swollen, red and tender.

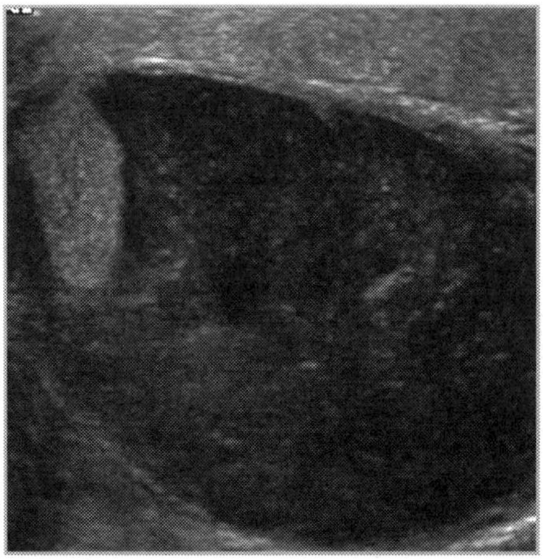

Fig 3.24a

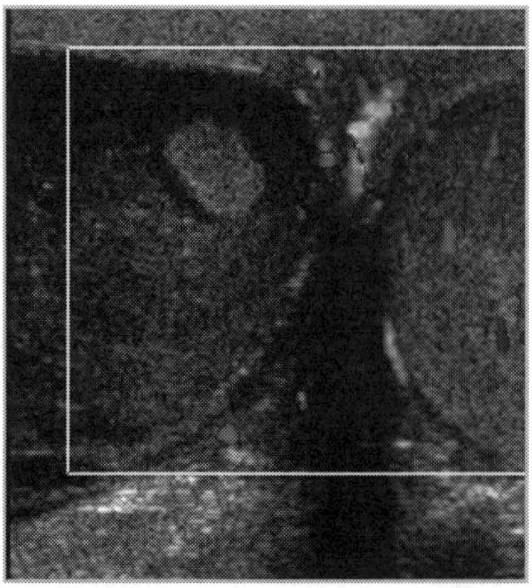

For colour version , see *Colour Images* section from page 411. Fig 3.24b

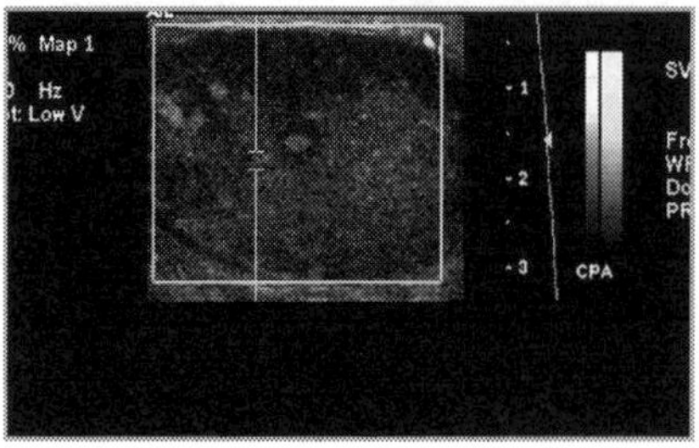

For colour version , see *Colour Images* section from page 411. Fig 3.24c

1. What do you see on the ultrasound scans of the scrotum?
2. What is the third scan and what do you see?
3. What is the diagnosis?
4. What are the predisposing factors?
5. What is the role of radiology and what is the most common differential diagnosis?
6. What are the complications?

Answers *on pages 183–211*

Case 3.25

A 2-year-old boy presents with pain, vomiting, incontinence, dribbling and abdominal distension. On examination there is a large, hard mass in the pelvis, extending to the lower abdomen.

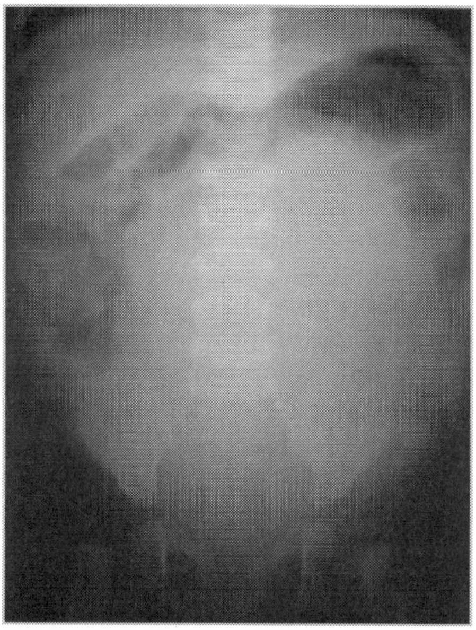
Fig 3.25a

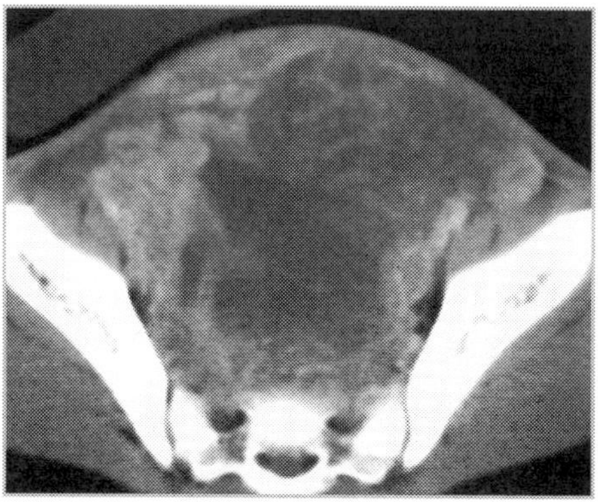
Fig 3.25b

1. What are the findings on the abdominal X-ray?
2. What are the findings on the abdominal CT scan?
3. What is the diagnosis?
4. What are the pathological and clinical features?
5. What is the organ of origin of this lesion?
6. What are the radiological features and differential diagnosis?

Answers *on pages 183–211*

Case 3.1: Answers

1. Ultrasonography of the right kidney shows a very large, cystic, anechoic area in the renal pelvis, which is the dilated pelvis. There is also blunting of the fornices.

2. On the IVU, the right collecting system and renal pelvis are grossly dilated. The distal ureter is not visualised.

3. Pelviureteric junction (PUJ) obstruction.

4. PUJ obstruction is the most common cause of obstruction in children. Causes:

(a) **Primary obstruction**:

– **intrinsic**: functional, excessive collagen, abnormal muscle orientation, abnormal conduction, high ureteral insertion, mucosal folds

– e**xtrinsic**: aberrant vessels, kinks, angulations, bands, cysts, aneurysm

(b) **Secondary obstruction**: stones, ischaemia, infection, trauma, iatrogenic.

It is more common in males, on the left side and presents with abdominal mass, pain, haematuria and a urinary tract infection (UTI).

Ultrasonography shows a large dilated anechoic renal pelvis, with no dilatation of the ureter. A dilated collecting system is seen. False-positive results may result from a large extrarenal pelvis, a peripelvic renal cyst, non-obstructive hydronephrosis or vesicoureteric reflux (VUR). False-negative results can be caused by patient dehydration, which is common in newborns. Skin defects, body habitus, bone, bowel gas and a poor technician can result in false-negative scans. An IVU can show non-functioning of a kidney. There might be delayed excretion of contrast. There is dilated renal pelvis without dilated ureters. Abrupt narrowing is seen at the PUJ.

5. PUJ obstruction can be diagnosed antenatally. If the AP diameter at the renal pelvis is > 4 mm at a gestational age of < 33 weeks and > 7 mm at a gestational age ≥ 33 weeks, obstruction is diagnosed. A follow-up postnatal ultrasound scan should be done, not before 48 hours after delivery. If there is persistent dilatation, follow-up ultrasonography and voiding cystoureterography (VCUG) are done to exclude VUR. Ultrasonic grading of PUJ obstruction:

Grade 0: normal kidney

Grade 1: minimal pelvic dilatation

Grade 2: greater pelvic dilatation without caliectasis

Grade 3: pelviectasis and caliectasis without cortical thinning

Grade 4: hydronephrosis with cortical thinning.

Occasionally, PUJ obstruction is an incidental finding on imaging studies.

Other tests that may be used for confirmation are diuresis urography (after injection of furosemide to differentiate obstructive and non-obstructive hydronephrosis), diuresis renography and a Whitaker pressure–flow urodynamic study. Mild grades are monitored every 6–9 months. For severe PUJ obstruction, a diuretic nuclear renogram to assess renal function is usually delayed until 1 month of age to allow for the physiological increase and stabilisation of the glomerular filtration rate (GFR). As reflux can cause hydronephrosis and coexists in 13–45% of cases of congenital PUJ obstruction, VCUG (voiding cycsourethrography) is performed in all patients, to assess for VUR. Pyeloplasty is done when the renal function worsens.

Case 3.2: Answers

1. The plain X-ray shows a large mass in the abdomen, which is causing inferior displacement of the bowel loops. The CT scan shows the heterogeneously enhancing mass in the right kidney, which is causing displacement of the adjacent vessels.

2. Wilms' tumour.

3. Wilms' tumour is the most common renal tumour in children (6–10% of all childhood malignancies); 80% occur between 1 and 5 years of age with peak incidence between 3 and 4 years. The tumour is bilateral in 4–13%, which occurs in a younger age group. Mutations in chromosome 11 are identified. It can be associated with cryptorchidism, hypospadias, hemihypertrophy, aniridia, Beckwith–Wiedemann syndrome, WAGR syndrome, Bloom syndrome and Drash syndrome. It usually presents as a palpable abdominal mass. Hypertension and microsopic haematuria are other presentations. Gross haematuria is rare. It arises from persistent primitive embryonal tissue (mesodermal blastema). Classic Wilms' tumour has a combination of epithelial, stromal and blastemal cell lines. The prognosis depends on the cell type and the presence of anaplasia.

4. The X-ray shows a large mass, with displacement of gas-filled bowel loops and effacement of the psoas shadow. Calcification is seen in 9–13%. Ultrasonography shows the mass, which is usually iso- or hyperechoic. Hypoechoic areas are seen as a result of necrosis and occasionally the tumour can be entirely cystic. Vascular invasion can be identified. CT and MRI are better in evaluation of perinephric extension, and the relationship to the great vessels, retroperitoneum and spinal canal. CT shows a heterogeneous, enhancing mass, with occasional specks of calcification, and splaying and displacement of blood vessels. Regional lymphadenopathy can be seen. Metastasis in the lung can be demonstrated on chest CT.

5. Neuroblastoma is the other most common tumour. It arises from the adrenal gland and causes inferior displacement of the kidney. It crosses the midline and encases the vessels (Wilms' tumour causes displacement of vessels, but not encasement). Bony metastasis is more common than Wilms' tumour.

6. A CT-guided biopsy is done for histological confirmation. The tumour is treated with chemotherapy followed by resection according to the surgical stage of the tumour and the histology. Some centres do a biopsy and chemotherapy before surgery, which facilitates later tumour resection and makes inoperable tumours operable.

Case 3.3: Answers

1. Axial contrast CT images are shown. The first picture shows normal contrast enhancing the left kidney. The right kidney appears normal anteriorly, but posteriorly there is a large hypodense area that is not enhancing, indicating a haematoma. The next picture done further inferiorly shows complete hypodensity in the renal parenchyma.

2. Renal trauma with haematoma and infarction. Blunt trauma accounts for 90% of renal injuries. It is associated with other organ injury in 75% and 95% have haematuria. Of those with gross haematuria 25% have significant renal injury, and 25% of those with renal vascular pedicle injury have no haematuria.

3. Renal trauma grading system:

Grade 1: subcapsular haematoma

Grade 2: superficial renal lacerations with perinephric haematoma

Grade 3: deep renal laceration without extension to collecting system

Grade 4: deep laceration with extension to collecting system/thrombosis of segmental artery with infarction

Grade 5: traumatic occlusion of main renal artery/renal artery avulsion/ shattered kidney.

4. Radiological features of various types of renal injury:

Contusions: high density in non-contrast, low density in contrast enhancement

Subcapsular haematoma: crescenteric fluid collection

Perinephric haematoma: surrounds kidney

Infarct: wedge-shaped hypoenhancement

Laceration: linear hypodensity

Fracture: laceration connects two cortical surfaces

Laceration with involvement of collecting system: extravasation of contrast in delayed images

Active haemorrhage: contrast enhancement within haematoma; active leak of contrast during arterial phase, same density as aorta

Shattered kidney: multiple renal lacerations

Occlusion of renal artery: no contrast in renal artery, hypodense kidneys

Avulsion of renal artery: haematoma in renal artery, no renal enhancement

Thrombosis of renal vein: hypodense filling defect in renal vein, hypodensity in kidney

Avulsion of PUJ: massive contrast extravasation from the PUJ.

Imaging is done only if the patient is haemodynamically stable. Ultrasonography is the fastest method of diagnosis, but CT is the most effective technique because it shows arterial bleed and collecting system injuries. Injury to other organs and bowel can also be assessed. Minor injuries can be followed up with renal ultrasonography.

5. Renal failure and Page kidney (post-traumatic renovascular hypertension) are the complications. Minor injuries and haemodynamically stable patients are observed without any intervention. Active bleeding can be managed by embolisation of the renal artery or surgery. Most of the urine leaks close spontaneously.

Case 3.4: Answers

1. The X-ray shows bilateral, small, punctate calcifications in the distribution of the medulla of both the kidneys. The kidneys are not enlarged. The IVU shows a striated nephrogram, with contrast radiating from the collecting system.

2. Nephrocalcinosis due to medullary sponge kidney.

3. Nephrocalcinosis refers to deposition of calcium salts in the renal parenchyma. Causes of medullary nephrocalcinosis: hyperparathyroidism, renal tubular acidosis, medullary sponge kidney, papillary necrosis, nephrotoxic drug (amphotericin), chronic pyelonephritis, TB, schistosomiasis, hypervitaminosis D, milk alkali syndrome, hyperoxaluria, hypercalcaemia, hypocalcaemia, Bartter syndrome, drugs such as furosemide, ACTH, vitamins E and D, sarcoidosis, hyperuricosuria

Causes of cortical nephrocalcinosis: chronic glomerulonephritis, cortical necrosis (pregnancy, shock, infection, toxins such as methoxyflurane, ethylene glycol), chronic rejection of a renal transplant, AIDS nephropathy, chronic hypercalcaemia, oxalosis, Alport syndrome.

4. Hyperparathyroidism, renal tubular acidosis and medullary sponge kidney are the three most common causes of medullary nephrocalcinosis. Medullary sponge kidney is a developmental disease characterised by dysplastic dilatation of the renal collecting tubules, usually seen in young adults. It is asymptomatic and detected incidentally. Occasionally it can produce stones, infections and haematuria with stasis. It can be unilateral, bilateral or segmental. Renal failure is seen in 10%.

5. Medullary nephrocalcinosis is seen as bilateral stippled calcifications of medullary pyramids, which are visualised as hyperechoic on ultrasonography and hyperdense on CT. A plain X-ray shows triangular calcifications conforming to the shape of the medullary pyramids. Cortical nephrocalcinosis is seen as a rim-like calcification of the renal cortex. In medullary sponge kidney, the X-ray shows medullary nephrocalcinosis. An IVU shows striated nephrogram in a brush-like configuration as a result of contrast radiating in the collecting ducts. This should be differentiated from papillary blush , which is amorphous contrast enhancement and a normal variant. There are cystic tubular dilatations, 1–3 mm, too small for ultrasonography and seen as hyperechoic lesions. It can be associated with hemihypertrophy, hypertrophic pyloric stenosis, Ehler–Danlos syndrome and horseshoe kidneys.

Case 3.5: Answers

1. The plain X-ray shows bilateral, dense areas of calcification in the retroperitoneum, above the level of the renal shadows.

2. Bilateral adrenal calcification, following an adrenal haemorrhage.

3. Adrenal haemorrhage is caused by physiological stress, trauma and hypercoagulopathy. It is more common in neonates, in whom the adrenal glands are large, well-vascularised organs; neonates are also prone to hypotension and/or asphyxia. Any condition leading to hypoxia may lead to shunting of blood flow to vital organs and damage of the endothelial cells, making them more prone to haemorrhage. The complexity of the adrenal vasculature may make it disproportionately susceptible to massive intraglandular haemorrhage. In times of physiological stress or shock, endogenous adrenocorticotrophic hormone (ACTH) release increases blood inflow rates to critical organs severalfold. As many patients with adrenal haemorrhage also have coexisting renal vein thrombosis, one theory is that the eccentric musculature of the adrenal vein encourages turbulence and local stasis, which, in turn, contribute to adrenal vein thrombosis.

4. In neonates haemorrhage is usually preceded by a palpable mass. Other clinical features are jaundice, hypotension and anaemia. Plain X-rays may show mass effect with anteromedial displacement of bowel loops and caudal displacement of kidneys. Calcifications are seen after resolution and can be seen as early as 1–2 weeks; they are peripheral or egg-shell shaped. Ultrasonography shows hyperechoic lesion. The CT scan shows adrenal enlargement with hyperdense haemorrhage. MRI can accurately characterise the stage. In the acute stage, the haemorrhage is an isointense low signal in T1 and a low signal in T2. In the subacute stage, there is initially a high signal rim in T1, followed by a complete high signal in T1. Fluid levels can be seen. High signal in T2 can be seen as a result of lysis and clots. On ultrasonography the adrenals are large, hyperechoic and mass like; later they reduce and become cystic, and eventually are not visualised at all.

5. Differential diagnoses for plain film appearances are hydronephrosis, multicystic dysplastic kidney, neuroblastoma and other retroperitoneal masses. There might be adjacent soft-tissue stranding. Bilateral adrenal calcification is seen in Wolman's disease, which is a lysosomal storage disease.

6. If there is suspicion of haemorrhage on ultrasonography, CT or MRI, the best course of action is to follow up with serial imaging, to exclude an underlying malignancy. Haemorrhage undergoes change in density, becomes cystic in 3–4 weeks and shows eventual resolution with or without residual calcification. Complications include adrenal insufficiency with volume loss and shock, adrenal pseudocysts and calcifications. Unilateral haemorrhage is rarely significant. It is more common on the right side. Abscess is a complication of haemorrhage. Underlying malignancy has to be excluded. Deaths are the result of massive blood loss in neonates and adrenal insufficiency in adults.

Case 3.6: Answers

1. There is no kidney on the right side. On the left side there is the left kidney and inferior to it another kidney facing the opposite direction. This is best seen on the IVU, where both the kidneys are seen on the same side and the collecting systems are facing opposite directions.

2. Crossed fused renal ectopia.

3. Crossed fused ectopia is fusion of both kidneys, with at least one kidney on the side opposite to its normal location. The fusion results from either failure of the primitive nephrogenic masses to separate or fusion of two metanephric blastemas during their abdominal ascent. The ectopic kidney usually forms the lower portion of the fused renal mass. Usually the lower kidney is malrotated, and both pelves point towards the midline. The ureter of the upper kidney descends on the same side to the bladder, whereas the ureter from the crossed ectopic kidney crosses the midline to enter the bladder on the contralateral side. The kidney is supplied by aberrant renal arteries.

4. The incidence is 1/500. Crossed renal ectopia is clinically silent, and is usually detected incidentally. False-positive diagnosis is a deformed kidney resulting from previous trauma or neoplasm in association with absent contralateral kidney, which can be confused for crossed fused renal ectopia.

5. UTIs, hydronephrosis and calculus are complications. Associated renal abnormalities such as reflux, megaureter, hypospadias, cryptorchidism, urethral valves, Wilms' tumour, multicystic dysplasia and ectopic ureterocele can occur in conjunction with ectopic kidneys.

Case 3.7: Answers

1. The IVU reveals bilaterally enlarged kidneys, which show a striated pattern of contrast in the kidneys. Ultrasonography of the abdomen shows bilateral enlarged kidneys, which are brighter than normal. There is no differentiation of the cortices and medulla. There is increased attenuation of sounds posteriorly. There is no hydronephrosis.

2. Autosomal recessive polycystic kidney disease (ARPKD).

3. Autosomal recessive polycystic kidney disease is caused by a chromosomal abnormality in chromosome 6p, characterised by dilated and elongated collecting tubules extending radially from the medulla into the cortex, associated with interstitial oedema. The epithelium becomes secretory instead of resorptive. The higher the percentage of abnormal tubules, the earlier the presentation and the worse the prognosis. Hepatic signs are more severe if renal findings are mild. There are four types depending on the age of presentation: perinatal, neonatal, infantile and juvenile. The **perinatal** type is very severe and most common and presents with oligohydramnios. Death is common as a result of renal or respiratory failure. The **neonatal** type results in death from renal failure/cardiac failure before their first year. The **infantile** form appears by 3–6 months and death is from chronic renal failure, hypertension or portal hypertension. The **juvenile** form appears from 6 months to 5 years and death is caused by portal hypertension.

4. X-rays can show enlarged renal shadows and central deviation of bowel loops. Hypoplastic lungs can be seen. Ultrasonography is the mainstay in diagnosis. Both the kidneys show smooth enlargement. Usually the cysts are not seen discretely as they are in the adult type. The kidneys appear very echogenic, as a result of multiple small cysts, which increases the number of acoustic interfaces. There is loss of corticomedullary differentiation. There is compression of the collecting system. The bladder is small. An IVU might show a sunburst nephrogram, which is striated as a result of radiating collecting ducts in delayed images. A CT scan shows a low density in kidneys and striated contrast excretion. MRI shows high intensity in the renal parenchyma. Differential diagnoses are medullary cystic disease (multiple medullary cysts) and medullary sponge kidney (cysts, hydronephrosis, calculi), multilocular cystic nephroma (cysts).

5. ARPKD is often associated with congenital hepatic fibrosis and pancreatic fibrosis. The older the presentation, the more involved the liver is, and the more likely is death from hepatic fibrosis and portal hypertension. Earlier presentations result in death by renal failure, respiratory failure or ventricular failure.

Case 3.8: Answers

1. This is voiding cystoureterography (VCUG). The child is catheterised with an 8 French feeding tube or 5 Fr in neonates. AP spot films of the bladder and abdomen are obtained. Contrast is introduced by drip infusion with the bottle held 40 cm above the table. The procedure is done under fluoroscopic screening. When the child indicates an urge to urinate or signs of voiding are seen, bilateral oblique views of the bladder are obtained including the catheter. When voiding begins, the catheter is removed. Two pictures of the urethra are obtained during voiding. Fluoroscopy of the renal area is done to observe reflux. After voiding is complete, AP spot views of the bladder and kidneys are carried out.

2. This patient shows reflux of contrast from the bladder into the right ureter and collecting system, which are mildly dilated, indicating a grade III reflux.

3. **Primary** VUR is caused by maldevelopment of the vesicoureteral junction with incompetence of the antireflux flap–valve action. Immaturity is a result of an underdeveloped longitudinal muscle of submucosal ureter. **Secondary** causes of reflux are ureterocele, ureteral duplication, bladder outlet obstruction and periureteral diverticulum. Reflux is seen in 30–50% of children with a UTI, and in 20% of siblings. Complications of reflux are cystitis, pyelonephritis and renal scarring, hypertension and end-stage renal disease.

4. Vesicoureteric reflux can also be assessed with Direct radionuclide cystogram (radioisotope introduced into bladder like conventional VCUG) or indirect radionuclide cystogram (intravenous injection of radioisotope and assessment once the isotope is excreted into bladder). MRI can also be used for this purpose. International grading system for VUR:

   I: reflux to ureter but not to kidney

   II: reflux into ureter, pelvis and calyces, without dilatation

   III: reflux to calyces with mild dilatation and blunt fornices

   IV: reflux to calyces with moderate dilatation and obliteration of fornices

   V: gross dilatation, tortuous ureters.

5. Imaging protocol for recurrent infections:

   Ultrasonography: for identifying any structural abnormality that is causing recurrent infections

   VCUG or radionuclide cystography is an imaging modality used for assessment of reflux; all children with infection, < 4 years, undergo VCUG. Even older children with an abnormal ultrasound scan and repeated infections undergo VCUG

   A **DMSA** (^{99m}Tc-labelled dimercaptosuccinic acid) scan is done for assessment of scarring of kidneys secondary to pyelonephritis.

Case 3.9: Answers

1. The IVU shows inferior displacement of the collecting system on the right side. The left collecting system is normal. The CT scan shows a large mass in the upper retroperitoneum, which completely encases the aorta and coeliac branches and crosses the midline. The mass is anterior to the right kidney, which seems to be distinct from the mass.

2. Neuroblastoma.

3. Neuroblastoma is the third most common malignancy in children after intracranial tumours and leukaemia. It arises from primitive sympathetic neuroblasts of the neural crest, in either the sympathetic ganglion chain or the adrenal medulla. Although it can occur anywhere along the sympathetic chain from the neck to the pelvis, the most common location is the adrenal gland. Seventy-five per cent are abdominal; thoracic lesions account for a further 10–15% and pelvic and cervical lesions make up the rest. It is usually seen below the age of 5 years, with most children presenting around 2 years. It affects both sexes equally. Unlike Wilms' tumour, the child is usually unwell, with lethargy, anaemia and reduced general status; 60% present with metastatic disease. Bone pain, limping, ecchymoses, pallor, black eyes, proptosis and facial swelling are signs. Symptoms caused by renal arterial compression (hypertension), spinal canal invasion and hormone activity can be seen. The prognosis depends on the staging at presentation and aggressiveness of the neoplasm as determined by cytogenetics. Stage IV disease and elevated numbers of the oncogene *NMYC* within chromosome 2 are associated.

4. Diagnosis is based on imaging and 24-hour urine collection of metabolites. X-rays can show an abdominal mass and skeletal metastasis. Ultrasonography is the initial examination, which shows a large adrenal mass, with displacement of the kidneys. It is usually a solid tumour with areas of calcification. Cystic tumours are rare. CT or MRI is required for a full assessment. MRI is better for demonstrating intraspinal extension, and CT shows calcification. MRI and CT are ideal for demonstrating encasement of coeliac/renal/mesenteric arteries, which is a characteristic feature of neuroblastoma, not seen in Wilms' tumour. Bony metastasis is seen as hot spots on an MDP (methylene diphosphonate) bone scan. Increased uptake is seen on an MIBG (*meta*-iodobenzylguanidine) scan as a result of chromaffin cell activity. Stage IV neuroblastoma occurs in children aged less than 12 months, with metastasis to the bone marrow and not bone; it has a good prognosis and spontaneous remission.

5. Children are initially treated with chemotherapy, after biopsy confirmation. This is followed by surgical excision depending on the stage.

Case 3.10: Answers

1. On the X-ray, there is a dense opacity in the left upper quadrant. On the IVU, there is a filling defect in the left renal pelvis. There is no hydroureteronephrosis.

2. Renal calculus.

3. The stones can be made up of calcium, magnesium or ammonium phosphate, cystine, uric acid, xanthine and matrix, and be drug induced. Causes of **calcium stones** are hyperparathyroidism, increased gut absorption of calcium, renal calcium leak, renal phosphate leak, hyperuricosuria, hyperoxaluria hypocitraturia and hypomagnesuria. **Struvite** stones are associated with chronic UTIs. **Uric acid** stones are caused by a high purine diet and cellular malignancies or after chemotherapy. **Cystine** stones are seen in cystinuria. **Drugs** causing stones include indinavir, guaifenesin, triamterene, silicate (overuse of antacids containing magnesium silicate), and sulfa drugs including sulfasalazine, sulfadiazine, acetylsulfamethoxazole, acetylsulfasoxazole and acetylsulfaguanidine.

4. Loin-to-groin pain caused by ureteric colic is the most common symptom. Flank tenderness and fever are present if there is a superimposed infection. X-rays show dense calculi. Stones are bright on ultrasonography, with acoustic shadowing behind them. Unenhanced helical CT is increasingly used in the diagnosis of ureteric colic. It can demonstrate small calculi and determine other causes of abdominal pain. Obstruction can be detected.

5. Infection, sepsis and obstruction are the complications. Hydration and analgesics are used in the management of acute ureteric colic. Of stones that are < 4 mm, 80% pass spontaneously. Only 20% of stones > 8 mm pass spontaneously. Percutaneous nephrostomy is done for emergency relief of obstruction. Percutaneous nephrolithotomy is done through the nephrostomy tract in stones > 2.5 cm in diameter, hard or cystine stones, staghorn calculi, lower calyceal stones, stones associated with obstruction, or in cases of ESWL failure or contraindication. ESWL is used in stones that are < 2.5 cm and lodged above the iliac crest. Anaesthesia or sedation is required. ESWL is contraindicated in untreatable bleeding disorders, pregnancy, weight > 135 kg, tightly impacted or cystine stones, or cases of ureteral obstruction distal to the stone.

Case 3.11: Answers

1. The ultrasound and CT scans show a fluid-filled lesion in the right ovary.

2. Right ovarian cyst.

3. An ovarian cyst is a fluid-filled sac in the ovary that can present at any age. Ovarian cysts can be **follicular** – in the first 2 weeks of the cycle (rupture of follicular cyst causes severe pain in mid-cycle); **corpus luteal** – the last 2 weeks of the cycle. Failure of corpus luteum degeneration leads to luteal cyst formation. These cysts may become inflamed or spontaneously haemorrhage, producing symptoms during the latter half of the menstrual cycle. **Endometriomas** are cysts filled with blood from ectopic endometrium. **Neoplastic:** complications are rupture, peritonitis, adnexal torsion, infertility, irregular vaginal bleeding, dysmenorrhoea, dyspareunia and underlying malignancy. At birth, 98% of newborn girls have small ovarian cysts as noted on ultrasonography, with 20% being < 9 mm in diameter. Larger cysts, which may occupy the entire fetal abdomen, are at increased risk of torsion or a mass effect, causing gastrointestinal obstruction, maternal polyhydramnios or pulmonary hypoplasia. Most neonatal cysts are asymptomatic and identified because of a palpable mass. Neonatal complex cysts are almost always the result of prenatal haemorrhage into a cyst or perinatal ovarian torsion. In a young girl found to have a symptomatic abdominopelvic mass, the ovary is the most common site of origin. Incidence of malignancy is higher than in the neonatal period. A single cyst < 1 cm in diameter in the prepubertal girl is considered normal with no further evaluation needed. Immature teratomas are the most common ovarian neoplasm in children.

4. Ovarian cysts are often asymptomatic and an incidental finding on ultrasonography or CT. Transabdominal and transvaginal ultrasonography are useful in assessing cystic size, structure and complexity (presence of internal septations and mural nodules). Cystic, unilocular, unilateral masses < 10 cm in diameter with regular borders are probably benign. Malignant ovarian cysts are associated with irregular borders, a size > 10 cm in diameter, papillary projections, solid areas, thick septa (> 2 mm), ascites and matted bowel. Colour Doppler ultrasonography aids in the diagnosis of an ovarian cyst or an ovarian torsion, where the blood flow is decreased. On a CT scan, simple ovarian cysts are fluid filled with no solid component. On MRI, the cyst is hypointense in T1- and hyperintense in T2-weighted images.

5. Functional cysts are followed up with ultrasonography at 6 weeks or at the conclusion of two menstrual cycles. A gynaecological follow-up examination is indicated to rule out any underlying malignancies or infertility, even in seemingly benign cysts. Follow-up is indicated on any cultures that have been sent and may indicate a subacute pelvic inflammatory infection.

Case 3.12: Answers

1. Ultrasound examination in axial and sagittal sections shows an enlarged uterus behind the bladder. There is a low-attenuation fluid collection with internal echoes present in the endometrial cavity and cervix. The adnexa are normal.

2. Haematometrocolpos.

3. Hydro-/haematometrocolpos is an accumulation of sterile fluid/blood in the uterus and vagina, secondary to distal outflow obstruction. Sterile fluid accumulates before menarche and blood accumulates after menarche. The causes of obstruction are:

   Congenital: imperforate hymen, transverse vaginal septum, segmental vaginal atresia, imperforate cervix, blind horn of bicornuate uterus, agenesis of uterus and vagina with active uterine anlage, persistent urogenital sinus, cloacal malformation

   Acquired: tumours, infection, attempted abortion, cervical stenosis, surgical scarring.

   Haematometra is caused by cervical dysgenesis, an obstructed bicornuate uterus or Rokitansky–Kuster–Hauser syndrome (agenetic uterus and vagina with active uterine anlage).

   This patient had an imperforate hymen. Although it is usually asymptomatic, it can present with cyclical abdominal pain, abdominal mass, amenorrhoea, urinary retention, constipation and hydronephrosis. An imperforate hymen can be confirmed by clinical examination. The hymen may bulge and show a bluish discoloration. Complications are endometritis, myometritis, parametritis, pelvic abscess, urinary infection and pelvic thrombophlebitis.

4. Ultrasonography shows a cystic retrovesical mass, with clear fluid or a fluid–fluid level (depending on whether clear fluid or blood). The bladder can by compressed by the distended uterus. In indeterminate cases, MRI can be done and the signal characteristics depend on the age of the haematoma. Clear fluid is dark in T1 and bright in T2. Haemorrhage is usually of high signal in T1 and T2. Treatment is surgical repair. Surgery of the transverse vaginal septum depends on its location.

5. Differential diagnoses are ovarian cyst, mesenteric cyst, duplication cyst, meningocele, trophoblastic tumour and cystic tumour.

Case 3.13: Answers

1. The coronal CT scan of the abdomen shows absence of a kidney on the right side. There is a hypertrophied kidney on the left.

2. Unilateral renal agenesis.

3. Unilateral renal agenesis is a result of failure of the ureteral bud either to form or to induce metanephric tissue. It has an incidence of 1:600–1000 pregnancies and has a male preponderance. It is more common on the left side. Coexisting anomalies are hypoplastic testis/vas/seminal vesicle cyst, uterine abnormalities (unicornuate/bicornuate/hypoplastic/aplastic), Turner syndrome, Fanconi's anaemia, Laurence–Moon–Biedl syndrome, Down syndrome and VATER anomalies. It is more commonly diagnosed in girls because of the associated congenital anomalies. It is diagnosed before age 1 year in 40% and 5 years in 75%. Bilateral renal agenesis is uncommon and is incompatible with life; it presents with Potters' facies, severe oligohydramnios and pulmonary hypoplasia. Absent urine in the bladder, absent renal arteries and skeletal abnormalities are also seen on ultrasonography.

4. An X-ray, IVU, ultrasonography and CT will show the absence of a kidney on one side and compensatory hypertrophy on the other. The adrenal glands are absent. The renal vessels are absent or rudimentary. An IVU shows no function. Colonic loops are seen in the renal fossa. Renal artery, ureteric bud and trigone are absent. Some 15% have a hypoplastic ureter.

5. Differential diagnoses for absent renal contour on a plain X-ray: agenesis, hypoplasia, nephrectomy, ectopic kidney, pelvic kidney and severe renal failure. Differential diagnoses for absent renal contour on CT or ultrasonography: agenesis, nephrectomy, severe renal failure and ectopic kidney.

Case 3.14: Answers

1. The first investigation is an MR angiography, which shows a normal right kidney supplied by a renal artery arising from the aorta. There is no kidney in the left renal fossa. The left kidney is seen in the pelvis and is supplied by a branch from the left common iliac artery. CT scan of the pelvis, shows the kidney located in the pelvis.

2. This is an ectopic pelvic kidney. The appearances of an ectopic kidney are the same as the normal kidney, except that it is in an abnormal place. There might be non-rotation of the collecting system and hence the renal pelvis can be situated anteriorly.

3. Pelvic kidney is the most common type of renal ectopia. During development the ureteral bud separates from the wolffian duct around week 4 and ascends towards the urogenital ridge. The metanephric blastema develops above the ureteric bud by week 5. A period of rapid caudal growth in the embryo assists in migration of this structure out of the pelvis and into its eventual retroperitoneal location in the renal fossa. The migration and rotation are complete by week 8. In a pelvic kidney, ascent is prevented, probably by the interior mesenteric artery. It is supplied by aberrant arteries, depending on the level of arrest – usually, by branches from the aorta or iliac arteries.

4. Ectopic kidney is associated with many other conditions such as renal agenesis, uterine abnormalities (unicornuate/bicornuate/aplastic uterus, duplicate/rudimentary vagina, undescended testis, hypospadias, duplicate urethra), adrenal cardiac and skeletal anomalies.

5. Hydronephrosis can occur as a result of alterations in the course of the ureter and there is increased risk of trauma, as a result of the pelvic location. Complications result from associated anomalies. VUR is also a feature.

Case 3.15: Answers

1. The X-ray of the abdomen shows a normal bowel appearance. The upper pole of the kidneys appears normal. The lower pole of the kidneys appears more medial than normal and fused.

2. The IVU shows fusion of the lower pole of the kidneys, consistent with horseshoe kidney.

3. Horseshoe kidney is seen in 1/400 children. Kidneys are formed by the union of the ureteric buds of the mesonephric ducts with the nephrogenic cords at the level of S1 and S2. Subsequently, they ascend as a result of straightening of the caudal end of the embryo and differential growth of pelvic structures. Horseshoe kidney occurs as a result of abnormal variation in growth, ventral flexion of the hind end of the embryo or variations in the growth of pelvic structures, which brings the developing kidneys abnormally close for a longer period, ending in fusion. The ascent of the fused kidney is limited at the level of the inferior mesenteric artery, so the isthmus is trapped under it. Hence the horseshoe kidney always lies lower than normal.

4. The kidneys can fuse at the upper or lower pole (90%). The region of fusion is called the isthmus, which can be fibrous or normal renal tissue and is situated at L4–5 between the aorta and inferior mesenteric artery. Occasionally it might pass between the aorta and the IVC or even posterior to these vessels. The long axis of the kidney is oriented medially and the pelvis and ureters are situated more anteriorly. The renal pelves are usually malrotated and lie anteriorly or laterally, depending on the severity of fusion. There are multiple renal arteries arising from the aorta, including the isthmus artery, which might arise from the renal artery, aorta, or mesenteric or iliac arteries. Boys are more commonly affected. IVU, ultrasonography, CT and MRI all detect horseshoe kidney. Differential diagnoses include crossed fused ectopia, where the fused kidneys are on the same side of the spine. In pancake kidney, the whole kidney is fused. Occasionally, in marked scoliosis, the axis of the kidneys is altered and it might mimic horseshoe kidney. Malrotated kidneys are another differential diagnosis.

5. There are lots of associated conditions in horseshoe kidney. Cardiovascular system (CVS), skeletal, CNS and anorectal malformations, hypospadias, undescended testis, bicornuate uterus, ureteral duplication, trisomy 18 and Turner syndrome are associated. Infections are common as a result of urine stasis and associated VUR. The PUJ obstruction is a common complication because of the high insertion of the ureter. Recurrent calculi are seen as a result of obstruction or infection. Increased risk of trauma is present, because of its position just anterior to the spine. The morbidity mainly depends on associated infections and stones. Most of them are asymptomatic and there is no reduction in the life span.

Case 3.16: Answers

1. This is a DMSA scan. The scan shows a normal looking right kidney. The left kidney is small and there are multiple filling defects, indicating a scar.

2. Scarring of the left kidney resulting from chronic atrophic pyelonephritis, secondary to VUR.

3. [^{99m}Tc]DMSA scan is used for morphological scanning of the kidneys. It is the best agent for visualising cortical tissue, evaluating renal function and diagnosing scars. It is used for imaging functional cortical mass and differentiating tumour from pseudotumours (such as the column of Bertin) and scars. This agent shows high protein binding and has a slow plasma clearance. Fifty per cent of the dose accumulates in proximal and distal renal tubular cells by 3 h; 5–10 mCi are injected and imaging is done after 1–3 h. A single photon emission CT (SPECT) scan is used to increase sensitivity. Pyelonephritis impairs renal tubular uptake of DMSA, resulting in cortical photopenic defects. Persistent photopenic defects on DMSA represent renal scarring and irreversible renal damage. The DMSA scan helps to confirm pyelonephritis and evaluate the effectiveness of VUR medical management. It also helps to differentiate infections and dysplastic kidneys, which have diffuse decreased uptake. Development of new photopenic areas indicates development of a new scar.

4. VUR results in intrarenal reflux of urine from the renal pelvis into the renal parenchyma. If the refluxed urine is sterile it does not produce any complications. If it is infected, bacterial endotoxins are released, resulting in release of free radicals and proteolytic enzymes; this causes fibrosis

and scarring of the renal parenchyma during healing. Initial scar distorts papillae and results in further reflux and scarring, triggering a vicious cycle.

5. VCUG and renal ultrasonography are performed in any child below age 5 years with a UTI, any child with pyelonephritis and any boy with a symptomatic UTI. If there is reflux, a DMSA scan is done to assess the extent of scarring. The aim of treatment is to allow normal renal growth, and to prevent UTI, pyelonephritis and renal failure. Prophylactic antibiotics are given for grade I–III reflux, so that the refluxed urine is sterile and does not cause renal damage. Surgical treatment of reflux is indicated for those children with grade IV–V reflux, persistent reflux despite medical therapy for 3 years, UTIs on prophylaxis, lack of renal growth, multiple drug allergies, etc. Ureteral reimplantation is performed. Ultrasonography is done yearly. A radionuclide cystogram is done yearly or every 18 months to monitor resolution. A DMSA scan is done if the child develops symptoms of pyelonephritis.

Case 3.17: Answers

1. The CT scan shows enlargement of both kidneys. There are multiple, large, wedge-shaped hypodensities in both kidneys, but no stone or hydronephrosis.

2. Acute pyelonephritis.

3. Acute pyelonephritis is inflammation of the upper urinary tract. It usually involves the pyelocalyceal lining and extends centrifugally along the medullary rays. Common organisms are *Escherichia coli*, *Proteus* and *Klebsiella* spp. *Enterobacter* and *Pseudomonas* spp. are other organisms. It is more common in females. VUR is a predisposing factor, as well as stasis and obstruction.

4. Acute pyelonephritis presents with fever, chills, nausea, vomiting, flank pain and tenderness. Leukocytosis, pyuria, bacteriuria and positive urine culture are seen, in addition to microscopic haematuria and bacteraemia. Imaging can be done, but it is not sensitive or specific:

IVU: normal in 75%; kidneys can be enlarged, immediately dense nephrogram, non-visualised kidneys, mucosal striations, compressed collecting system, delayed opacification of collecting system

Ultrasonography: normal, enlarged kidney, oedematous and hypoechoic, loss of central sinus complex, wedge-shaped hypoechoic areas, loss of corticomedullary differentiation, thick wall of renal pelvis

CT: enlarged kidneys, hypodense wedge-shaped areas from papilla to capsule, which enhance on delayed scans, striated nephrogram, loss of corticomedullary differentiation, effaced calyces

MRI: wedge-shaped increased signal intensity in T2

Scintigraphy: focal areas of decreased uptake.

5. Complications of acute pyelonephritis are renal abscess, perinephric abscess, pyelonephrosis and scarring with recurrent infections. Prompt treatment with antibiotics results in resolution without scars. Delayed treatment can result in chronic pyelonephritis with scarring, decreased renal function, hypertension and renal failure.

Case 3.18: Answers

1. Ultrasonography of the transplanted kidney reveals a bright, echogenic cortex. Doppler ultrasonography of the transplanted kidney shows a high resistive index and low pulsatility index, with no diastolic flow. (Doppler ultrasonography of normal renal transplant shows good diastolic flow and low resisitive index due to low resistance circulation.)

2. The X-ray shows calcification in the transplanted kidney.

3. Rejection of renal transplant. Rejection is the most common cause of renal transplant failure. Almost all transplants have some degree of rejection. **Hyperacute rejection** occurs within a few minutes of transplantation. **Accelerated acute** occurs in 2–5 days, **acute** in 5 days–6 months, and **chronic** after a year. Acute rejection occurs at least once in the first year in 50% of patients.

4. Ultrasonography shows an enlarged kidney, with heterogeneous cortical echoes and loss of corticomedullary differentiation, hypoechoic renal pyramids and thickening of renal collecting system. Doppler ultrasonography shows decreased diastolic flow, which is characterised by a high resistance index and low pulsatility index. MRI shows increased cortical intensity and loss of corticomedullary differentiation. A scintigram shows normal initial perfusion, but eventually the renal perfusion and function are decreased. Ultrasonography can be used to assess other complications such as hydronephrosis, peritransplant collections such as haematoma, abscess and lymphoceles. Doppler ultrasonography can also assess complications such as renal artery stenosis, renal vein thrombosis and other vascular complications. Failed renal transplantation and rejection result in a calcified transplant.

5. The ultrasound and Doppler appearances are not specific for rejection. Other conditions that produce reduced diastolic flow are acute tubular necrosis (develops in first few days, if scintigram perfusion is normal or only slightly decreased, but function is decreased), cyclosporine and other immunosuppressant toxicity, acute pyelonephritis, obstruction and renal vein thrombosis. The acute complications are the most common cause of acute graft failure after a transplantation. Nuclear medicine is very sensitive but not specific. Ultrasonography, Doppler ultrasonography and other imaging modalities can be used to find other complications, but they might not be very sensitive. Often a biopsy is needed to differentiate these conditions. Toxic levels of ciclosporin will confirm diagnosis of ciclosporin toxicity.

Case 3.19: Answers

1. This is a VCUG. An oblique view shows a bladder distended with contrast. The posterior urethra is dilated and there is a smooth narrowing of the midurethra.

2. Posterior urethral valve. This is seen in boys and usually presents on antenatal ultrasonography or in the neonatal period or later childhood. Children present with recurrent UTIs, hesitancy, straining, dribbling, enuresis, palpable kidneys and bladder, failure to thrive or rarely haematuria.

3. Posterior urethral valve is a congenital fold or mucous membrane located in the posterior urethra, which is the prostatic and membranous portion. There are three types:

Type I: mucosal folds extend anteriorly and inferiorly from the verumontanum of the urethra and fuse at a lower level

Type II: mucosal folds extend anterosuperiorly from the verumontanum towards the bladder neck

Type III: diaphragm-like membrane, located below the level of the verumontanum.

VCUG shows fusiform dilatation and elongation of the posterior urethra which persists throughout voiding. Occasionally it is seen as a filling defect in the urethra. The distal urethra appears collapsed. The bladder is distended and might show prominent trabeculations or sacculations as a result of obstruction. VUR can be seen. After voiding, post-void residual urine is seen.

4. Complications are urinary obstruction, VUR, UTIs, renal dysplasia (obstruction during gestation), prune-belly syndrome, neonatal pneumothorax/pneumomediastinum and neonatal urine leak. Posterior urethral valve can be diagnosed on antenatal ultrasound scans, with oligohydramnios, bilateral hydroureteronephrosis, distended urinary bladder, thick-walled bladder, posterior urethral dilatation and dilated utricle in urethra. Urinary leak and dysplastic kidneys can be seen.

5. Differential diagnoses for prominent ureters include obstruction, VUR, primary megaureter and megacystic microcolon, intestinal hypoperistalsis syndrome.

Case 3.20: Answers

1. Ultrasonography of the abdomen shows an enlarged left kidney, which is replaced by multiple cysts of varying sizes. There are some patchy areas of normal renal parenchyma. The right kidney is normal.

2. Multicystic dysplastic left kidney.

3. Multicystic dysplastic kidney is the second most common cause of abdominal mass in neonates (after hydronephrosis) and the most common cause of a cystic renal mass in infants. It is a sporadic disease that is caused by obstruction or atresia of the ureter during the metanephric stage, before 8–10 weeks of gestational age, which results in interference with ureteric bud division and inhibits induction and maturation of nephrons. The collecting tubules develop into cysts. The most common type is the unilateral form, which is more common on the left side and secondary to pelvi-infundibular atresia. In the segmental type there is focal renal dysplasia that is produced by high-grade obstruction of the upper pole moiety of a duplex kidney. A bilateral multicystic dysplastic kidney is fatal and caused by urethral obstruction.

4. The appearance of the multicystic dysplastic kidney depends on the level of obstruction during development. If the obstruction is at the level of the PUJ, the kidney is enlarged and there are multiple medium-sized cysts or a single large cyst in the kidney. If the obstruction is lower down in the ureter, the kidney is small and there might be small or no cysts in the kidneys. If the insult was earlier in gestation (< 11 weeks), the kidneys are small with loss of reniform appearance and there are 10–20 cysts. If the obstruction is later (hydronephrotic form), there is a large central cyst communicating with smaller cysts and there might be some function. Ultrasonography shows a large lobulated kidney. Occasionally it presents as a small kidney in adults. The ureter is atretic with atretic hemitrigone. The opposite kidney is large. Calcification can be seen in the cysts. A scintiscan shows no function. The cysts are of varying size and shape, with the largest cyst in the peripheral non-medial location. They are separated by septa and there is no communication between cysts. Cysts disappear in infancy. The central sinus complex is absent. No renal parenchyma is identified. Unilateral multicystic dysplastic kidney is associated with abnormalities on the opposite side such as PUJ obstruction, VUR, horseshoe kidney, ureteral anomalies, renal agenesis, megaureter and malrotation. Reflux and ectopic ureteric insertion on the same side can be seen. The renal artery is absent or hypoplastic in angiography.

5. Complications of this condition include renal failure, renin-dependent hypertension and malignancy. Differential diagnosis is hydronephrosis (the largest cyst is situated medially and there is communication between cysts), obstructive renal dysplasia with cysts (associated with partial obstruction), multilocular cystic renal tumour (solitary cystic tumour with normal renal parenchyma), cystic Wilms' tumour, cystic mesoblastic nephroma, cystic renal cell carcinoma (older children) and clear cell sarcoma.

Case 3.21: Answers

1. The IVU shows a duplicated collecting system and ureters on both sides.

2. This is a duplex collecting system. The patient's symptoms are caused by ectopic ureteric insertion, below the level of bladder sphincter.

3. Ureteral duplication can be complete or incomplete. Complete duplication is caused by a second ureteral bud arising from the mesonephric duct. Partial duplication results from early division of the ureteral bud.

   Partial duplication: the ureter may be blind ending if there is no contact with the blastema. There might be a bifid ureter or a bifid pelvis. The duplicated ureter enters the main ureter at a distinct angle and there is characteristic ureteroureteral/yo-yo reflux, with the urine moving between the upper and lower pole ureters as a result of peristalsis. It can be associated with PUJ obstruction of the lower pole.

   Complete duplication: there are two ureters draining as per the Weigert–Meyer rule.

   The upper ureter can insert above or below the bladder sphincter. In boys the insertion is always above the sphincter. They may present with urge incontinence or epididymo-orchitis. In girls insertion can be below the level of the sphincter, into the urethra or vagina, vestibule, cervix, uterus, fallopian tube or rectum, and they present with bedwetting or intermittent dribbling. It is more common in girls and bilateral in 15–40%.

   The **Weigert–Meyer rule** applies to complete duplication of the ureter. The upper pole moiety inserts ectopically, medial and inferior to the lower pole ureter, below the level of the trigone, into any of the wolffian duct derivatives. The lower pole ureter inserts orthotopically. An IVU shows a normal appearance of the lower pole. The upper pole can be seen normally or there might be poor visualisation. In this case the upper pole may be obstructed and can have a drooping lily sign (hydronephrotic upper pole causing downward displacement of lower pole calyces), enlarged kidney, nubbin sign (scarring and decreased function of lower moiety mimicking a mass) and displacement of proximal urine upwards. Ultrasonography shows two separate renal sinuses and absent connection between the upper and lower pole collecting system. MCUG can detect complications such as reflux in the lower moiety and ureterocele.

5. VUR (common in the lower pole as a result of a shortened ureteral tunnel), obstruction (upper resulting from ectopic insertion/ureterocele or aberrant artery crossing), ectopic ureteral insertion, ectopic ureterocele (upper), renal dysplasia (upper) and infections (partial duplication) are the complications.

Case 3.22: Answers

1. There is a large heterogeneous mass in the right testis. The mass has solid and cystic components.

2. Teratoma of the testis.

3. Testicular cancers are the most common tumours in males between age 15 and 35 years, accounting for 1.5% of all male cancers.

Classification:

(a) **Germ cell tumours:**

– seminoma

– non-seminomatous: embryonal cell carcinoma, teratoma, epidermoid cyst, yolk sac tumour, choriocarcinoma

(b) **Sex cord and stromal tumours**: Leydig cell tumour, Sertoli cell tumour, gonoblastoma

(c) **Secondary tumours**: metastasis, lymphoma, leukaemia.

4. Testicular tumours present with a painless enlarging testis, with mass or pain and heaviness in the lower abdomen. They can present with gynaecomastia or virilisation or with metastasis. α-Fetoprotein is elevated in yolk sac tumours. β-Human chorionic gonadotrophin (β-hCG) is elevated in choriocarcinoma and seminoma; LDH correlates with the bulk of the tumour. There is increased risk in an undescended testis, and with gonadal dysgenesis and a family history. Peak age is 25–35 years. Metastasis spreads along the testicular lymph drainage to the left para-aortic nodes, interaortocaval node, lungs and left supraclavicular nodes. Haematogenous metastasis is seen early in choriocarcinoma. Seminomas are seen in older adults. The tumours seen in children are teratomas, embryonal cell carcinoma, yolk sac tumour, Sertoli cell tumour (oestrogen secreting) and Leydig cell tumour (androgen secreting).

5. Testicular tumours are best diagnosed by ultrasonography, which shows homogeneous or heterogeneous soft-tissue tumours with increased vascularity. The tumour staging is done by CT scan, which is useful for finding enlarged retroperitoneal nodes. CT of the chest is done for pulmonary metastasis. Occasionally MRI is done in indeterminate cases. Treatment is with orchiectomy and chemotherapy, depending on the stage.

Case 3.23: Answers

1. Ultrasonography shows a swollen and oedematous epididymis.

2. The second and third scans are colour Doppler scans, which show intense vascularity in the epididymis and testis.

3. Acute epididymo-orchitis.

4. *E. coli, Staph. aureus, Neisseria gonorrhoeae, Chlamydia trachomatis* and *Proteus mirabilis* are common organisms that cause epididymitis. It usually results from an ascending UTI, but can also result from haematogenous spread. Initially the epididymis is involved, which is followed by global or focal involvement of the testis. Clinical features are fever, pain, swelling, tenderness, erythema, pyuria, dysuria and frequency. Leukocytosis, pyuria and bacteriuria can be seen. The most common clinical condition that can be confused with epididymitis is a testicular torsion. **Phren sign** (relief of pain on elevation of testis) is positive (unlike torsion, where there is no relief). Elevated WBCs are seen. Differentiation of these two entities is crucial, because torsion requires emergency surgery and epididymo-orchitis is managed.

5. On ultrasonography, the epididymis is enlarged and shows low echoes. If the head is enlarged it suggests a haematogenous spread. If the tail is enlarged, it suggests an ascending infection with reflux from the urine. The spermatic cord is enlarged. Thick tunica albuginea can be seen. The testis also shows low echoes when it is involved. Reactive fluid collection can be seen. Colour Doppler shows an increased number and concentration of vessels in the affected region. The peak systolic velocity is increased. Ultrasonography helps in differentiation from torsion, which has no vascular flow within it. A scintiscan shows increased perfusion of the spermatic cord vessels and increased activity of the scrotal contents, which can be curvilinear and lateral if only the epididymis is involved and central if the testis is also involved. There is no uptake if there is torsion. Other differential diagnoses are testicular abscess (increased perfusion, no uptake centrally), tumours (increased perfusion, decreased uptake, raised tumour markers, ultrasonography shows focal mass) and hydrocele (no uptake).

6. Complications are orchitis, abscess, testicular infarction, chronic epididymo-orchitis, atrophy, hydrocele, pyocele and Fournier's gangrene.

Case 3.24: Answers

1. Ultrasonography of the scrotum shows an enlarged testis that is diffusely of low echogenicity. The second picture is an axial view that compares it with the normal left testis, which has normal echogenicity.

2. The third scan is a colour Doppler picture, and does not show any flow in the testis or epididymis.

3. Acute testicular torsion

4. Acute testicular torsion is a urological emergency and the most common scrotal disorder in boys. It is common in the neonatal period and puberty. Predisposing factors are a bell-and-clapper deformity (high insertion of tunica vaginalis on the cord), loose meso-orchium between the testis and epididymis and loose attachment of testicular tunics to the scrotum. There is a tenfold increased incidence in undescended testis. Trauma, sexual activity, exercise, active cremasteric reflex and cold weather are other factors. Torsion presents with sudden severe pain, swelling, erythema, tenderness, low-grade fever, nausea and vomiting. The testis is swollen, oedematous and erythematous. It lies horizontally and there is loss of the normal cremasteric reflex.

5. Usually testicular torsion is a clinical diagnosis. Ultrasonography can be done if clinical examination is indeterminate. It is normal in the early stages (< 6 h), but after that shows diffuse hypoechogenicity. The testis and epididymis are enlarged. A twisted spermatic cord is rarely seen. Scrotal skin is thickened and there is a reactive hydrocele. Doppler ultrasonography does not show any flow within the testis or epididymis. Loss of spermatic cord Doppler flow is demonstrated. A false negative is seen in incomplete torsion < 360°, or torsion–detorsion sequence. A nuclear scan shows decreased perfusion and there is a round cold area in the region of the testis. Occasionally the nubbin sign is positive – a bump of activity extending medially from the iliac artery as a result of increased

blood flow in the spermatic cord with abrupt termination. The most common differential diagnosis is epididymo-orchitis. **Phren sign** (relief of pain on elevation of testis) is negative (in epididymitis the pain is relieved). FBC may be normal or show elevated WBCs. Differentiation of these two entities is crucial, because torsion requires emergency surgery and epididymo-orchitis is managed with antibiotics. Doppler ultrasonography shows a swollen testis and epididymis, with increased vascular flow.

6. Testis usually turns medially up to 108°. Diminished blood flow is seen in < 180° torsion after 1 h. Absent blood flow is seen in any degree of torsion after 4 h. Testicular atrophy is the major complication. Other complications are infection, infertility and cosmetic deformity. Analgesics are administered. Manual detorsion is attempted, which involves twisting the testicle

Case 3.25: Answers

1. The X-ray shows a large mass arising from the pelvis, extending into the abdomen, displacing the bowel loops superiorly.

2. The CT scan of the pelvis shows a large mass with heterogeneous contrast enhancement, arising behind the bladder and extending into the lower abdomen. The bladder has been compressed anteriorly.

3. Pelvic rhabdomyosarcoma.

4. Rhabdomyosarcoma is a tumour arising from primitive embryonal mesenchyme. The histological types are embryonal, botyroid, alveolar and pleomorphic. It is the fourth most common malignant solid tumour in children after CNS tumours, neuroblastoma and Wilms' tumour. It is more common in boys and presents at a mean age of 7 years.

5. This tumour probably arises from the prostate gland. In boys, pelvic rhabdomyosarcomas arise from the prostate or bladder. In girls they can arise from the vulva, vagina or cervix. Symptoms are abdominal pain, distension, urinary frequency, dysuria, palpable bladder and haematuria.

6. Ultrasonography shows a heterogeneous mass with areas of haemorrhage and necrosis. The tumour is very vascular with a high diastolic component. The CT scan also shows a heterogeneous, enhancing mass. MRI shows a mass hyopointense in T1 and hyperintense in T2, with contrast enhancement. Although the appearances can be non-specific, the appearance of an aggressive mass in a child's pelvis is characteristic of pelvic rhabdomyosarcoma. An IVU might show elevation of the bladder floor with obstruction of the bladder neck and a large post-void residual urine. Metastasis can be seen in retroperitoneal lymph nodes, bones, lungs and liver (10–20% at time of presentation). Differential diagnoses include sacrococcygeal chordoma, metastatic neuroblastoma, Ewing's sarcoma, synovial cell sarcoma, fibrosarcoma, haemangiopericytoma and primitive neuroectodermal tumour. The tumour is aggressive and needs surgery with chemo- and radiotherapy. Local recurrence is common.

4

MUSCULOSKELETAL RADIOLOGY QUESTIONS

Case 4.1

An 11-year-old girl presents with pain and deformity of the back. On examination she has difficulty in lateral bending and there is tenderness in her mid-thoracic and lumbar spine.

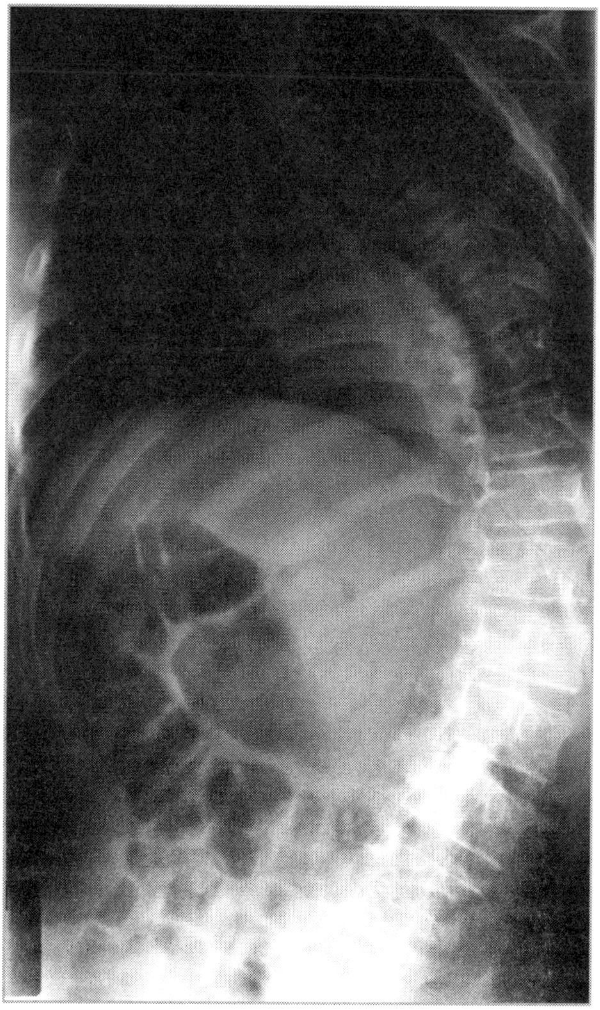

Fig 4.1

1. What does the X-ray show?
2. What is the diagnosis?
3. What are the types of this disease?
4. What is the role of radiology?
5. Does this patient need treatment?

Answers *on pages 273–334*

Case 4.2

An 11-year-old boy presented with severe pain, tenderness and limitation of movement of the left shoulder. On examination the proximal portion of the left shoulder was warm and tender, with a bony swelling and restriction of joint movements.

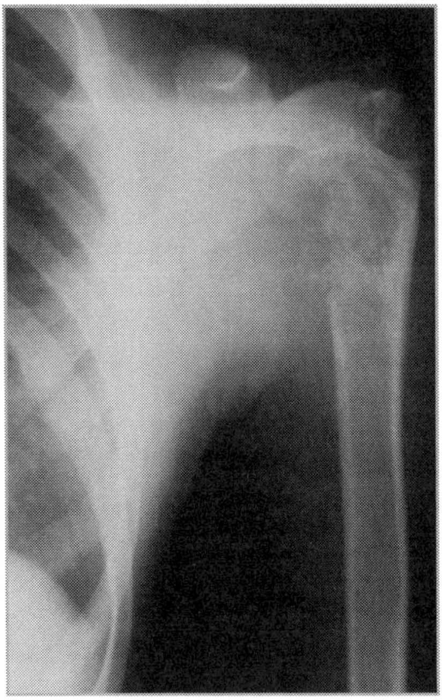

Fig 4.2a

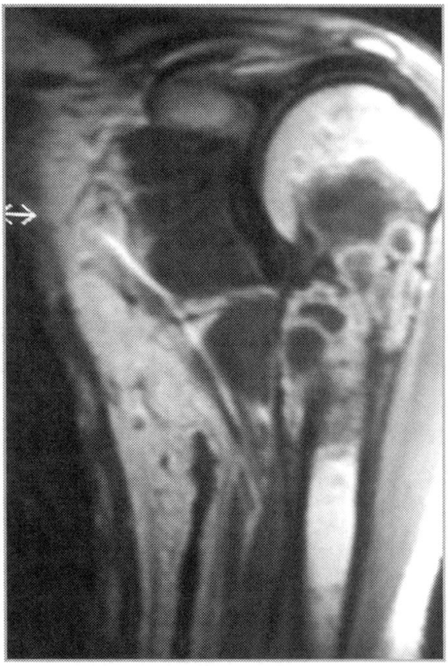

Fig 4.2b

1. What do you observe on the plain film and MRI of the left shoulder?
2. What is the diagnosis?
3. What are the clinical features?
4. What are the radiological features and differential diagnosis?
5. What are the prognostic factors and treatment?

Answers *on pages 273–334*

Case 4.3

A 15-year-old girl presents with severe pain in her left shoulder. On examination the shoulder is very warm, red and tender. Lab analysis shows an elevated WBC. A series of radiological tests was ordered.

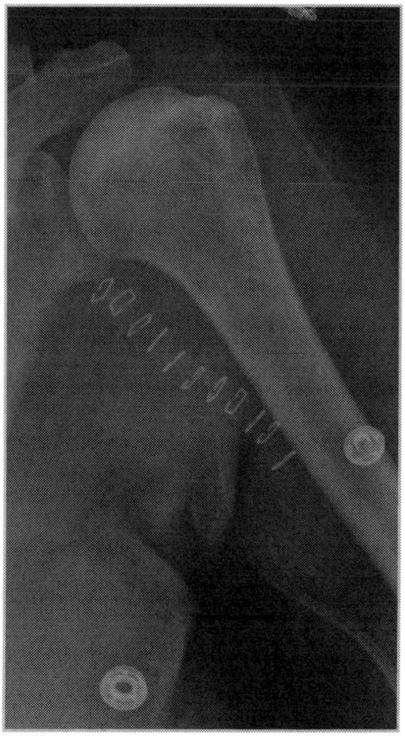

Fig 4.3a

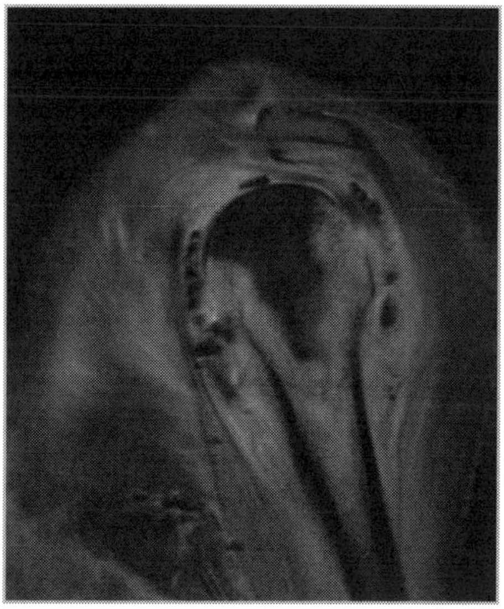

Fig 4.3b

1. What do you see on the X-ray of the left shoulder?
2. What are the findings on MRI?
3. What is the diagnosis?
4. What are the causes of the disease and the clinical course?
5. What are the radiological features and the treatment?

Answers *on pages 273–334*

Case 4.4

A 13-year-old boy presents with malaise, diffuse body ache and pain around the knee joints. Clinical examination revealed no restriction of joint movements, but mild tenderness around the knee joints.

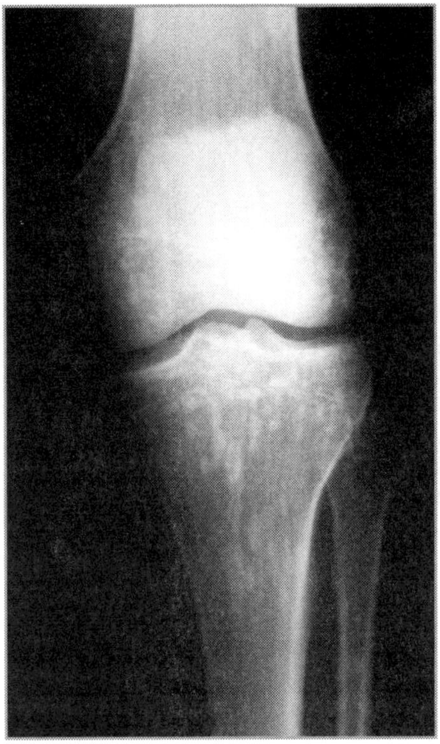

Fig 4.4a

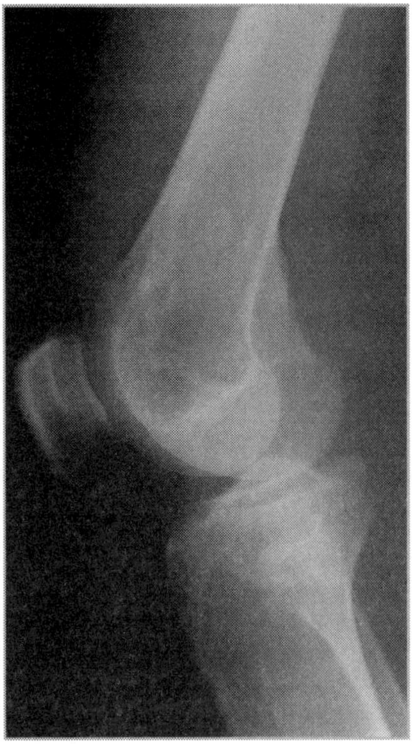

Fig 4.4b

1. What do you see on the plain X-ray?
2. What is the diagnosis?
3. What are the radiological features?
4. What is the differential diagnosis?
5. What is it associated with?

Answers *on pages 273–334*

Case 4.5

A 12-year-old boy presents with fatigue, loss of weight, anorexia and abdominal pain.

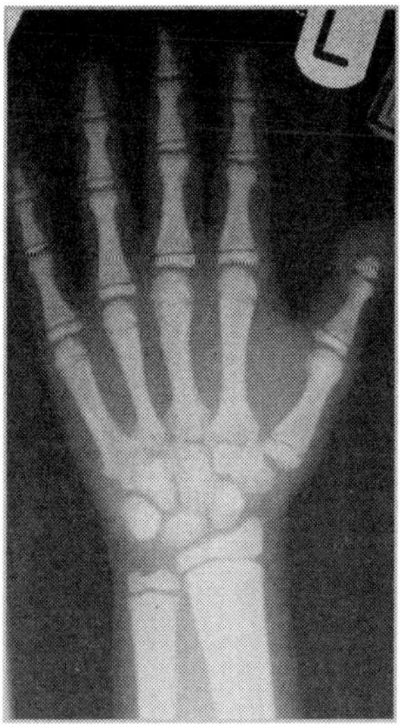

Fig 4.5a

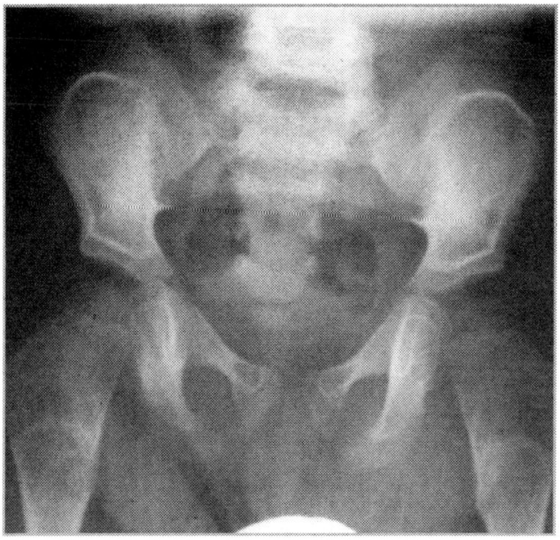

Fig 4.5b

1. What do you observe on the plain X-rays of the hands and pelvis?
2. What is the diagnosis?
3. What the differential diagnosis for this radiological appearance?
4. What the clinical features of this disease?
5. What are the radiological features?

Answers *on pages 273–334*

Case 4.6

A 2-year-old boy is brought to A&E with a history of falling out of bed. On examination there are bruises on his arms and legs in varying stages of development.

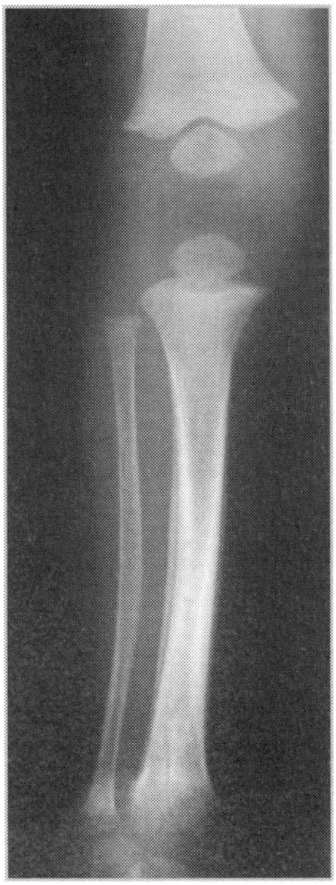

Fig 4.6a

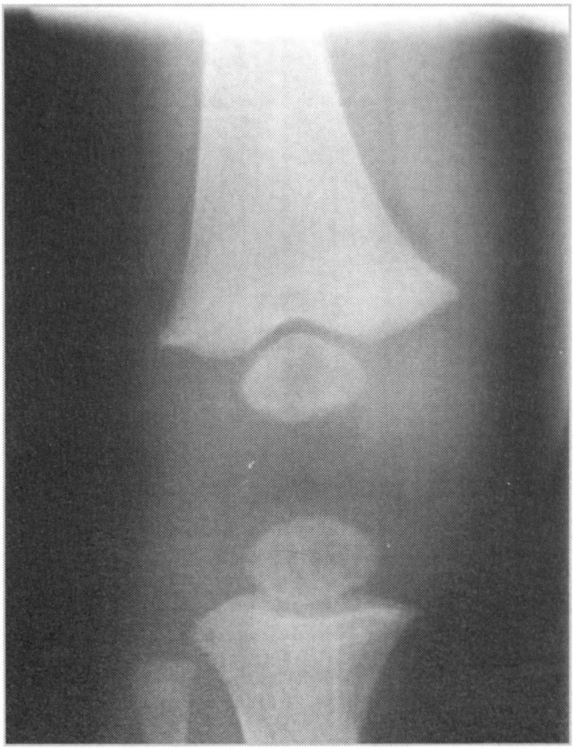

Fig 4.6b

1. What do you observe on the plain X-ray?

2. What is the diagnosis?

3. What the differential diagnosis for this radiological appearance?

4. What are the clinical features of this disease?

5. What are the most suspicious findings?

Answers *on pages 273–334*

Case 4.7

A 15-year-old boy with a chronic medical condition presents with low back pain. On examination he had tenderness in the lumbar and dorsal spine and restriction of joint movements.

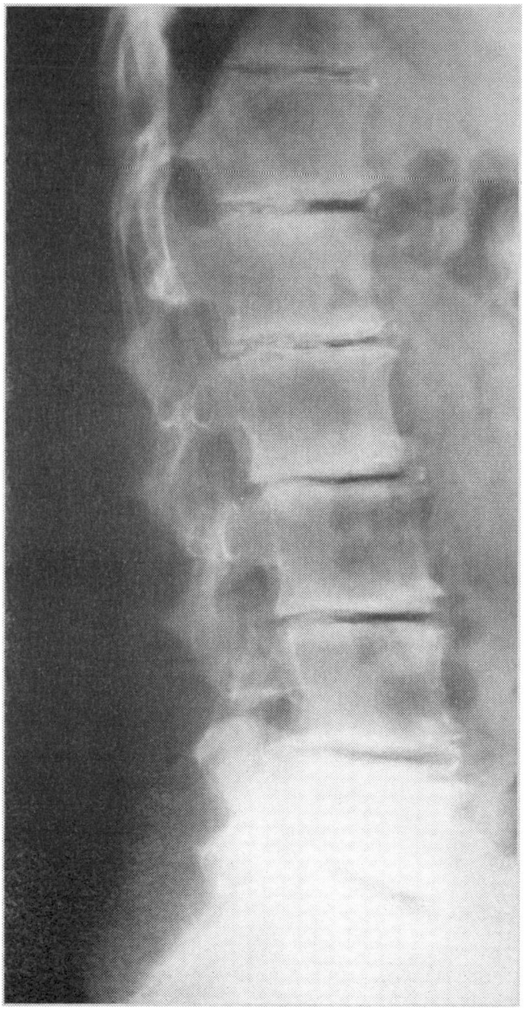

Fig 4.7

1. What do you observe on the plain film of the spine?
2. What is the diagnosis?
3. What are the radiological features?
4. What is the radiological differential diagnosis for this appearance?
5. What are the clinical features and treatment?

Answers *on pages 273–334*

Case 4.8

A 12-year-old girl presented with pain in the right shoulder. On examination, tenderness was elicited over the proximal humerus, with limitation of joint movements. No warmth or tenderness was noticed. The lab tests were normal.

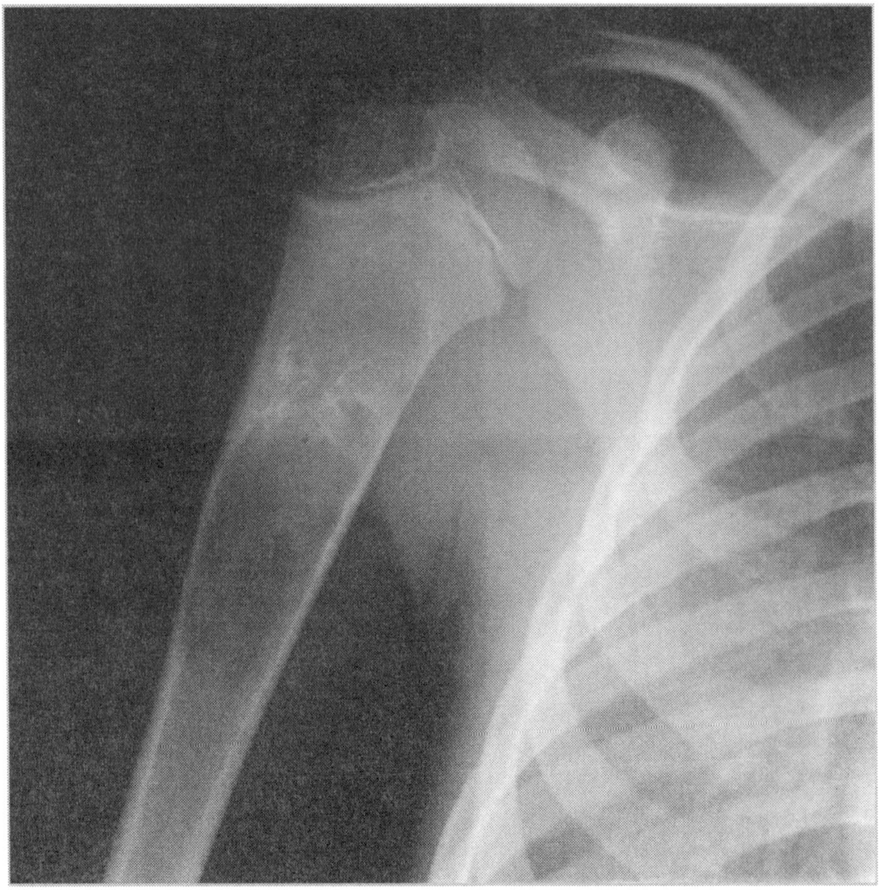

Fig 4.8

1. What do you observe on the plain film of the humerus?
2. What is the diagnosis?
3. What is the pathology of this lesion and what are the clinical features?
4. What are the common locations and radiological features?
5. What are the differential diagnosis and the treatment?

Answers *on pages 273–334*

Case 4.9

An 11-year-old girl presents with pain in the right hip and knee. On examination there is no swelling or redness of the hip joint, but there is pain and restricted abduction and external rotation of the hip. The knee joint appears normal.

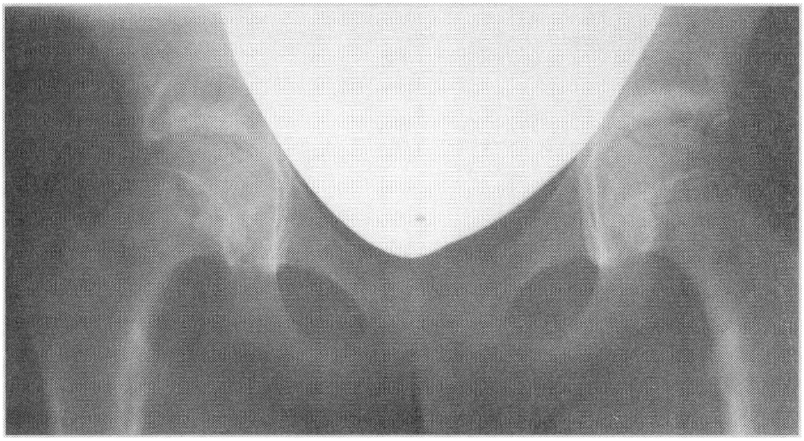

Fig 4.9a

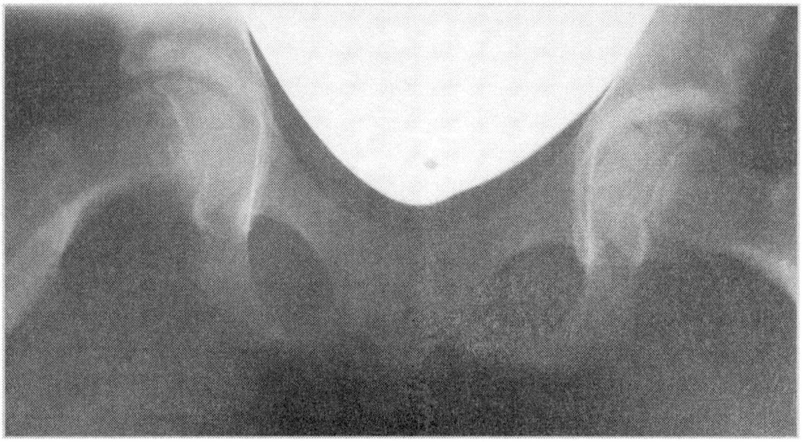

Fig 4.9b

1. What are the two views and what do you observe on the plain films?
2. What is the diagnosis?
3. What are the aetiology, predisposing factors and clinical features of this condition?
4. How do you diagnose this condition with X-rays?
5. How do you grade this disease?
6. What are the complications?

Answers *on pages 273–334*

Case 4.10

An 11-year-old boy presents with intermittent right knee pain, locking on running and limitation of joint movements. On examination his right knee joint is very tender and there is limitation of flexion movements.

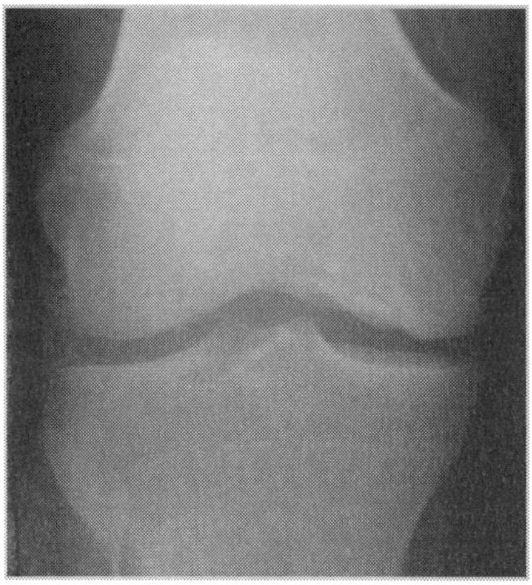

Fig 4.10a

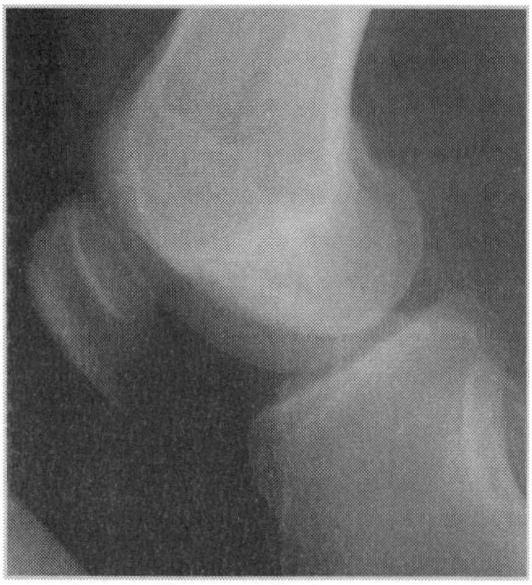

Fig 4.10b

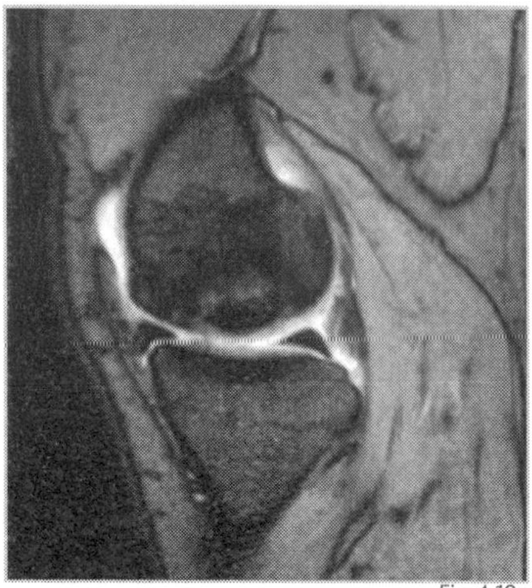

Fig 4.10c

1. What do you observe on the X-ray of the knees?
2. What do you observe on the MRI of the knee?
3. What is the diagnosis?
4. What is the pathophysiology?
5. What are the stages?
6. What is the differential diagnosis?

Answers *on pages 273–334*

Case 4.11

A newborn girl shows positive Barlow's test and Ortolani's test. X-rays and ultrasound scan were done.

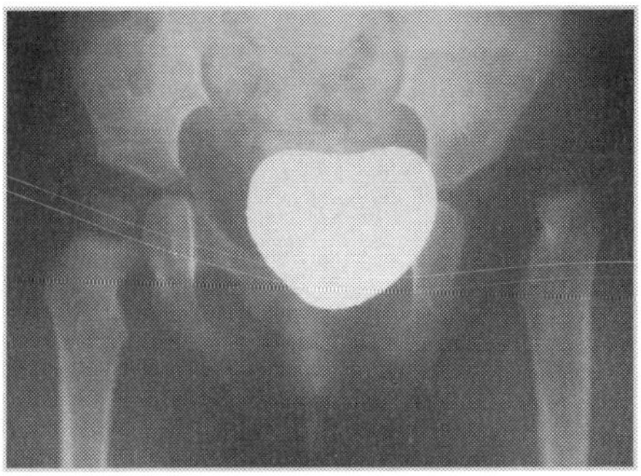

Fig 4.11a

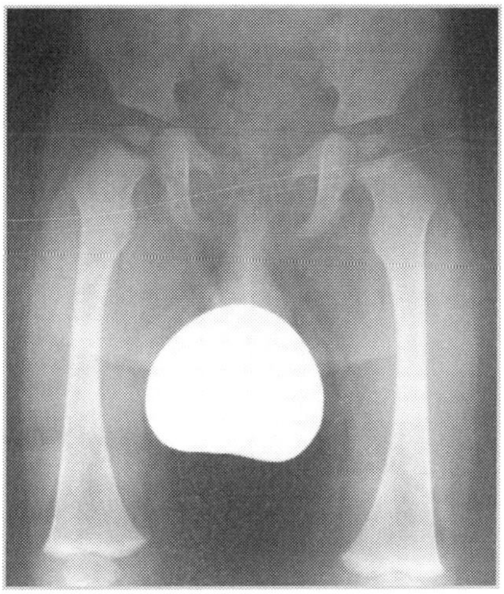

Fig 4.11b

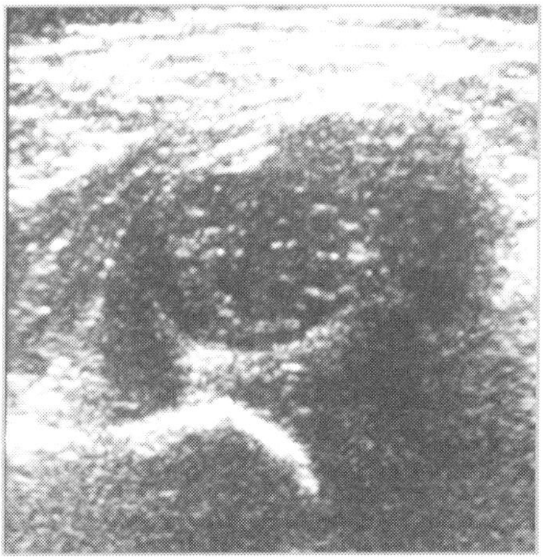

Fig 4.11c

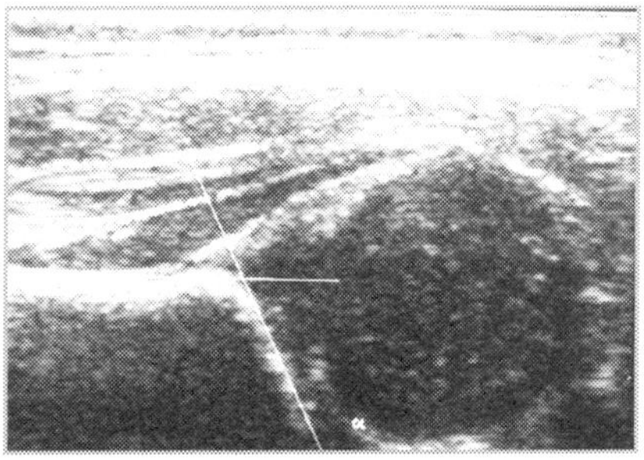

Fig 4.11d

1. What do you find on the plain X-ray of the pelvis? The figure on the right shows the normal alignment.
2. What is the second investigation and what do you observe? The figure on the right is a normal scan for comparison
3. What is the diagnosis?
4. What are the radiological features of this disorder?
5. What are the sonographic findings?
6. What are the complications of this disorder?

Answers *on pages 273–334*

Case 4.12

A 15-year-old boy presents with a dull aching pain in the left arm. On examination there is no swelling or redness of the arm but there is pain and restricted abduction. The elbow joint is normal.

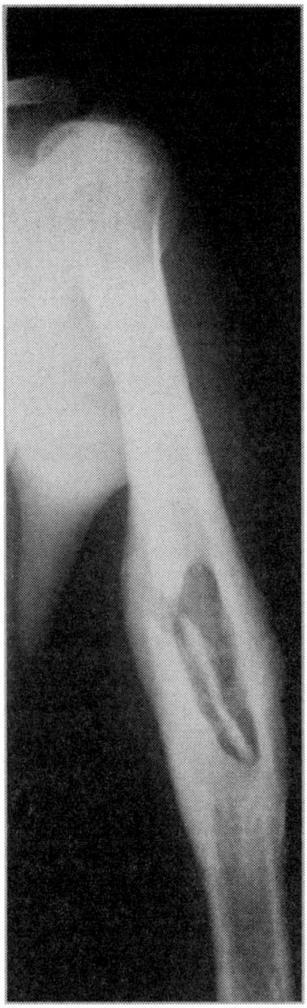

Fig 4.12a

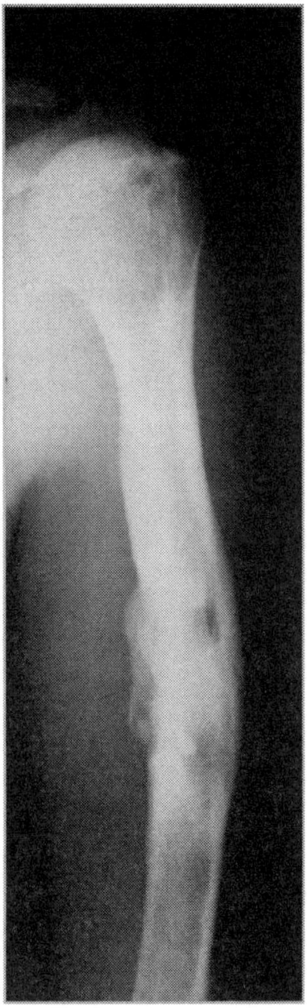

Fig 4.12b

1. What do you observe on the plain films?
2. What is the diagnosis?
3. What are the aetiology, predisposing factors and pathological features of this condition?
4. How do you diagnose this condition with X-rays?
5. What are the variants of this disease and the complications?

Answers *on pages 273–334*

Case 4.13

A 12-year-old girl presents with pain, tenderness and restricted movement of the right arm. She also has precocious puberty. On examination, she has severe tenderness on the proximal shaft of the right humerus and excessive pigmentation of the skin.

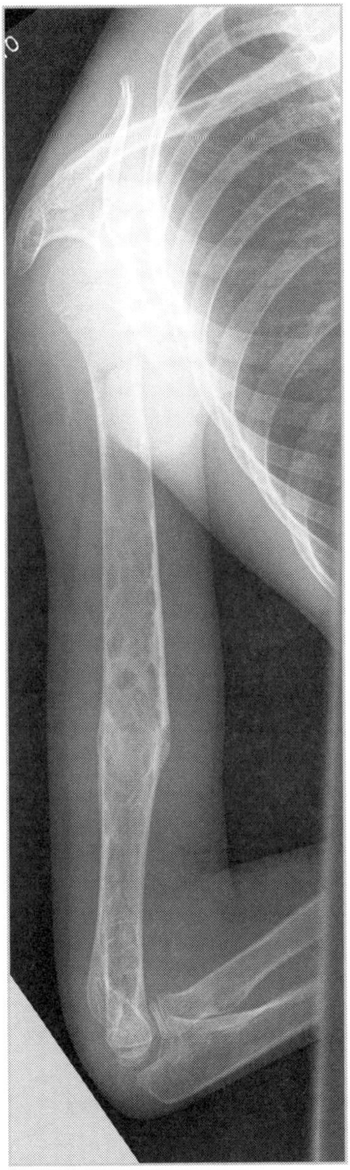

Fig 4.13

1. What are the findings on the X-ray?
2. What is the diagnosis?
3. What are the pathology and clinical features?
4. What are the radiological features?
5. What is the differential diagnosis?
6. What are the complications?

Answers *on pages 273–334*

Case 4.14

A 7-year-old boy presents with left shoulder and neck pain. On examination there is limitation of movement of the left shoulder and spine. There is no tenderness.

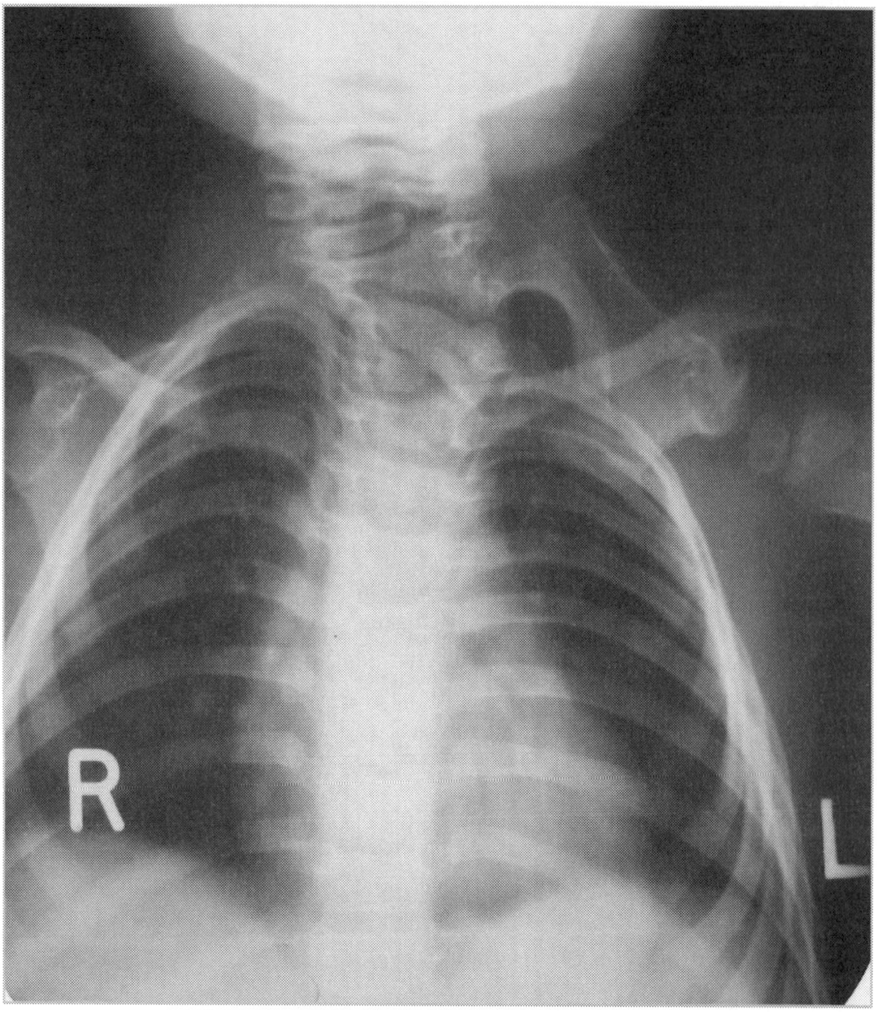

Fig 4.14

1. What do you observe on the plain film of the chest?
2. What is the diagnosis?
3. What are the development and clinical presentations of this disorder?
4. What are the clinical features?
5. What are the associations?

Answers *on pages 273–334*

Case 4.15

A 15-year-old boy presents with non-specific bone pain. A bone scan was normal. X-rays were taken.

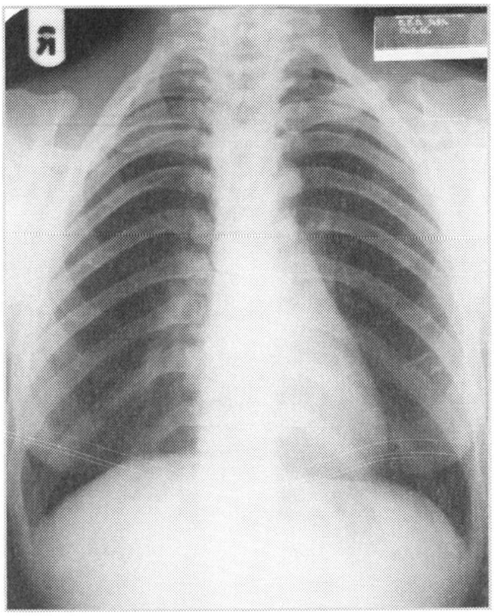

Fig 4.15a

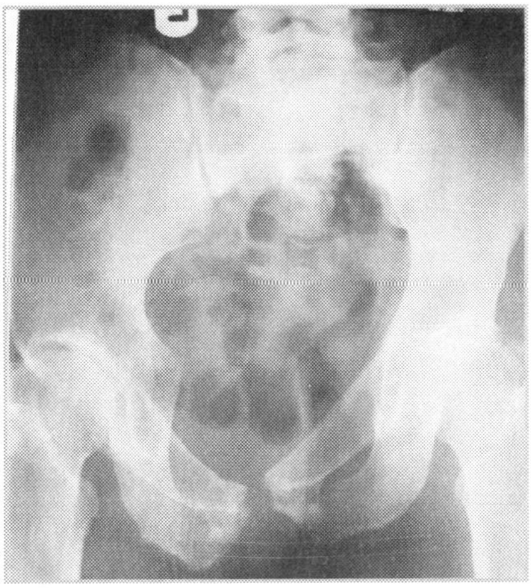

Fig 4.15b

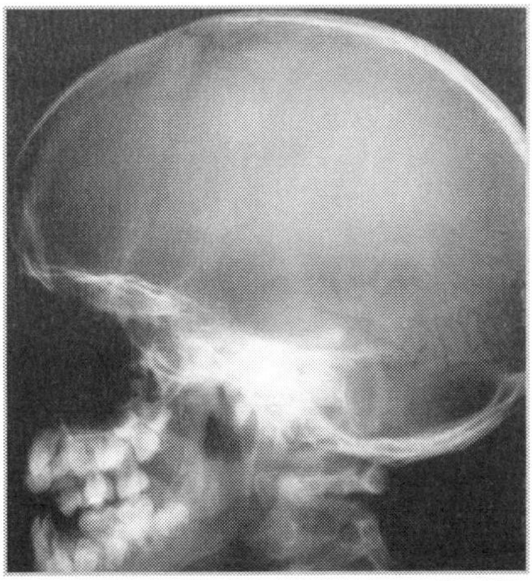

Fig 4.15c

1. What are the findings on the chest X-ray?
2. What is abnormal on the pelvis and skull X-rays?
3. What is the diagnosis?
4. What is the aetiology of this disease?
5. What are the radiological features?
6. What is the differential diagnosis?

Answers *on pages 273–334*

Case 4.16

A 12-year-old boy has severe defects in the arms and legs from birth. X-rays of the arms and legs were taken.

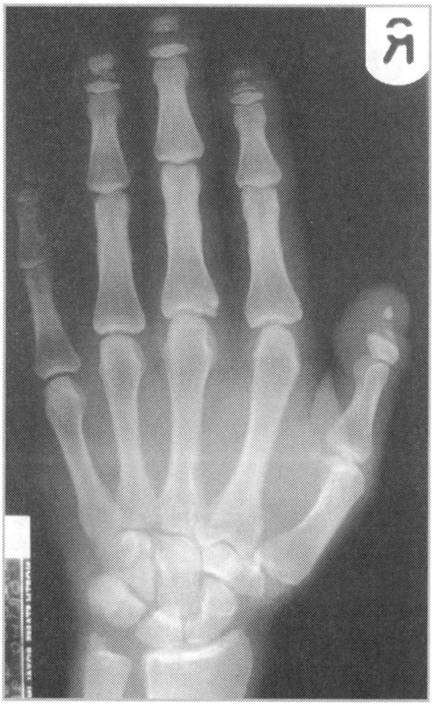

Fig 4.16a

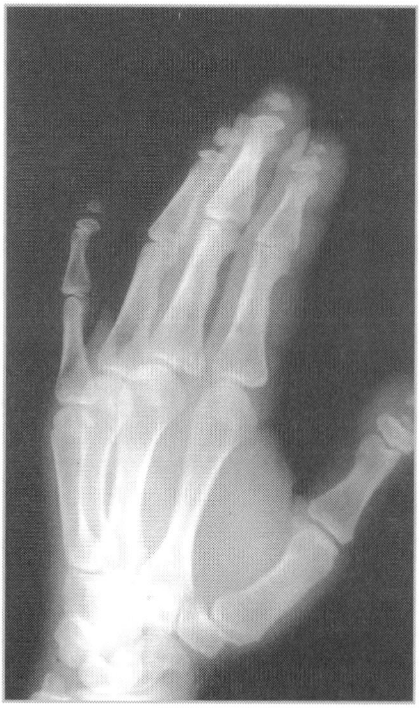

Fig 4.16b

1. What do you observe on the X-rays of the hand?
2. What is the diagnosis?
3. What is the differential diagnosis?
4. What is the aetiology of this condition?
5. How is this condition managed?

Answers *on pages 273–334*

Case 4.17

Whole body X-ray was done on a stillborn male baby, delivered in the third trimester.

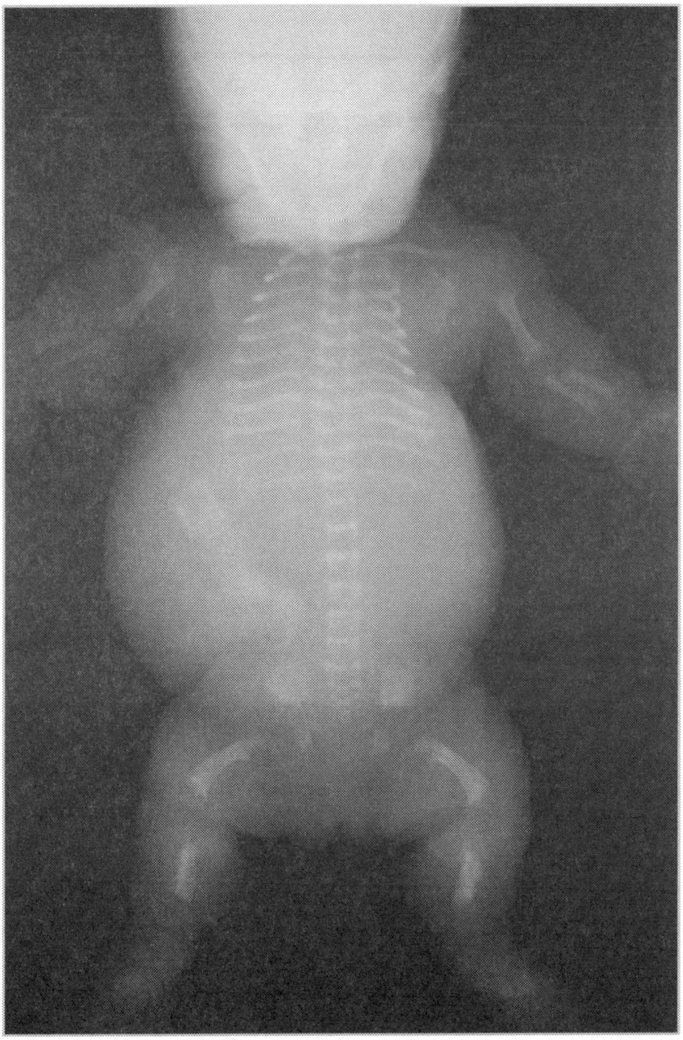

Fig 4.17

1. What do you see on the plain X-ray?
2. What is the diagnosis?
3. What are the radiological features?
4. What is the differential diagnosis?
5. What is the prognosis?

Answers *on pages 273–334*

Case 4.18

A 14-year-old boy with a chronic renal problem presented with fatigue, anorexia, nausea and generalised bone pain.

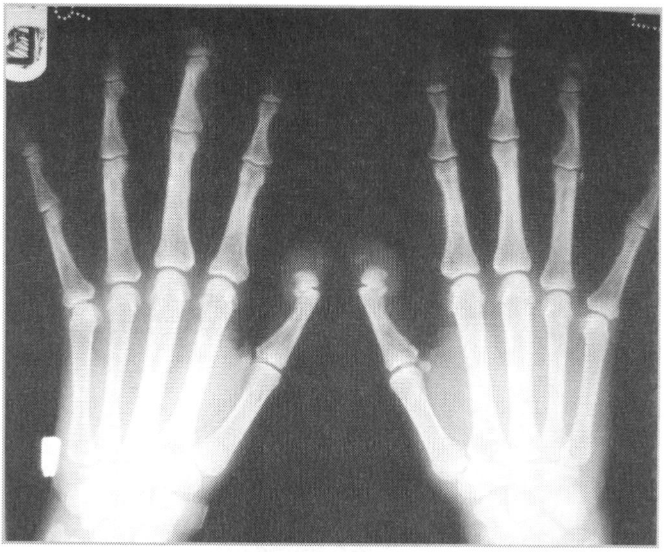

Fig 4.18a

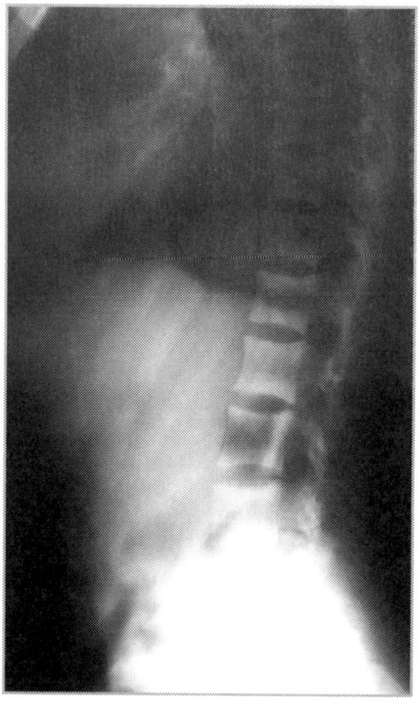

Fig 4.18b

1. What do you observe on the plain films of the spine and the hands?
2. What is the diagnosis?
3. What are the mechanism and pathophysiology of this disease?
4. What are the radiological features?
5. What are the complications?

Answers *on pages 273–334*

Case 4.19

An 8-year-old girl presents with pain in her right shoulder and palpable bony swelling. There is no history of trauma. On examination there is no warmth or tenderness. Slight restriction of movement at the shoulder joint was noted.

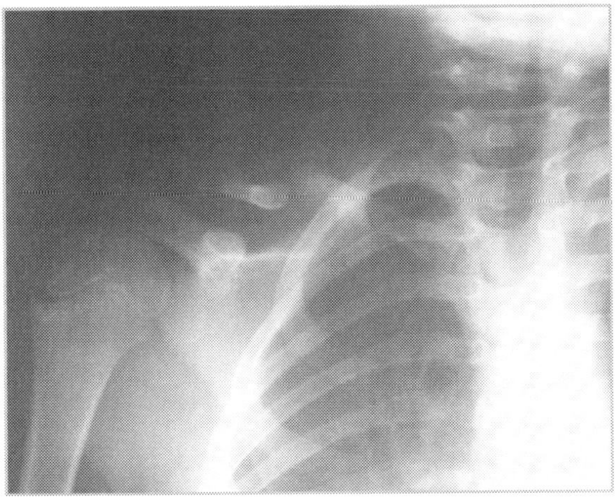

Fig 4.19a

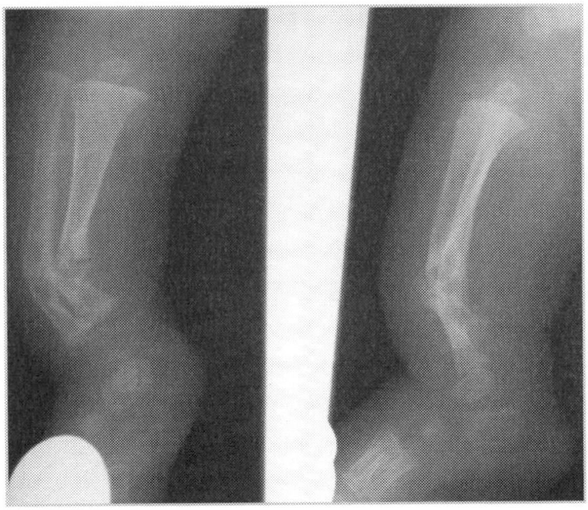

Fig 4.19b

1. What are the findings on the X-ray?
2. What do you see on the X-ray of the leg?
3. What is the diagnosis?
4. What are the causes of this abnormality?
5. What is the development of this condition and what are the radiological features?
6. What is the treatment for this condition?

Answers *on pages 273–334*

Case 4.20

An 8-year-old girl presents with bone pain and growth retardation.

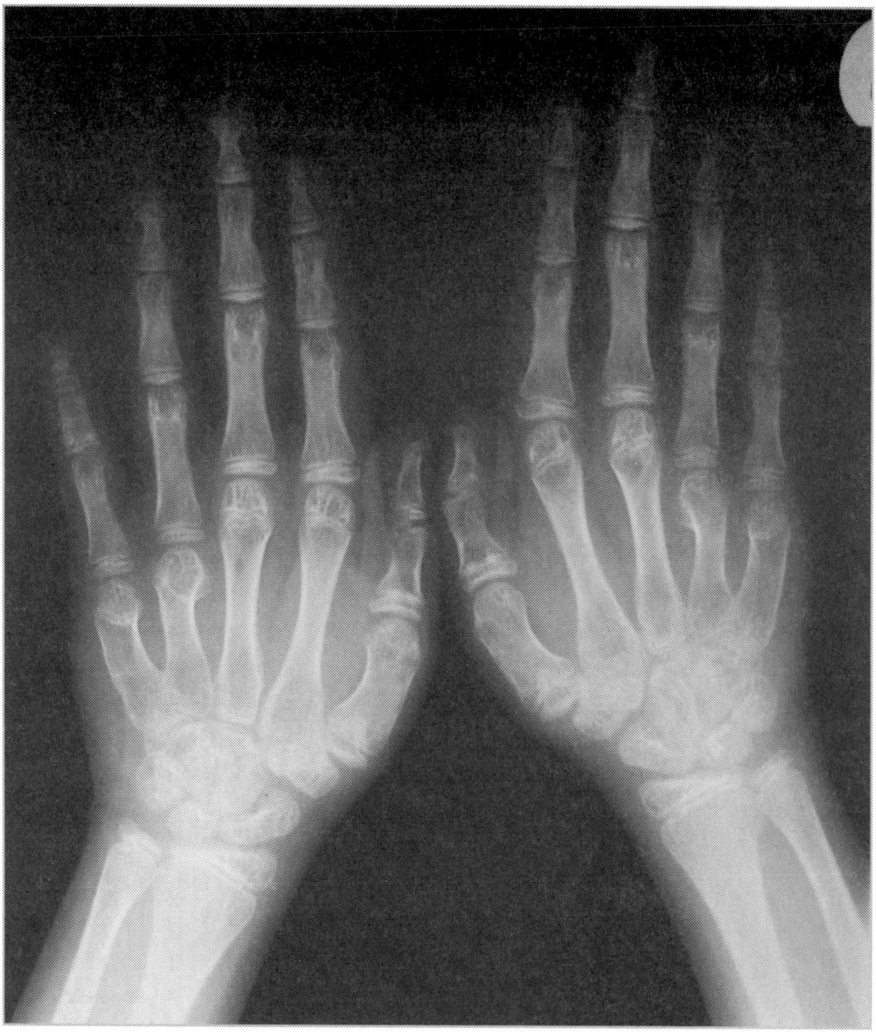

Fig 4.20

1. What do you observe on the plain X-ray?
2. What is the diagnosis?
3. What is the differential diagnosis for this radiological appearance?
4. What are the clinical features of this disease?
5. What are the radiological features?

Answers *on pages 273–334*

Case 4.21

A 9-year-old boy presents with spinal deformity, bone pain, loss of weight, nausea and vomiting. On examination he has scoliosis and generalised bone tenderness.

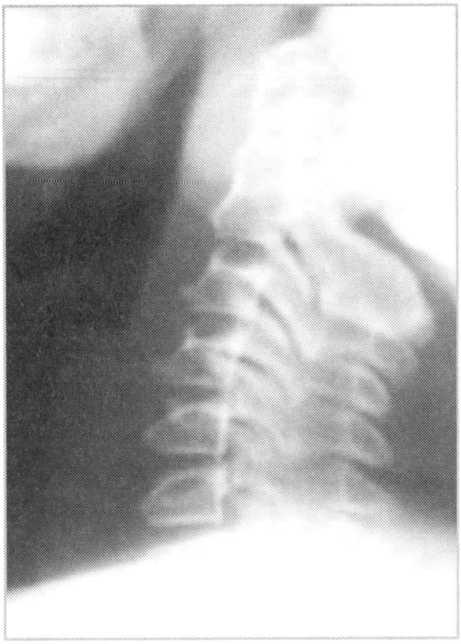

Fig 4.21a

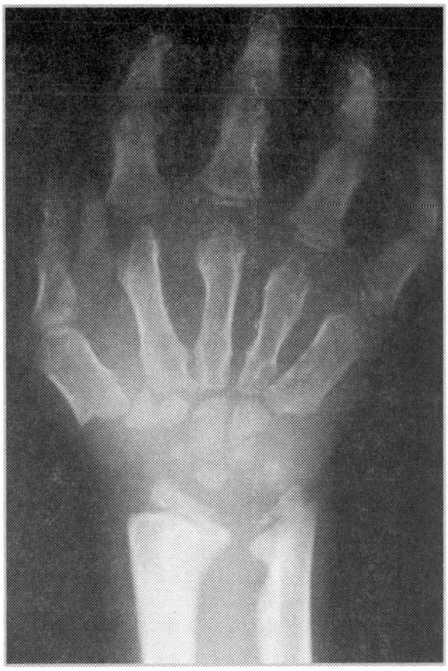

Fig 4.21b

1. What do you observe on the plain films of the spine and hands?
2. What is the diagnosis?
3. What are the types of the disease?
4. What are the radiological features?
5. What are the differential diagnosis and treatment?

Answers *on pages 273–334*

Case 4.22

A 14-year-old boy presents with failure to thrive, generalised bone pain and vomiting.

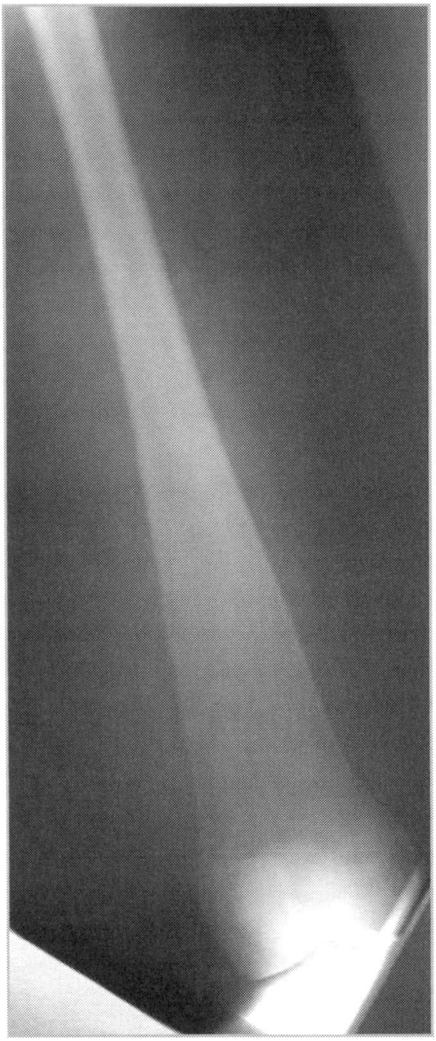

Fig 4.22a

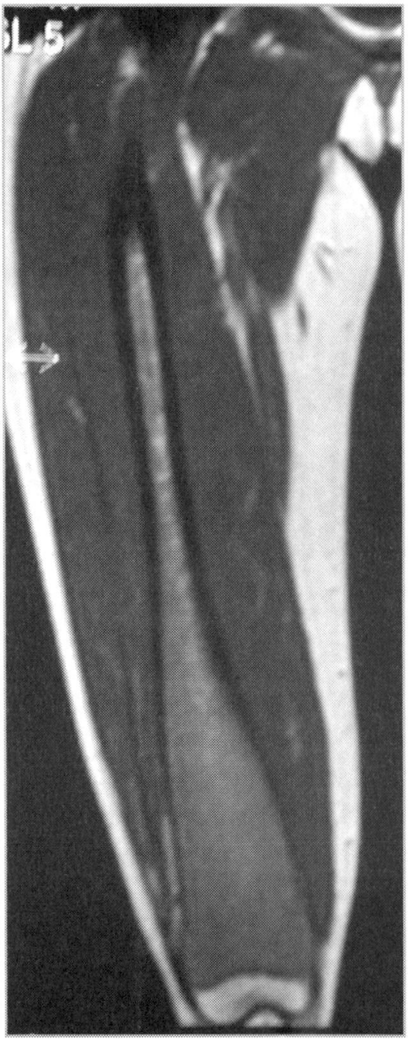

Fig 4.22b

1. What do you note on the X-ray and MR scan?
2. What is the diagnosis?
3. What is the mechanism of development of this deformity?
4. What are the causes of this abnormality?
5. What are the clinical and radiological features of this disorder?

Answers *on pages 273–334*

Case 4.23

A 9-year-old boy presents with pain, failure to thrive and chest infections. Clinical examination revealed generalised tenderness, worse in the knee joints.

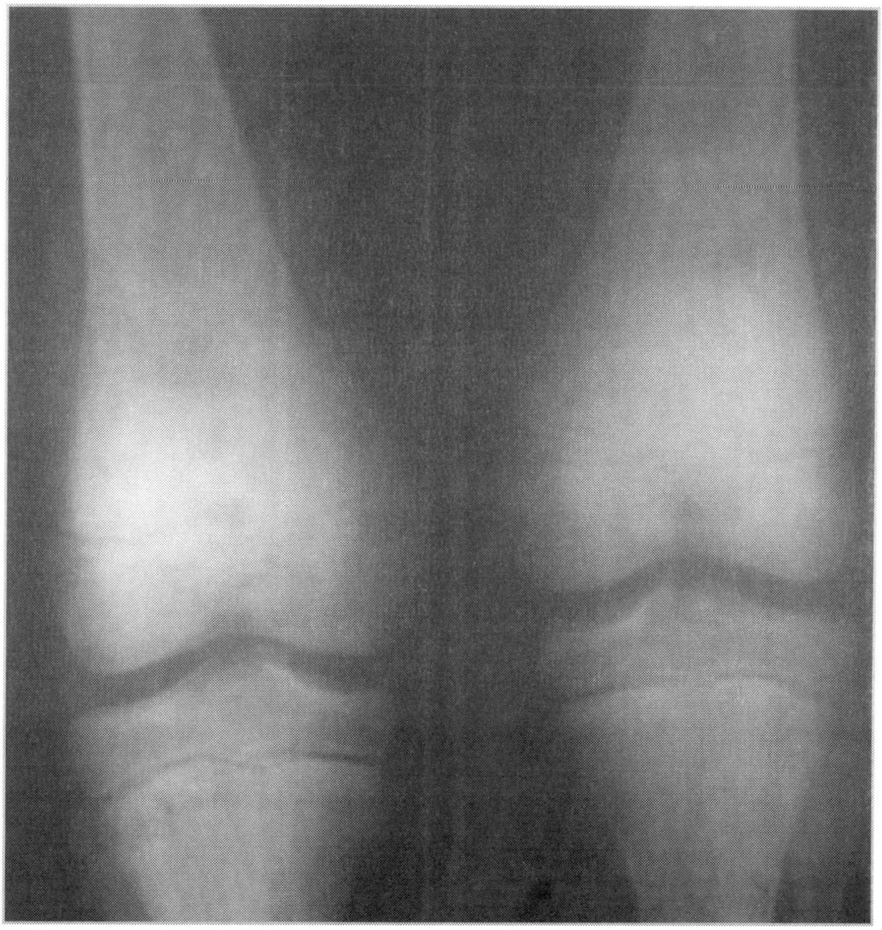

Fig 4.23

1. What do you observe on the plain X-ray?
2. What is the diagnosis?
3. What is the differential diagnosis for this radiological appearance?
4. What are the clinical features of this disease?
5. What are the radiological features?

Answers *on pages 273–334*

Case 4.24

A 4-year-old boy presents with failure to thrive, irritability and bowed legs. On examination he has bilateral knocked knees and an abnormal skull.

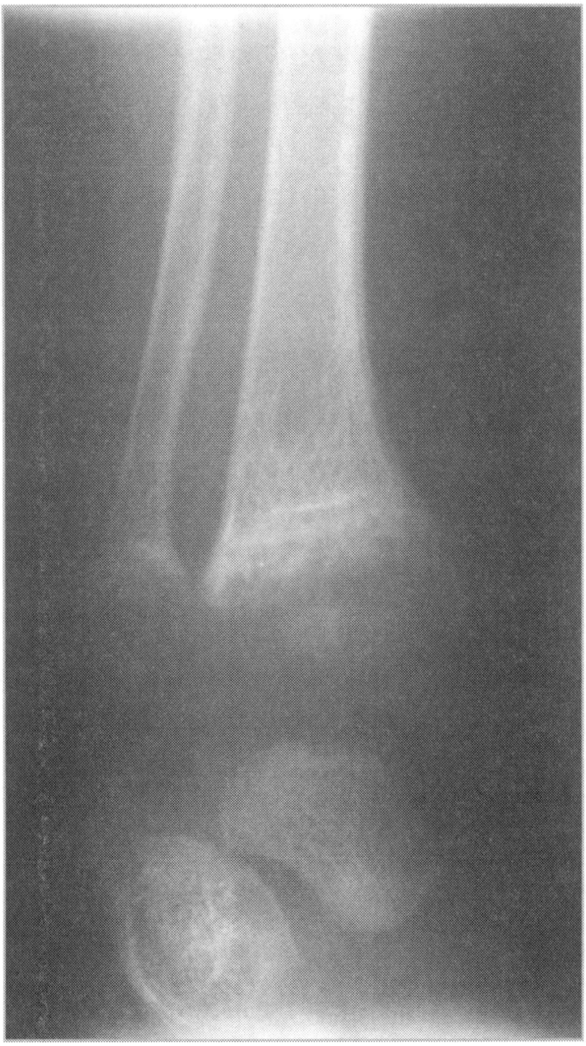

Fig 4.24

1. What are the findings on the ankle X-ray?
2. What is the diagnosis?
3. What is the pathophysiology of this disease?
4. What are the causative factors?
5. What are the radiological features and differential diagnosis?

Answers *on pages 273–334*

Case 4.25

A 13-year-old boy presented with severe low back pain and fever. On examination spinal tenderness was noted in the L4–5 region. An urgent X-ray and MRI were performed.

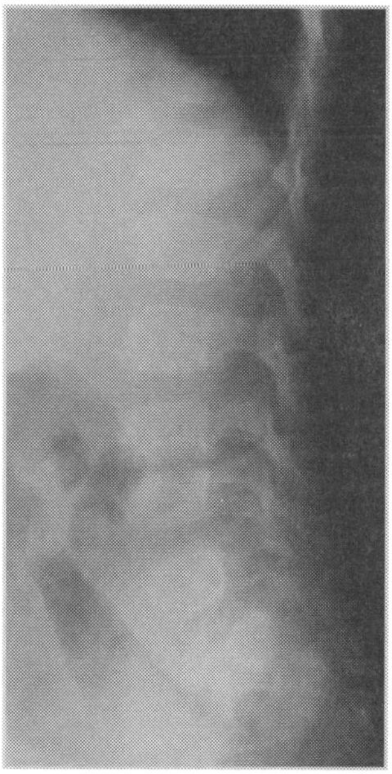
Fig 4.25a

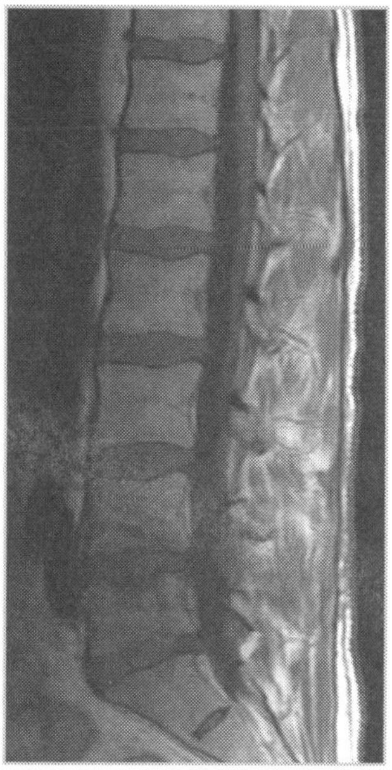
Fig 4.25b

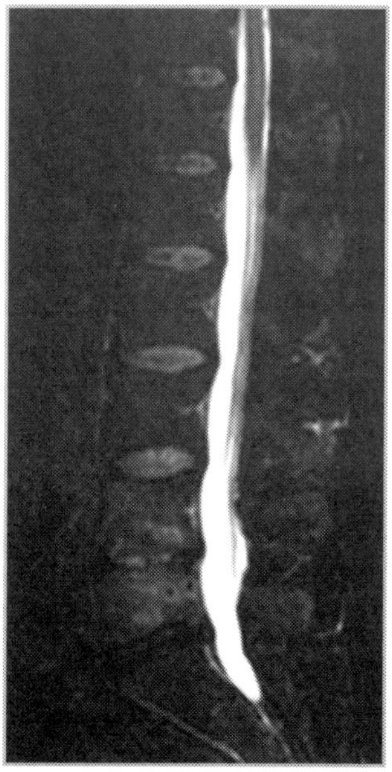
Fig 4.25c

1. What are the observations on the X-ray and MRI?
2. What is the diagnosis?
3. What are the clinical features of this condition?
4. What are the radiological features?
5. What is the management of this condition?

Answers *on pages 273–334*

Case 4.26

A 14-year-old girl presents with intermittent backache and stiffness. On examination she has tenderness at many levels in the dorsal vertebrae.

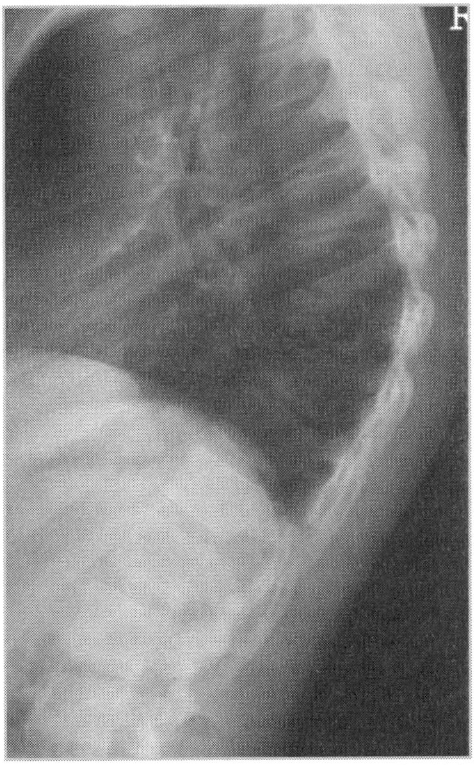

Fig 4.26a

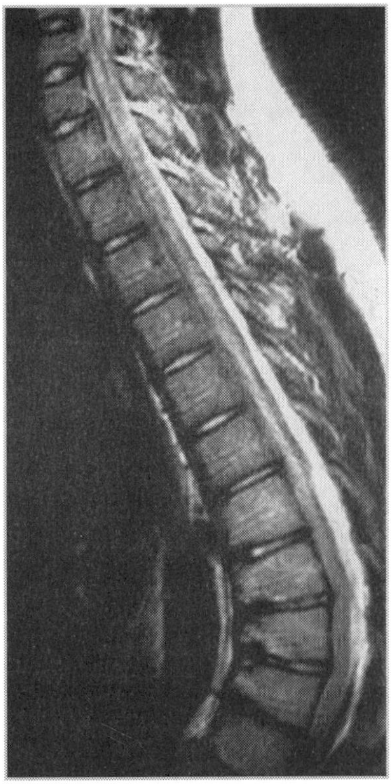

Fig 4.26b

1. What do you observe in the X-ray and the MRI scan of the spine?
2. What is the diagnosis?
3. What is the aetiology of this condition?
4. What are the radiological features?
5. What is the differential diagnosis?
6. What is the treatment?

Answers *on pages 273–334*

Case 4.27

An 11-year-old boy presents with dull pain in his left leg, which is worse in the night. On examination, there is a red, tender swelling in the medial aspect of the left tibia.

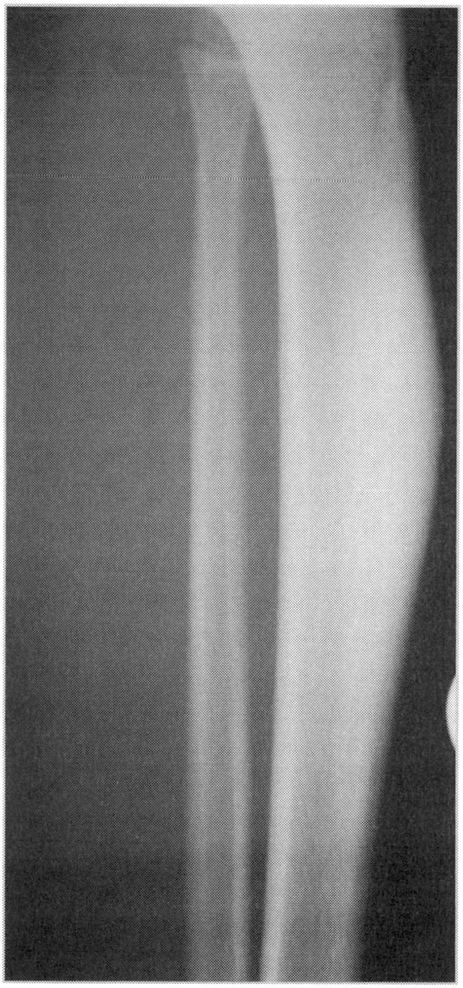

Fig 4.27

1. What are the findings on the X-ray?
2. What is the diagnosis?
3. What are the clinical features and pathology?
4. What are the radiological features?
5. What is the differential diagnosis?
6. What is the treatment?

Answers *on pages 273–334*

Case 4.28

A 15-year-old boy presents with backache that is worse in the night, paraesthesiae in the leg and a decreased range of motion. On examination, there is tenderness in the lumbar spine and a restriction of flexion and extension.

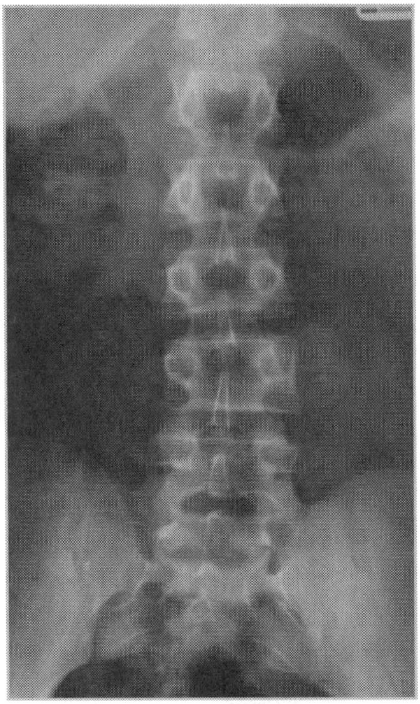

Fig 4.28a

1. What are the findings on the X-ray and the CT scan?
2. What is the diagnosis?
3. What are the radiological features?
4. What is the differential diagnosis?
5. What are the complications and the treatment?

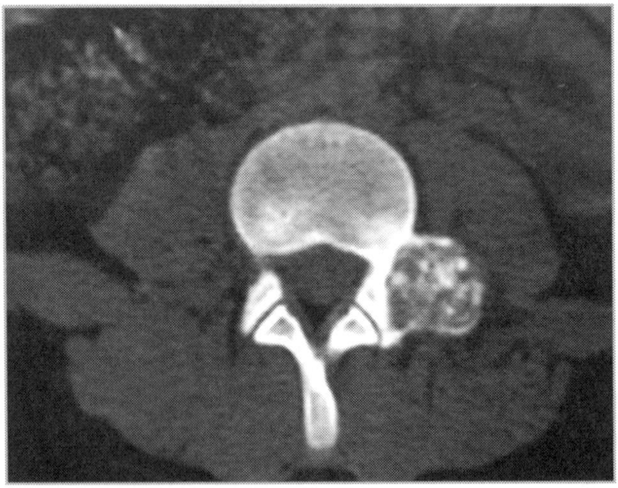

Fig 4.28b

Answers *on pages 273–334*

Case 4.29

A 10-year-old boy presented with pain in the right leg, which limits his movements. On examination, tenderness was elicited over the proximal tibia, with limitation of joint movements. No warmth or tenderness was noticed. The lab tests were normal.

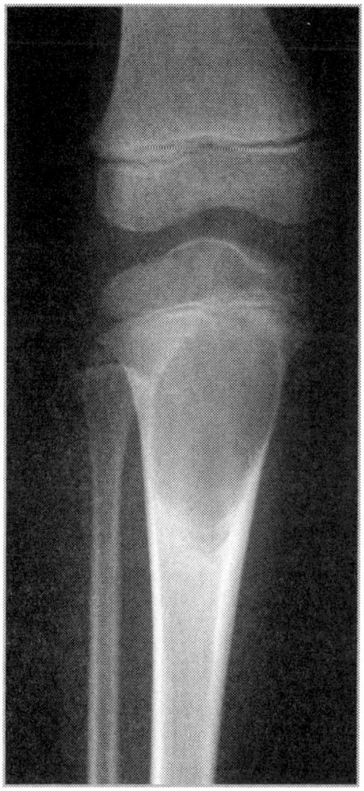

Fig 4.29a

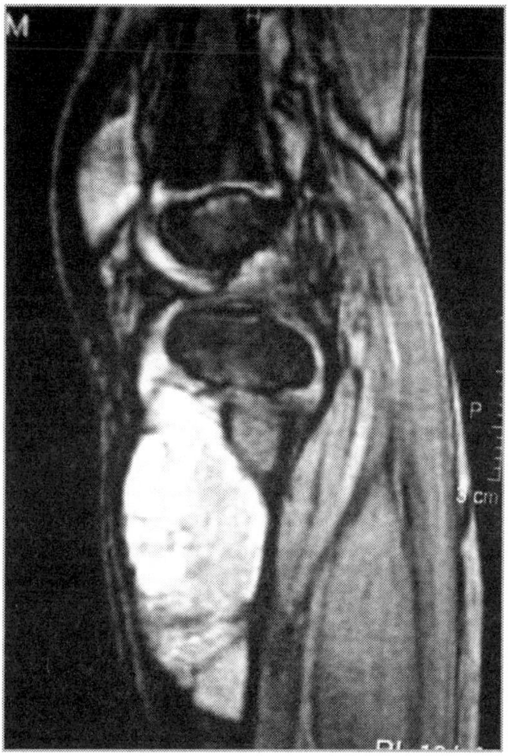

Fig 4.29b

1. What do you observe on the plain film of the leg?
2. What is the second investigation and what do you observe?
3. What are the diagnosis and the clinical features?
4. What are the common locations and the radiological features
5. What are the complications and the differential diagnosis?

Answers *on pages 273–334*

Case 4.30

A 10-year-old girl presents with delayed development and growth retardation.

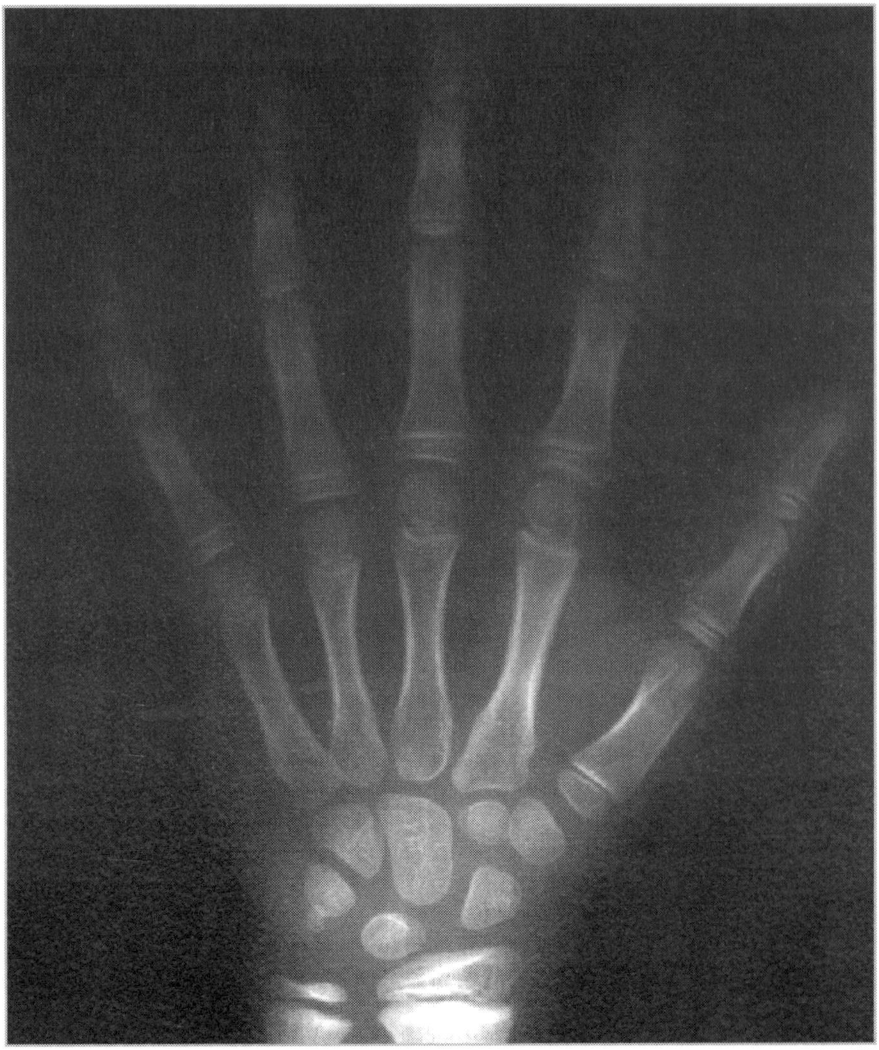

Fig 4.30

1. What is this investigation?
2. What is the purpose of this X-ray?
3. What is the system used for this procedure?
4. What is the rationale for using this side?
5. What are the causes of delayed bone age?

Answers *on pages 273–334*

Case 4.31

An 11-year-old boy presents with fever, severe pain and swelling of his right leg. On examination he is febrile. His right leg is swollen, red and tender. The swelling is bony hard on palpation and there is severe restriction of the right knee joint movements.

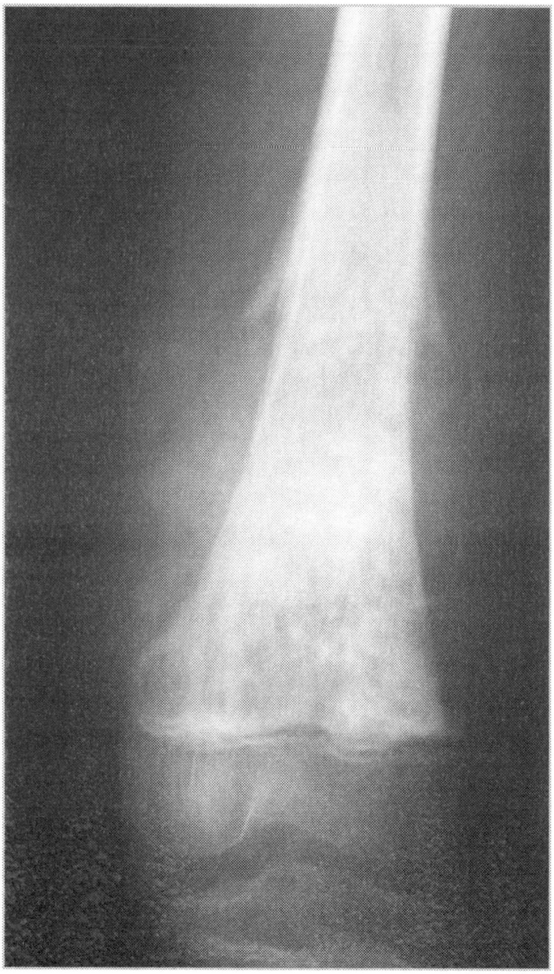

Fig 4.31

1. What are the findings on the plain film?
2. What is the diagnosis?
3. What are the clinical features, the complications and the treatment?
4. What are the radiological features and the differential diagnosis?
5. What are the variations in the presentation?

Answers *on pages 273–334*

Case 4.32

A 15-year-old girl presents with pain, tenderness and swelling in her neck. On examination there is a tender bony protuberance in the lower cervical spine. There is no abnormal reflex or altered sensation in the upper limbs.

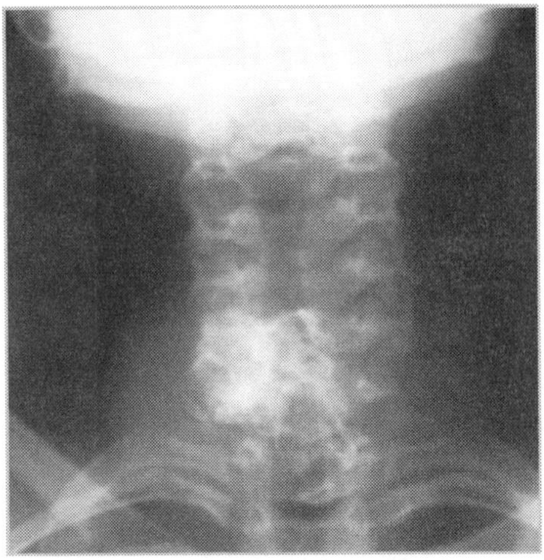

Fig 4.32a

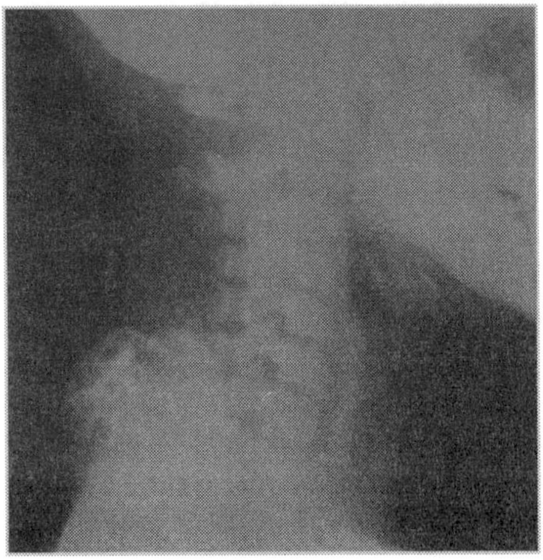

Fig 4.32b

1. What are the findings on the X-ray?
2. What is the diagnosis?
3. What are the pathology and variants of this disease?
4. What are the radiological features?
5. What is the differential diagnosis?
6. What are the complications and treatment?

Answers *on pages 273–334*

Case 4.33

A 2-year-old boy presents with irritability and inability to walk. On examination there is tenderness over the left hip joint and there is restriction of movement of his left hip joint.

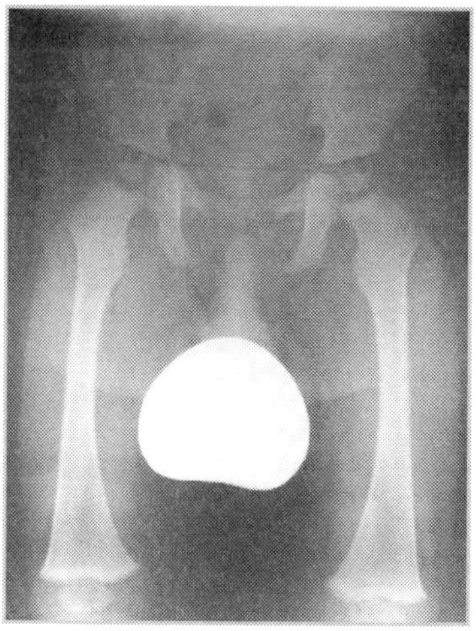

Fig 4.33a

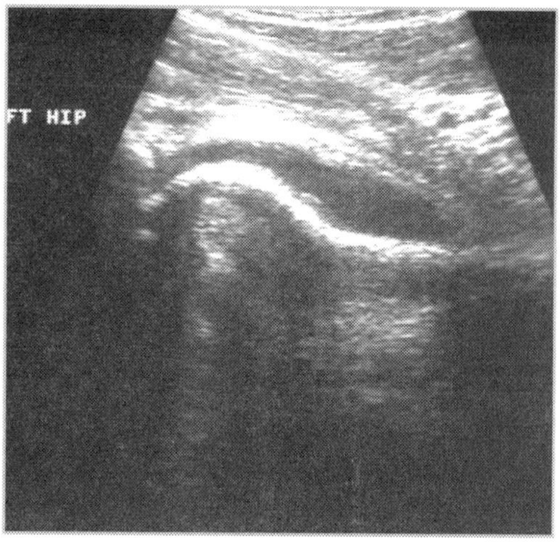

Fig 4.33b

1. What do you see on the plain X-ray?
2. What is the second investigation and what are the findings?
3. What is the diagnosis?
4. What are the causes of this appearance and what are the radiological features?
5. What is the next step?

Answers *on pages 273–334*

Case 4.34

A 6-year-old boy presents with severe pain and limp in the right leg. The patient was afebrile, with restriction of movement in the right hip joint.

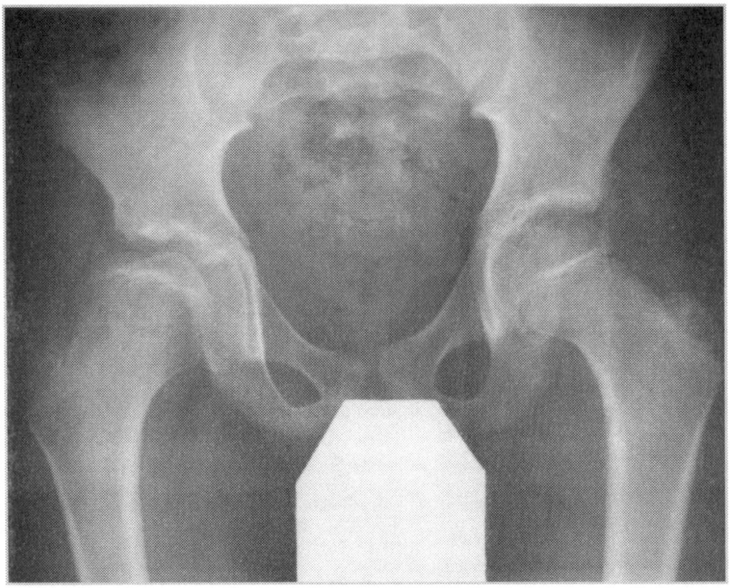

Fig 4.34a

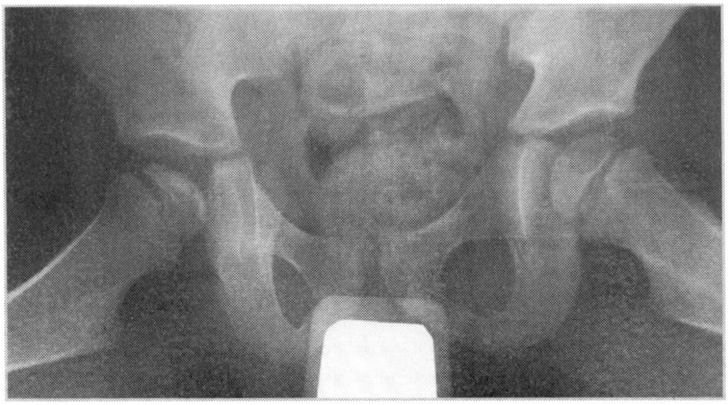

Fig 4.34b

1. What are the findings on the plain film?
2. What is the diagnosis?
3. What are the clinical features?
4. What are the radiological features and stages?
5. What is the differential diagnosis?
6. What are the complications?

Answers *on pages 273–334*

Case 4.35

A 2-year-old boy presents with failure to thrive, delayed milestones and bony deformities. A skeletal survey was ordered.

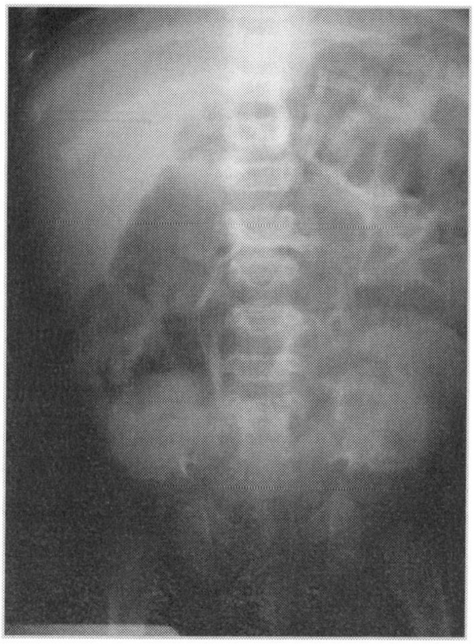

Fig 4.35a

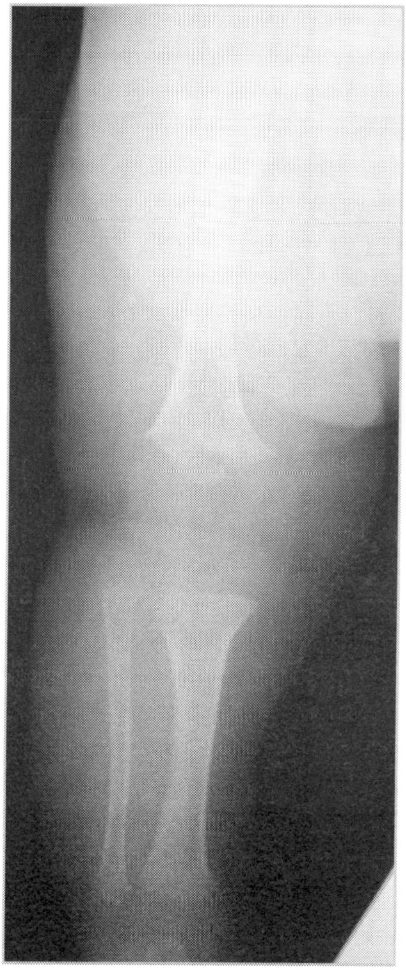

Fig 4.35b

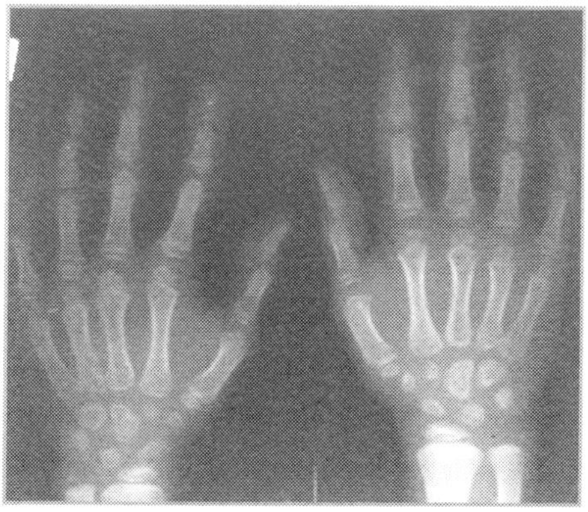

Fig 4.35c

1. What do you see on the X-rays of the abdomen, pelvis and hands and legs?
2. What is the diagnosis?
3. What are the aetiology, clinical features and prognosis of this disease?
4. What are the radiological features?
5. What are the serious complications and treatment of this disease?

Answers *on pages 273–334*

Case 4.36

A 14-year-old boy presents with pain on the right side of the neck and pain and paraesthesiae in his arm and forearm. The elevated arm stress test is positive.

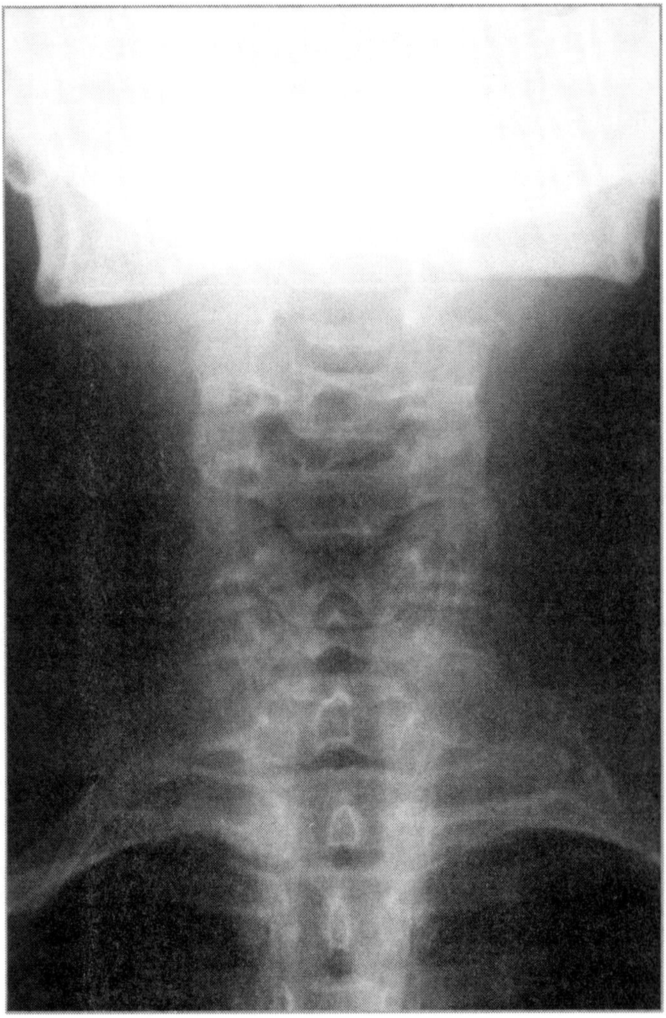

Fig 4.36

1. What do you observe on the chest X-ray?
2. What is the diagnosis?
3. What are the clinical features of this condition?
4. What are the types and the radiological features?
5. What are the complications and the treatment?

Answers *on pages 273–334*

Case 4.37

A 9-year-old boy presents with pain and deformity of the back. On examination he has difficulty in lateral bending and there is tenderness in the midthoracic spine.

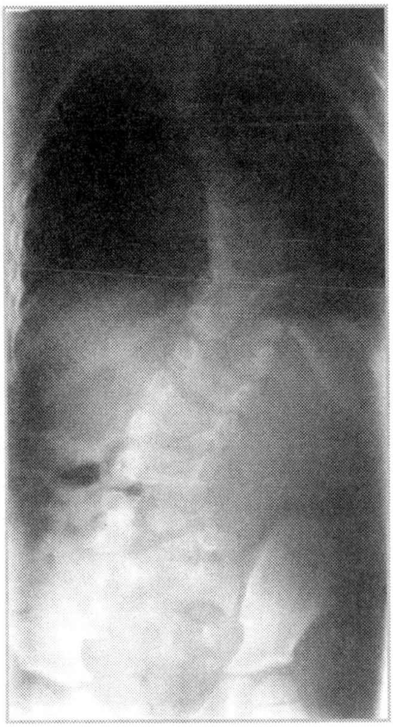

Fig 4.37a

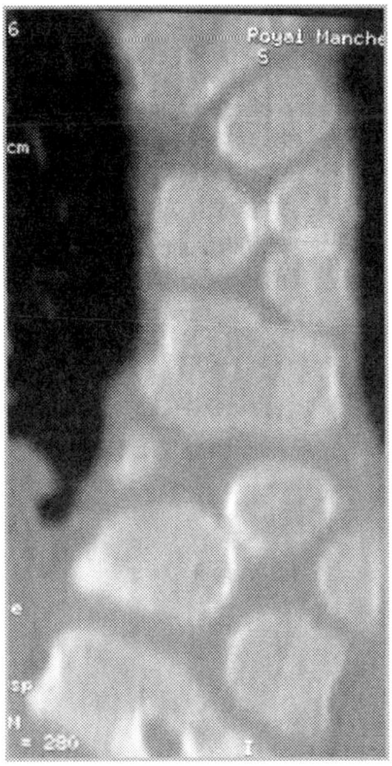

Fig 4.37b

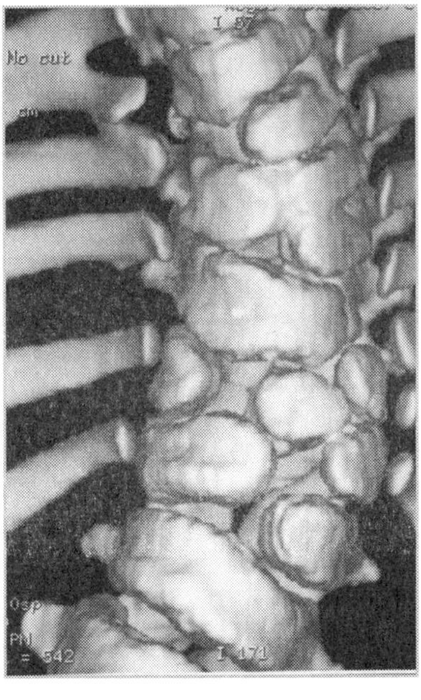

Fig 4.37c

1. What does the X-ray show?
2. What do the CT scans show?
3. What is the diagnosis?
4. What are the types of this disease?
5. What is the most common differential diagnosis?
6. What is the treatment?

Answers *on pages 273–334*

Case 4.38

A 10-year-old girl presents with multiple swellings and pain in her hand. Clinical examination revealed multiple lumps and tenderness in both hands. A large lump was present in the ulnar aspect of the left hand.

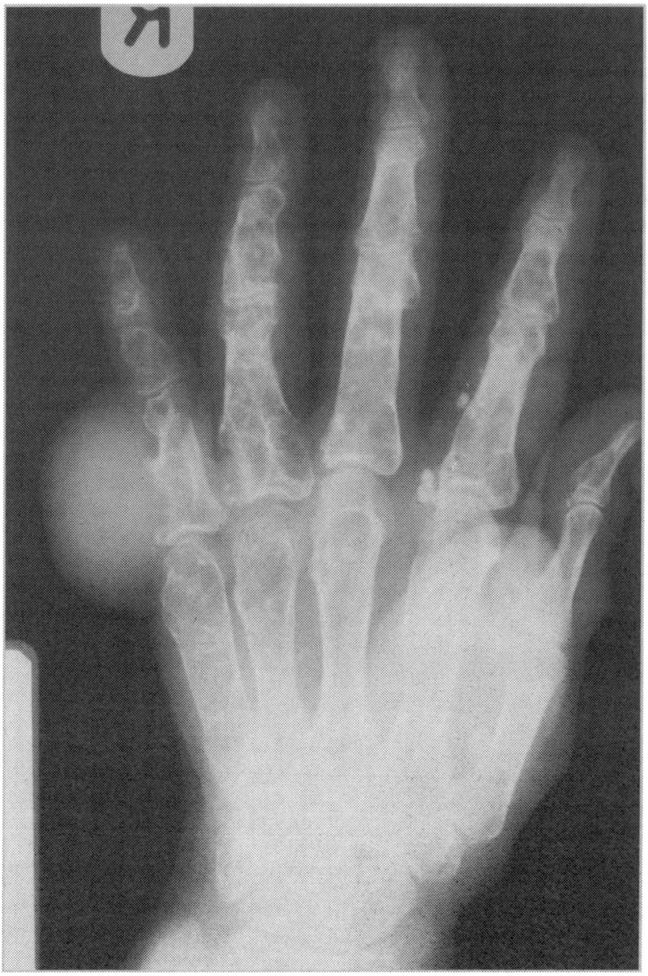

Fig 4.38

1. What are the findings on the X-ray?
2. What is the diagnosis?
3. What are the clinical features and variations in disease?
4. What are the radiological features?
5. What are the differential diagnoses?
6. What are the complications?

Answers *on pages 273–334*

Case 4.39

A 14-year-old girl presents with pain, tenderness and swelling in the right leg.

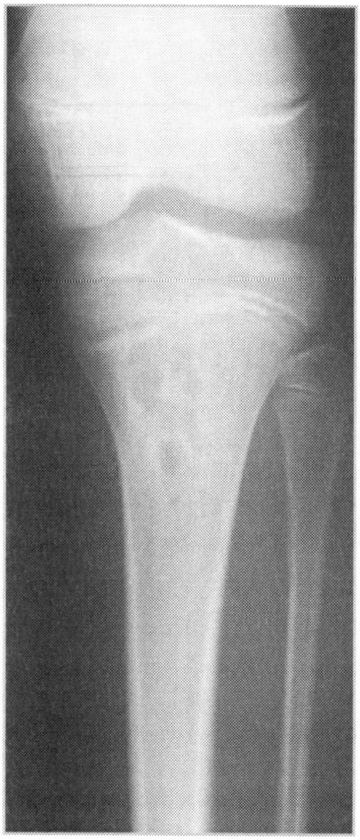

Fig 4.39a

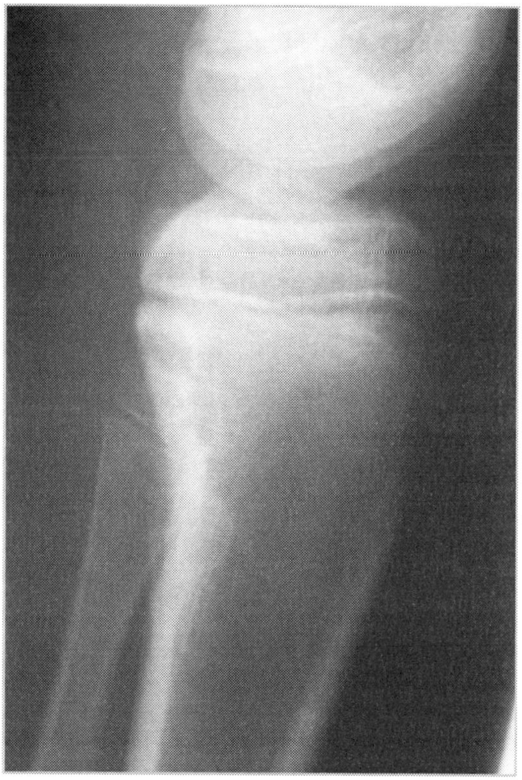

Fig 4.39b

1. What are the findings on the X-ray?
2. What is the diagnosis?
3. What are the clinical features and pathology?
4. What are the radiological features?
5. What is Jaffe–Campanacci syndrome?
6. What is the differential diagnosis?

Answers *on pages 273–334*

Case 4.40

A 9-year-old girl injured her left hand, when playing. On examination the thumb is painful and tender, with limited movement.

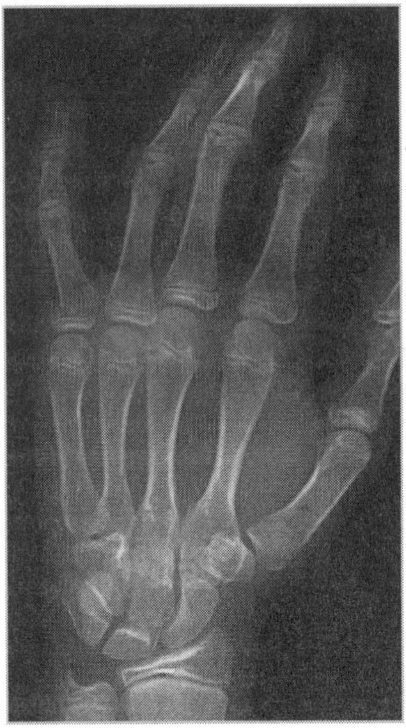

Fig 4.40a

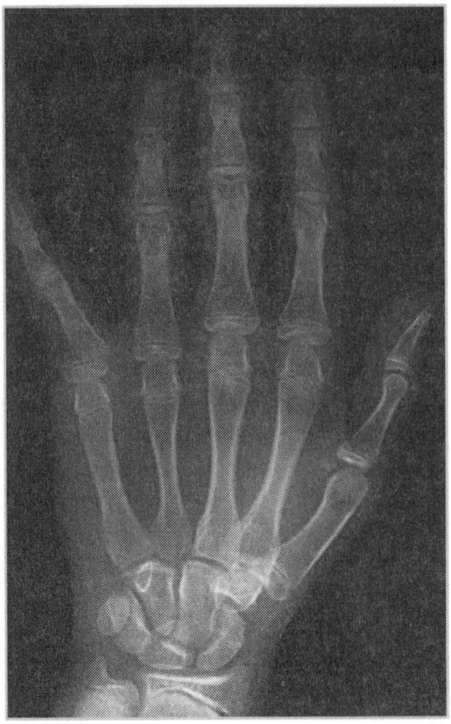

Fig 4.40b

1. What are the findings on this X-ray?
2. What is the diagnosis?
3. What is the mechanism of injury?
4. What are the types of this injury?
5. What is the treatment?

Answers *on pages 273–334*

Case 4.41

A 9-year-old girl presents with a deformed wrist and limitation of joint movement. There is no history of trauma. On examination there is no tenderness, but there is deformity of the wrist. There is limitation of flexion and extension at the wrist joint.

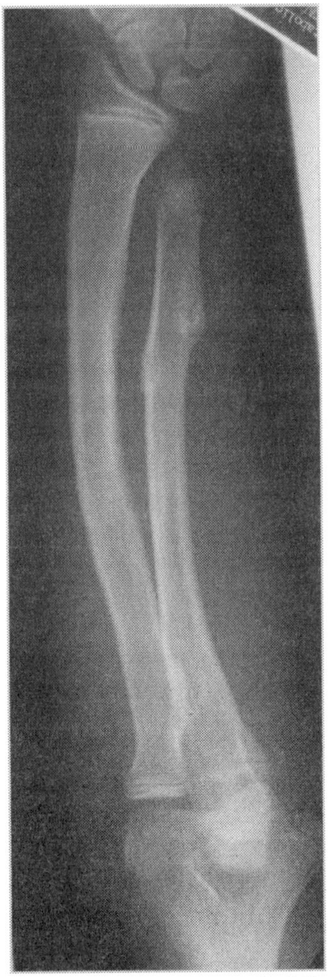

Fig 4.41a

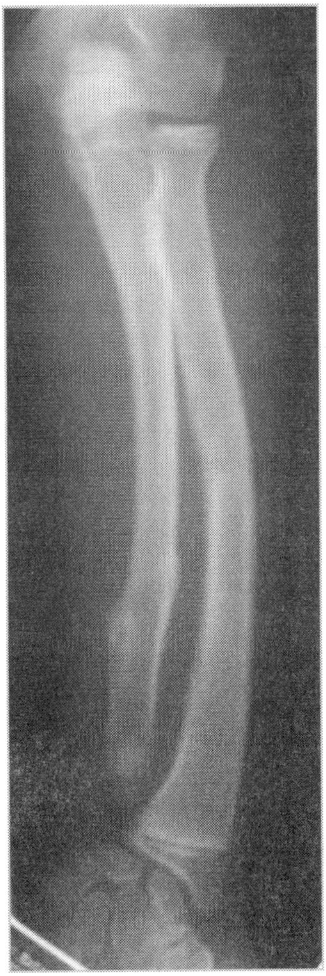

Fig 4.41b

1. What are the findings on the X-ray?
2. What is the diagnosis?
3. What is the development of this condition?
4. What are the causes?
5. What are the radiological features?

Answers *on pages 273–334*

Case 4.42

A 7-year-old boy with a chronic medical problem presents with pain and deformity of his hip joint with restricted abduction and external rotation.

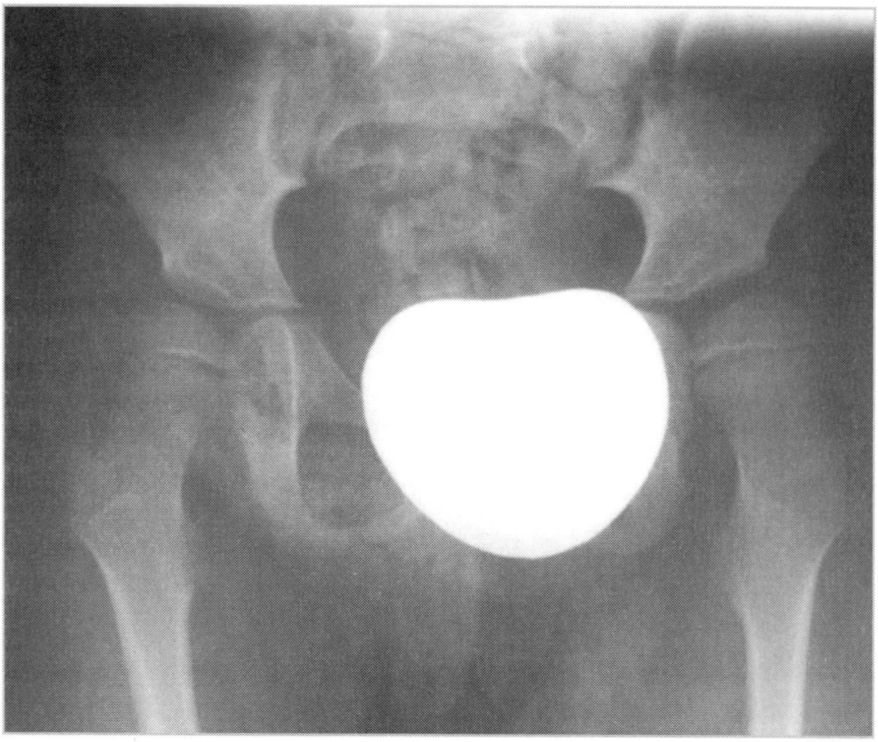

Fig 4.42

1. What do you see on the plain X-ray of the pelvis?
2. What is the diagnosis?
3. What is the underlying medical problem?
4. What are the radiological features of this condition?
5. What are the treatment options for this condition and what is the differential diagnosis?

Answers *on pages 273–334*

Case 4.43

A 15-year-old boy presents with severe pain in his right foot after a crush injury. On examination, his foot is tender on the lateral aspect and there is severe limitation of movement. An X-ray was taken.

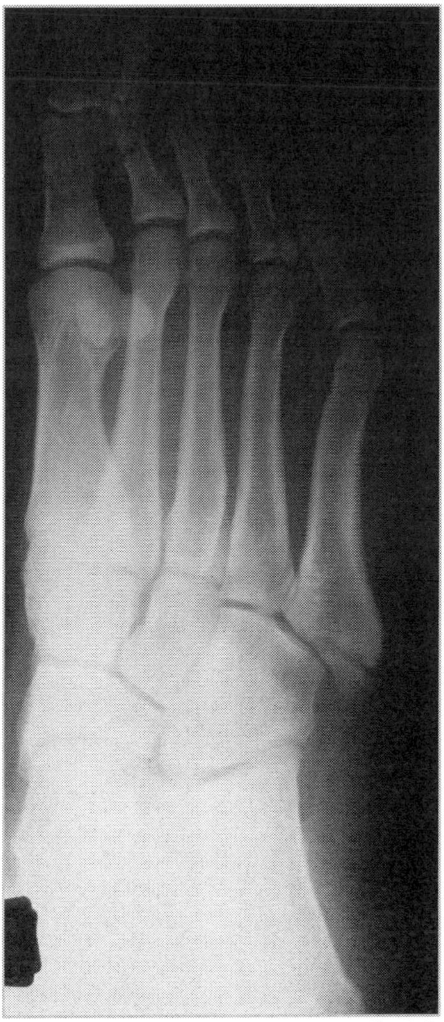

Fig 4.43

1. What are the findings on this X-ray?
2. What is the diagnosis?
3. What are the types and the mechanisms of injury?
4. What are the clinical features and the treatment?
5. What is the most common mistake made in this location?

Answers *on pages 273–334*

Case 4.44

A 4-year-old boy falls from a swing and presents to A&E with a painful and swollen left wrist. On examination there is tenderness and swelling of the left wrist, which has restricted motion.

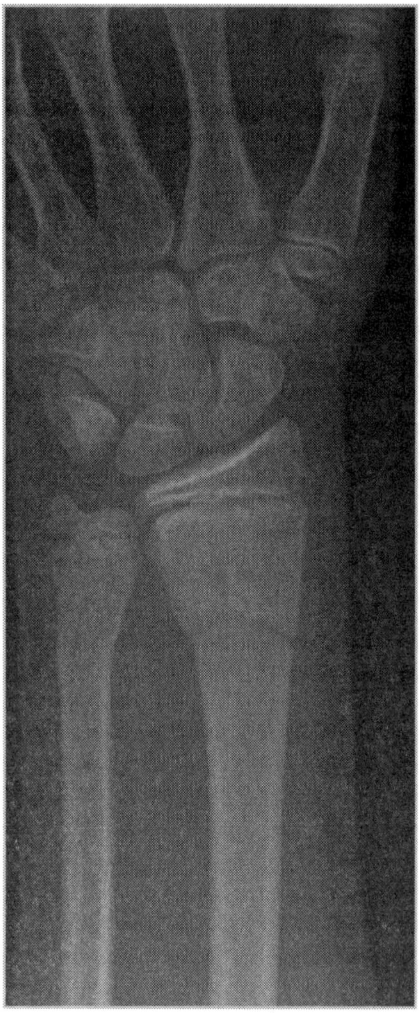

Fig 4.44a

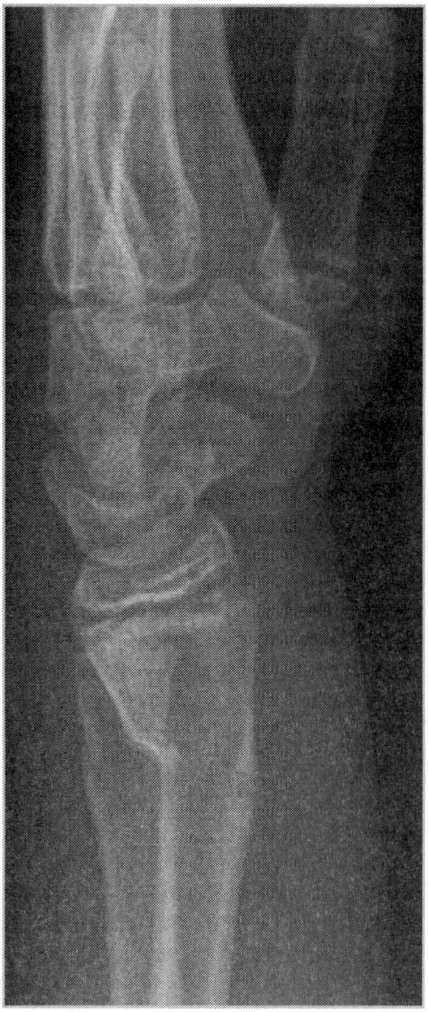

Fig 4.44b

1. What are the findings on this X-ray?
2. What is the diagnosis?
3. What is the mechanism of injury?
4. What are the things to look for on the X-ray to confirm the diagnosis?
5. What is the treatment?

Answers *on pages 273–334*

Case 4.45

A 9-year-old boy presented with severe pain in her knees and hips. On examination the hip and knee joints are tender and movement limited.

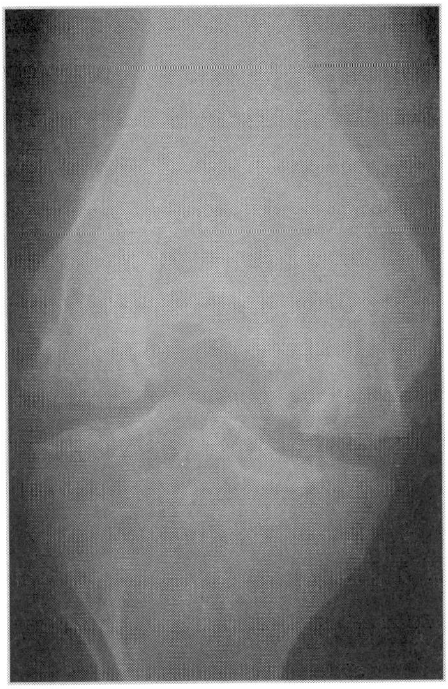

Fig 4.45a

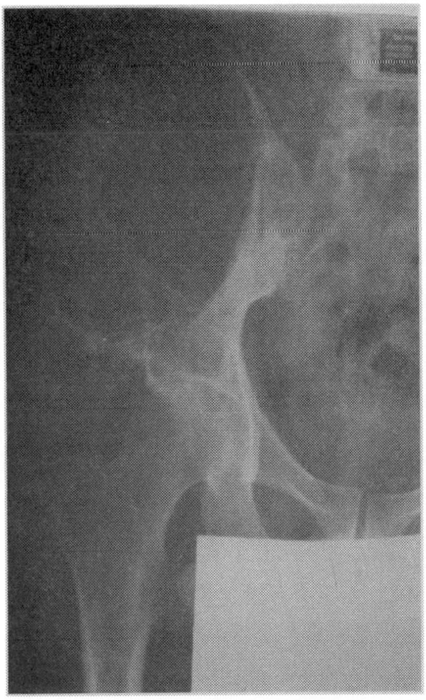

Fig 4.45b

1. What do you observe on the plain X-rays of the right knee and pelvis?
2. What is the diagnosis?
3. What are the clinical features of this disease?
4. What are the radiological features?
5. What is the differential diagnosis?

Answers *on pages 273–334*

Case 4.46

A 16-year-old boy presents with bowed legs and a tender bony lump on the medial aspect of his left leg. On examination he has leg length discrepancy and bilateral bowed legs, with the left leg shorter than the right.

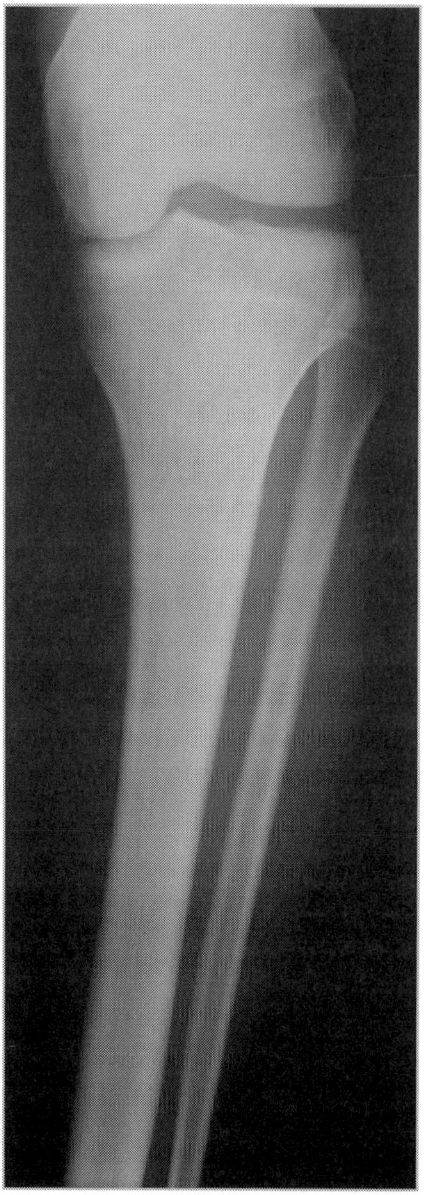

Fig 4.46

1. What are the findings on the X-ray?
2. What is the diagnosis?
3. What is the development of this disorder?
4. What is the mechanism of development of this condition and what are the predisposing factors?
5. What are the radiological features of this disorder?
6. What is the differential diagnosis?

Answers *on pages 273–334*

Case 4.47

A 6-year-old boy falls from a tree on outstretched hands. He presents with severe pain in his arm and forearm; his arm is flexed and there is swelling, tenderness and limitation of movement about the elbow joint.

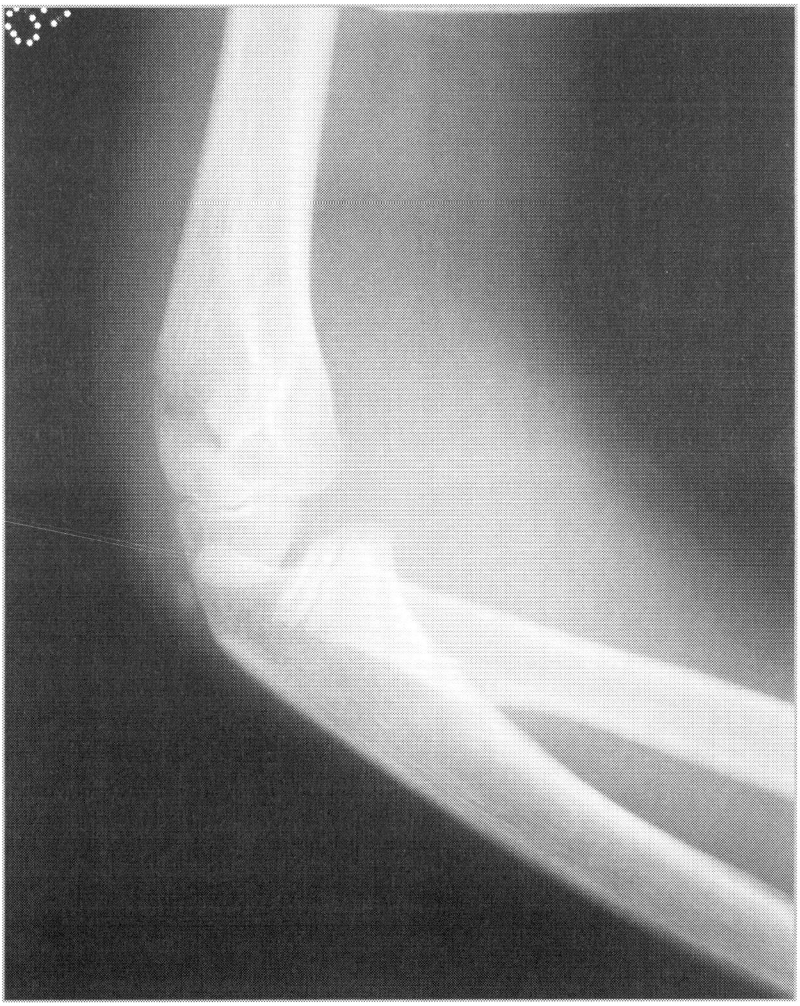

Fig 4.47

1. What are the findings on this X-ray?
2. What is the diagnosis?
3. What is the mechanism of injury?
4. What are the important things to look for on an X-ray?
5. What is the treatment of this condition?

Answers *on pages 273–334*

Case 4.48

A 2-year-old boy presents with deformity in his foot.

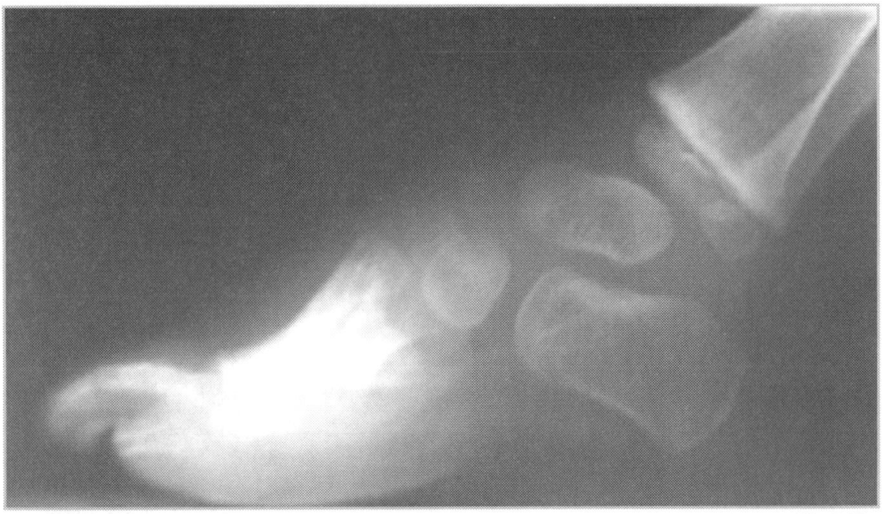

Fig 4.48a

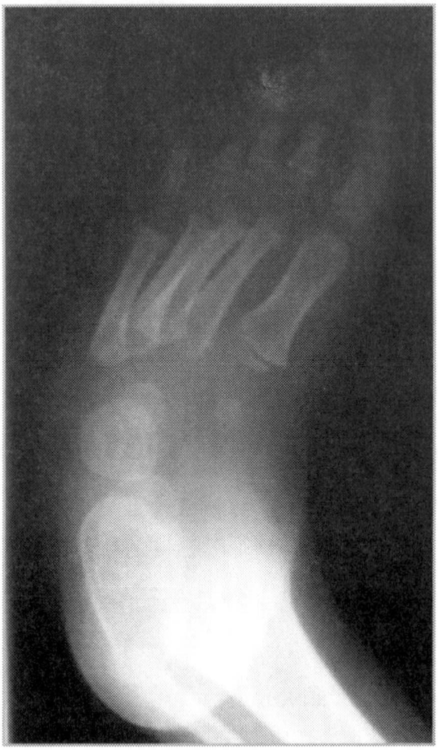

Fig 4.48b

1. What do you observe on the plain film of the foot?
2. What is the diagnosis?
3. What is the development of this disease?
4. What are the radiological features?
5. What are the associations of this disease and the treatment?

Answers *on pages 273–334*

Case 4.49

A 13-year-old boy presents with skin rashes, muscular weakness and pain.

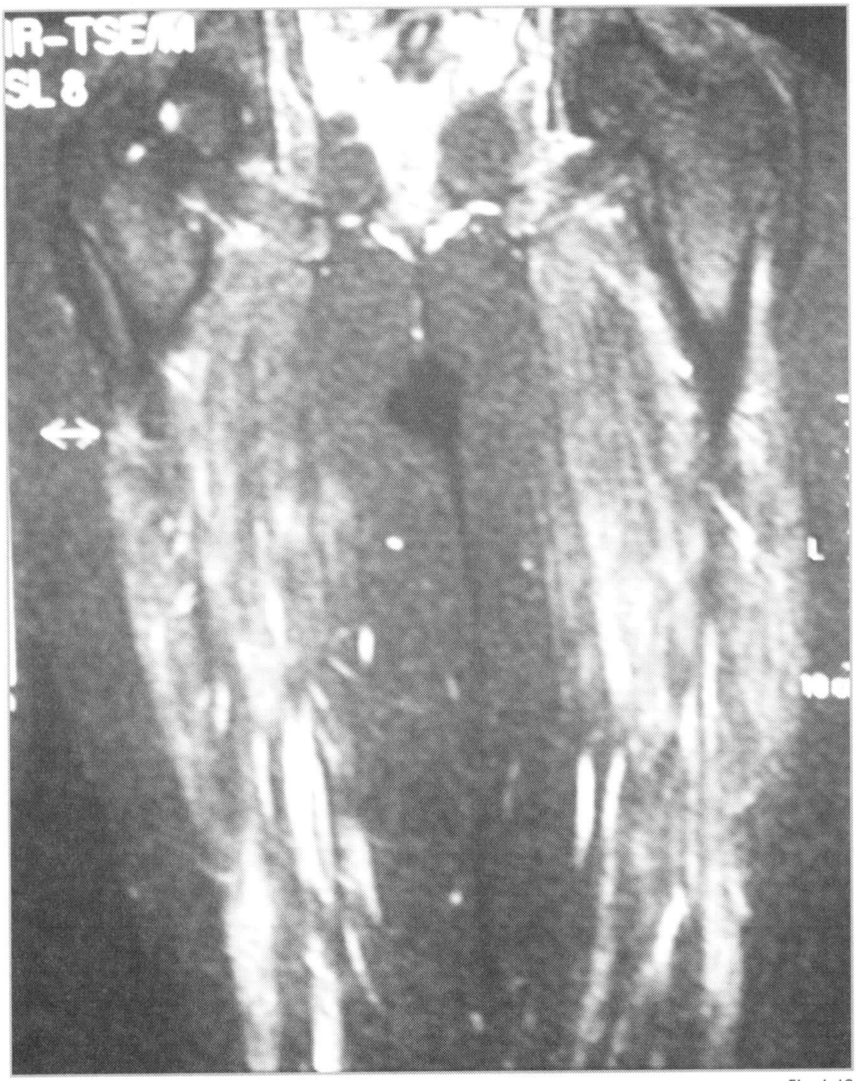

Fig 4.49

1. What do you see on the MR scan of the thigh?
2. What is the diagnosis?
3. What other investigations are needed?
4. What are the clinical features and what are the serum abnormalities?
5. What are the radiological features?

Answers *on pages 273–334*

Case 4.50

A 14-year-old boy presents with fever, pain and stiffness of multiple joints, especially the knee and wrist joints. On examination, there is tenderness and restricted movements of multiple joints.

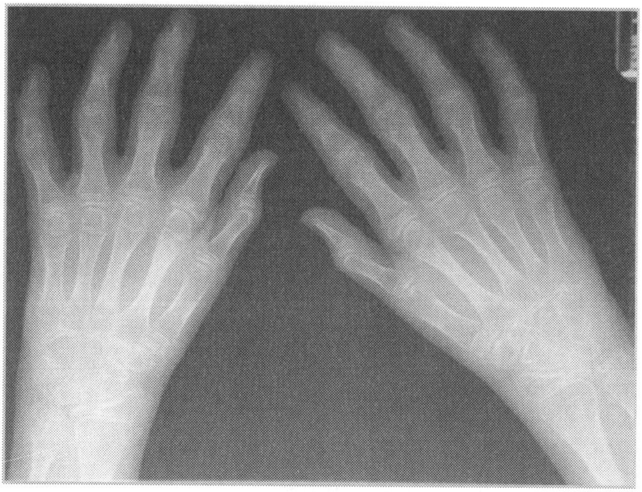

Fig 4.50a

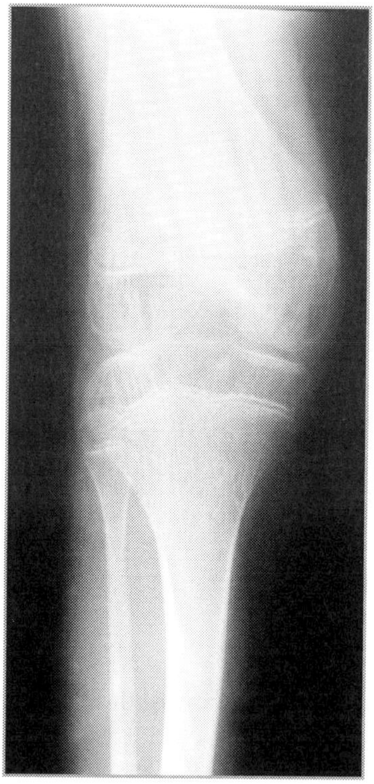

Fig 4.50b

1. What do you see on the plain X-ray of the wrist and knee joints?
2. What is the diagnosis?
3. What are the clinical features?
4. What are the radiological features?
5. What is the differential diagnosis?

Answers *on pages 273–334*

Case 4.51

A 6-year-old girl presented with failure to thrive, recurrent infections and headache.

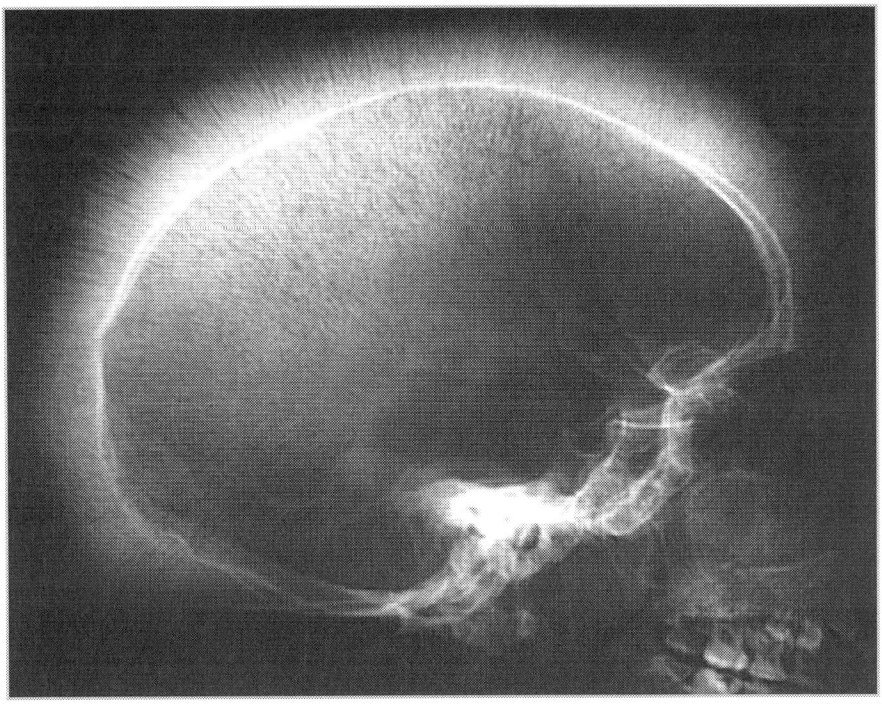

Fig 4.51

1. What do you observe on the plain X-ray?
2. What is the diagnosis?
3. What is the differential diagnosis for this radiological appearance?
4. What are the clinical features of this disease?
5. What are the radiological features of this disease?

Answers *on pages 273–334*

Case 4.52

A 3-year-old girl, sitting in the front seat of the car, was involved in a high-velocity motor vehicle accident and brought to A&E.

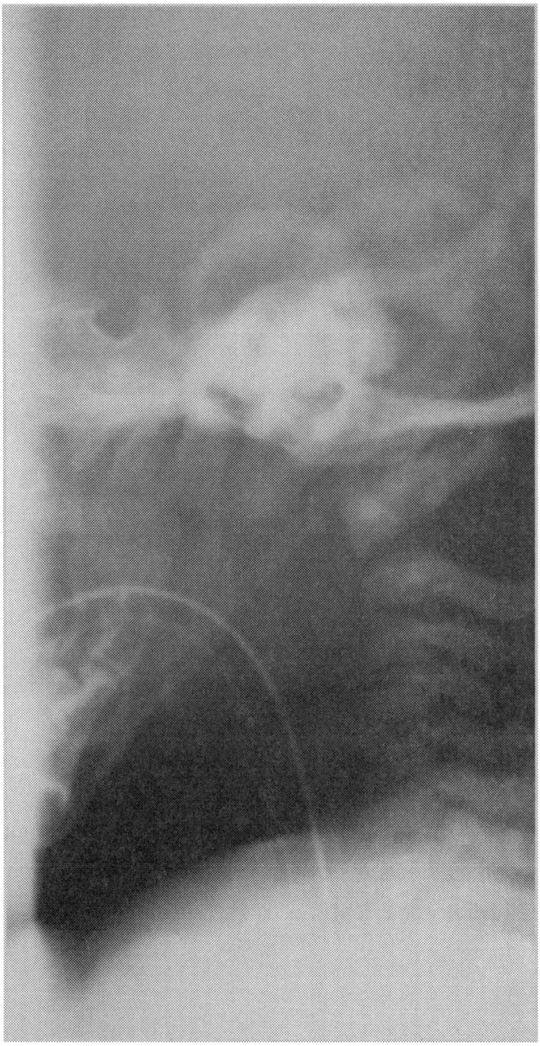

Fig 4.52

1. What do you observe on the X-ray of the cervical spine?
2. What is the diagnosis?
3. What are the types of this injury? What is the mechanism of injury?
4. What are the radiological features and the management?
5. What is the differential diagnosis?

Answers *on pages 273–334*

Case 4.53

A 5-year-old boy with severe growth retardation and deformities had a skeletal survey.

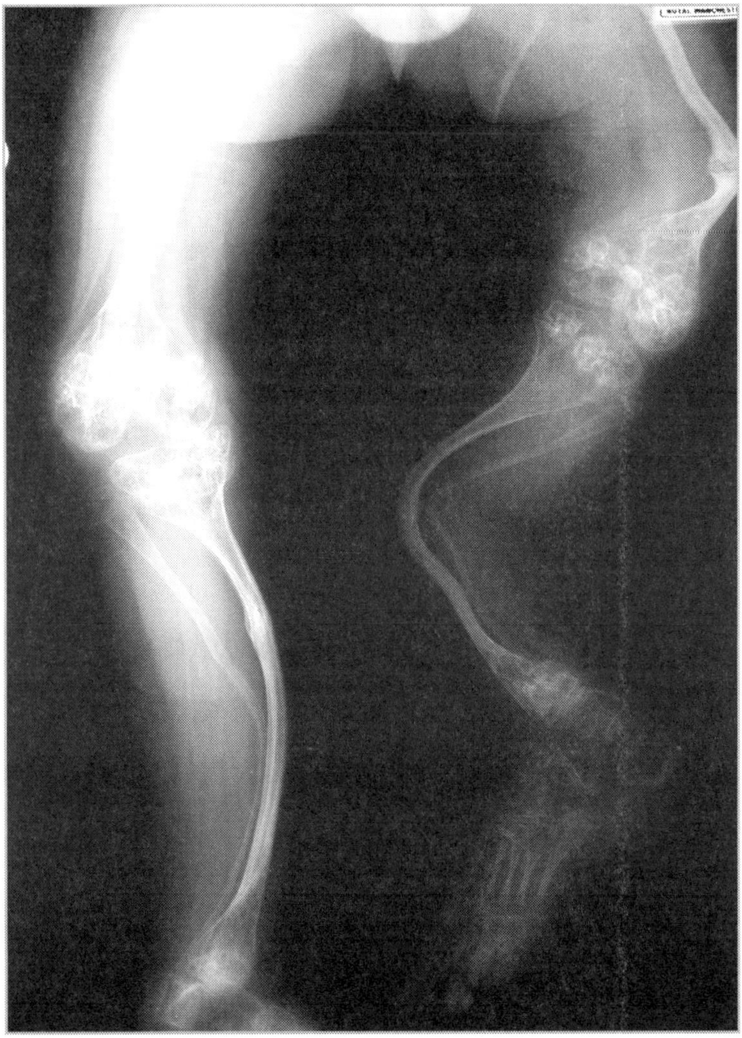

Fig 4.53

1. What are the findings on the X-ray?
2. What is the diagnosis?
3. What are the types of this disease?
4. What are the radiological features?
5. What are the complications and the differential diagnosis?

Answers *on pages 273–334*

Case 4.54

A 16-year-old girl presents with back pain, fever, night sweats and weight loss. On examination, severe tenderness was elicited from the dorsolumbar junction.

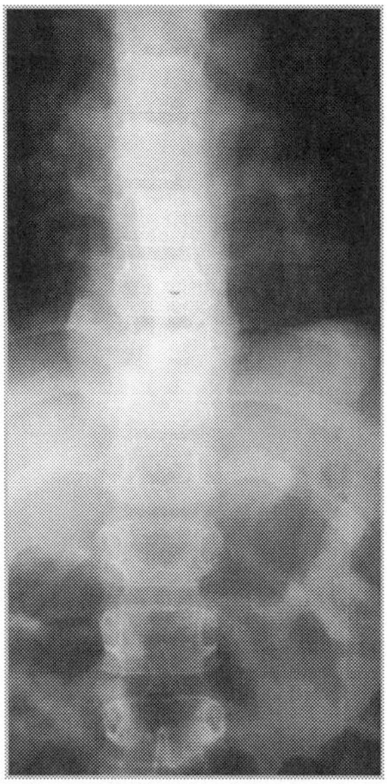

Fig 4.54a

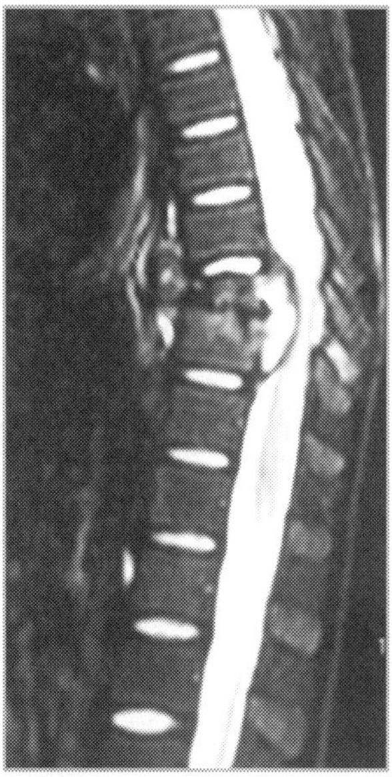

Fig 4.54b

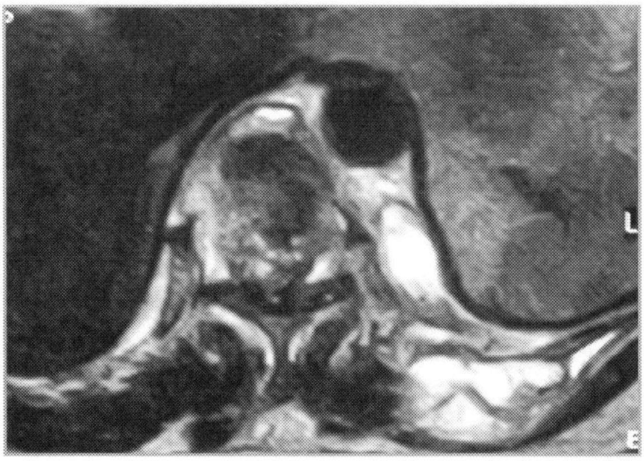

Fig 4.54c

1. What do you see on the X-ray of the spine and MRI?
2. What is the diagnosis?
3. What are the pathophysiology and the mode of spread?
4. What are the common locations and the clinical features?
5. What are the radiological features and the differential diagnosis?

Answers *on pages 273–334*

Case 4.55

A 6-month-old boy was referred with fever, irritability and a palpable lump in the legs. On examination he had tender swellings in both the legs and the arms. A skeletal survey was ordered.

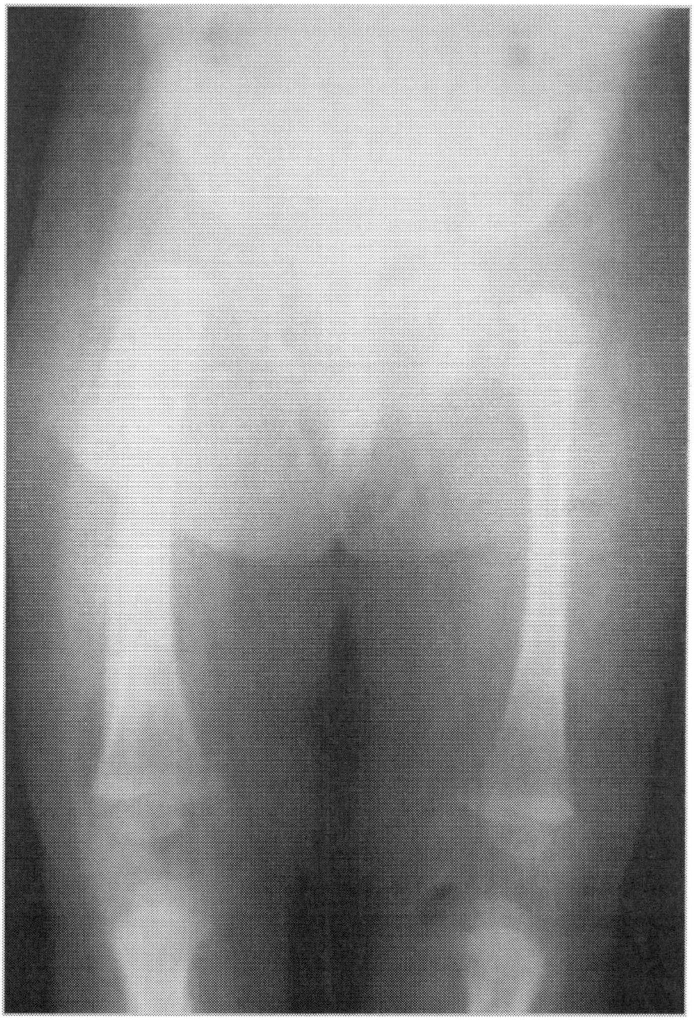

Fig 4.55

1. What are the findings on the X-ray?
2. What is the diagnosis?
3. What is the pathophysiology of this condition?
4. What are the radiological features?
5. What is the differential diagnosis?

Answers *on pages 273–334*

Case 4.56

A 3-month-old infant presents with fever, loss of appetite and swelling of the right hip joint. Clinical examination revealed a red, swollen and tender right hip joint with restriction of movement. The WBC count is elevated.

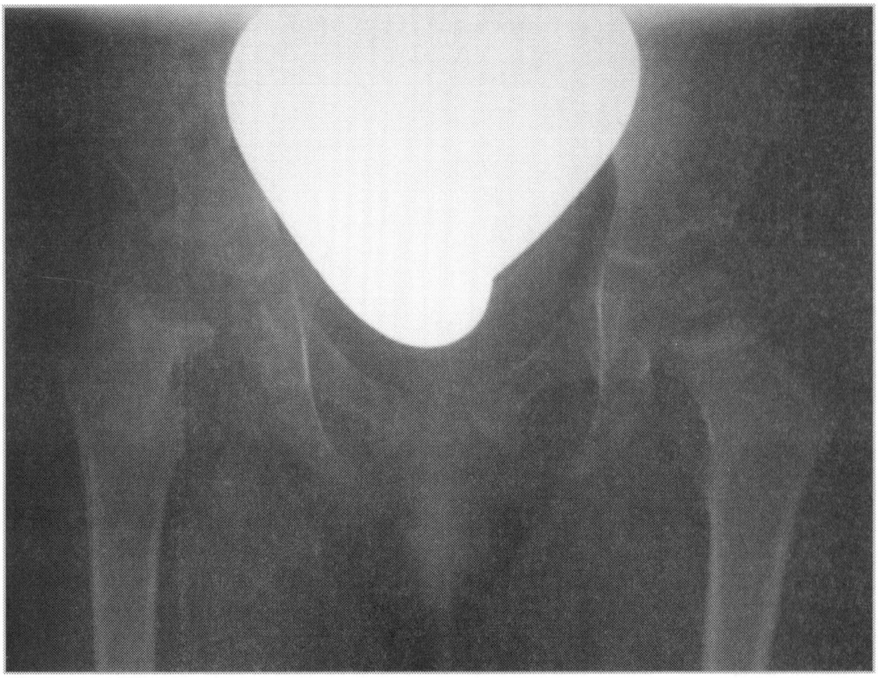

Fig 4.56

1. What do you observe on the X-ray of the pelvis?
2. What is the diagnosis?
3. What are the causes and the pathophysiology of this lesion?
4. What are the radiological features?
5. What is the differential diagnosis?

Answers *on pages 273–334*

Case 4.57

A 17-year-old presents with pain in his knee joint. On clinical examination, multiple, bony swellings are palpated around the knee joint.

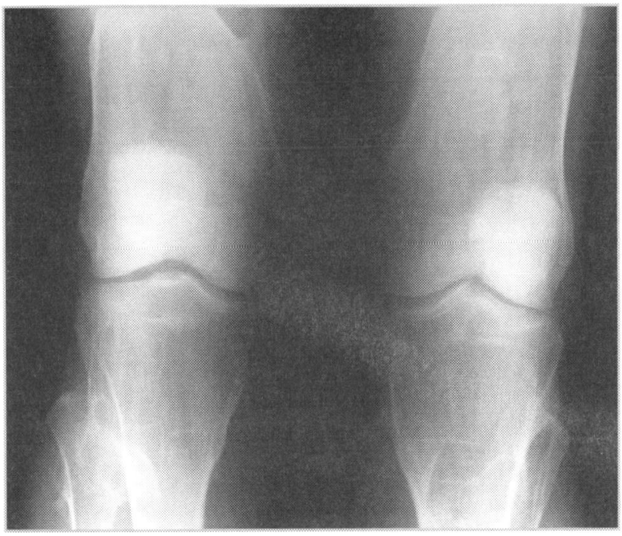

Fig 4.57a

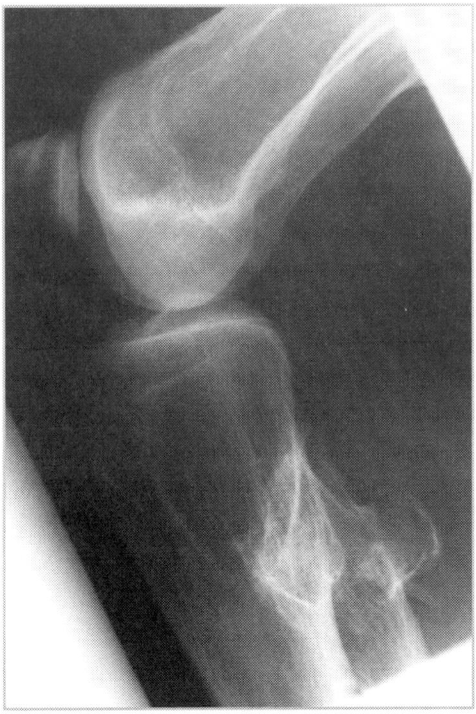

Fig 4.57b

1. What do you find on the X-ray of the knee?
2. What is the diagnosis?
3. What are the cause and the clinical features of this condition?
4. What are the radiological features and the differential diagnosis?
5. What are the complications?

Answers *on pages 273–334*

Case 4.58

A 12-year-old boy presents with low backache, which is severe on bending. Clinical examination showed point tenderness of the L3 vertebra. There is restriction of spinal movements.

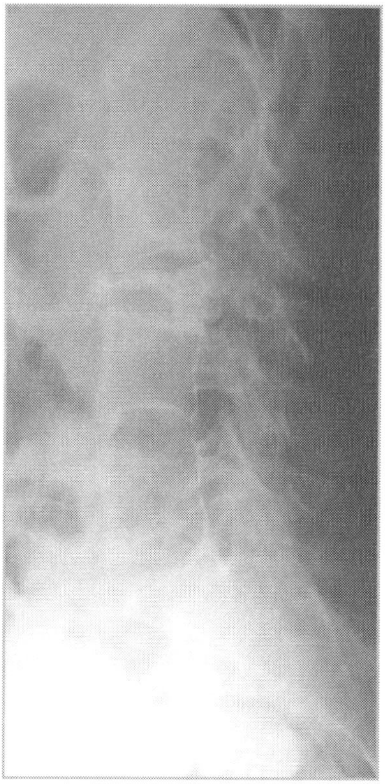

Fig 4.58a

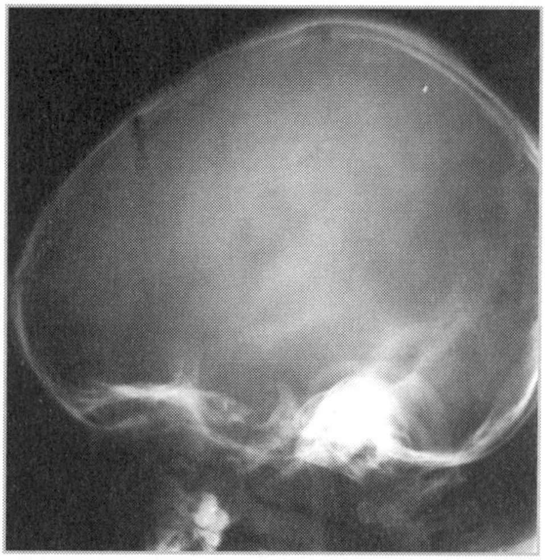

Fig 4.58b

1. What can you observe on the plain films of the spine and skull?
2. How is this radiological appearance described and what is the diagnosis?
3. What are the other causes for the appearance on the spinal X-ray?
4. What are the clinical and the radiological features?
5. What is the management of this disease?

Answers *on pages 273–334*

Case 4.1: Answers

1. The AP X-ray of the spine shows an extensive lateral bending deformity in the dorsolumbar region, which is concave to the right side.

2. Idiopathic scoliosis. Scoliosis is the presence of one or more lateral rotatory curves of the spine in a coronal plane > 10°. Scoliosis can be postural or structural. Structural scoliosis can be **congenital** (failure of formation, failure of segmentation, combination), **idiopathic, mesodermal** (neurofibromatosis, osteogenesis imperfecta, mucopolysaccharidosis [MPS], Marfan syndrome) **neuromuscular** (spinal dysraphism, myelomeningocele, syringomyelia, Chiari, polio, arthrogryposis, motor neuron disease, congenital hypotonia), or result from **radiation**, **dysplasia**, **infections** or **tumours.**

3. Idiopathic scoliosis is the most common type (80%). There are three types:

Infantile: up to 3 years, boys, thoracic, convex to left

Juvenile: 4–9 years, dorsolumbar, convex to left

Adolescent: 10 years, maturity, most common, girls, thoracic, convex to right.

4. The X-ray is used to confirm diagnosis, exclude underlying causes, assess the severity of curves, monitor progression, assess skeletal maturity and determine suitability for surgery. Bone scans are useful for painful scoliosis to exclude underlying tumours or infections. CT with sagittal and coronal reconstructions is useful for assessing segmentation anomalies and to find the true extent of rotation and rib deformities. MRI is used for assessing spinal and neurological diseases, which might preclude surgery. On an X-ray, an apical vertebra refers to the vertebra that is displaced most. End-vertebrae are the superior and inferior vertebrae in the curve. A neutral vertebra is not rotated. The primary curve is the structural curve and the secondary one is the non-structural curve that develops as compensation for the primary curve. There are many indices used to grade scoliosis. The common one is the Cobb–Webb technique (lines are drawn tangential to the superior and inferior end-vertebrae). The Cobb angle is formed at the intersection of these lines; Cobb classification gives:

I: < 20°

II: 21–30°

III: 31–50°

IV: 51–75°

V: 76–100°

VI: 101–125°

VII: > 125°.

Vertebral rotation is assessed by the Nash–Moe technique. Skeletal maturity is assessed by the Risser technique, which evaluates the level of ossification of the iliac wing apophysis. If the apophysis is completely fused, the patient is skeletally mature and the curve unlikely to progress further. Routine views obtained are posteroanterior (PA) and lateral views of the entire spine, including the pelvis, to visualise the iliac apophysis, with lateral bending views for assessing compensatory curves.

5. Scoliosis produces cosmetic deformity, disability, pain, cardiovascular compromise, respiratory failure and restrictive lung disease. Scoliosis progresses with age; the rate of progression depends on the cause and the patient's growth. Progression stops when maturity is attained, especially if the curve is < 30°. When the curve is < 25° in an immature skeleton or 30° in mature, management is regular follow-up and radiographs. Curves < 25° require treatment when they are rapidly progressive. Curves 25–50° are managed with orthotic device. Spinal fusion is required for curves > 50°.

Case 4.2: Answers

1. The X-ray of the left shoulder shows a destructive lytic lesion in the proximal humerus, which is associated with bony destruction, multilamellated periosteal reaction and soft-tissue swelling. MRI shows intense contrast enhancement in the bone marrow and the soft tissue medial to the humerus.

2. Ewing's sarcoma of the left humerus.

3. Ewing's sarcoma is the second most common primary malignant bone tumour of childhood. It is more common in boys and seen between age 5 and 15 years. Pain, swelling, tenderness, mass, fever, weight loss and irritability are the common clinical features and these can mimic a systemic infection.

4. It is more common in the lower limbs, around the knee in the mid-diaphyseal location. It is also seen in flat bones, especially in older children. Five per cent are seen in the vertebrae, where it is seen in posterior elements and occasionally purely in extraskeletal soft tissue. The X-ray shows a permeative or moth-eaten pattern of bone destruction with a wide zone of transition, indicating its aggressive nature. It contains both sclerotic and lytic elements. A soft-tissue component is seen and is often very large. It can be seen without visible cortical destruction as a result of spread through the haversian canals. Periosteal reaction is of the onion-skin type (lamellated) or spiculated with a perpendicular sunburst pattern. Codman's triangles are seen as a result of elevation of the periosteum and central destruction of the periosteal reaction caused by the tumour. A CT scan demonstrates the destructive lesion and soft-tissue component. It gives an accurate extent of the mass. MRI scan shows low signal in T1 and high signal in T2. Accurate delineation of the intramedullary extent is best seen in T2. After treatment, bone marrow shows low signal because of fibrosis. High signal is seen on a bone scan. Metastasis is seen in 25%. A PET scan is very sensitive in diagnosis and for follow-up of a therapeutic response. Differential diagnoses of an aggressive lesion with periosteal reaction and soft-tissue swelling in long bones include acute osteomyelitis, metastatic neuroblastoma, leukaemia, osteosarcoma, fibrosarcoma, lymphoma and eosinophilic granuloma. It might be difficult to differentiate from acute osteomyelitis, which also has Codman's triangle, destruction and soft-tissue swelling. Osteosarcoma has a bone matrix.

5. Bad prognostic factors are male sex, age > 12 years, anaemia, elevated LDH, radiotherapy only for local control and poor chemotherapeutic course. As most patients have occult metastatic disease, multidrug chemotherapy as well as local disease control with surgery and/or radiation are indicated in treatment of all patients. Treatment consists of neoadjuvant chemotherapy followed by wide or radical excision and includes radiotherapy. Complete excision at the time of biopsy is performed if a malignancy is confirmed.

Case 4.3: Answers

1. The X-ray of the left shoulder shows a subtle area of lucency and patchy areas of sclerosis in the head of the humerus.

2. Post-contrast MRI shows intense, patchy uptake of contrast into the bones. Extensive enhancement is also seen in the surrounding soft tissue.

3. Acute osteomyelitis.

4. Acute osteomyelitis is infection of bone caused by an infecting organism, usually *Staphylococcus aureus.*

Children < **1 year:** group B streptococci, *Staph. aureus, Haemophilus influenzae* (5–50%) and *E. coli.*

Children > **1 year**: *Staph. aureus, E. coli, H. influenzae, Serratia marcescens* and *Pseudomonas aeruginosa.*

It can be acquired through the haematogenous or exogenous route. It is common in long bones, starting in metaphyseal sinusoidal veins and resulting in focal oedema, which leads to local tissue necrosis, breakdown of the trabecular bone structure, and removal of bone matrix and calcium. Infection spreads along the haversian canals, through the marrow cavity and beneath the periosteal layer of the bone. Subsequent vascular damage causes the ischaemic death of osteocytes, leading to the formation of a sequestrum. Periosteal new bone formation on top of the sequestrum is known as involucrum. Clinically there is bone pain, fever, malaise, irritability, restricted limb movement, swelling, tenderness, warmth and regional lymphadenopathy. Complications include chronic osteomyelitis, metastatic infection, septic arthritis caused by the transphyseal spread of the infection, angular deformity of bones as a result of arrest of bone growth, pathological fractures, bacteraemia, septicaemia, soft-tissue infection, persistent sinuses and premature epiphyseal fusion. Primary treatment is a combination of a penicillinase-resistant synthetic penicillin and a third-generation cephalosporin. In patients with sickle cell anaemia and osteomyelitis, the primary bacterial causes are *Staph. aureus* and salmonellae. Thus, the primary choice for treatment is a fluoroquinolone antibiotic (not in children). A third-generation cephalosporin (eg ceftriaxone) is an alternative.

5. X-rays are normal in the earlier stages. Subtle soft-tissue swelling and displacement of fat planes can be noted. Within 10–14 days, a longitudinal lucent destructive lesion with areas of sclerosis and periosteal reaction appears. The X-ray excludes other causes of bone pain such as septic arthritis, Ewing's sarcoma, osteosarcoma, juvenile arthritis, sickle cell crisis, Gaucher's disease and stress. A three-phase ^{99m}Tc-labelled diphosphonate bone scan (perfusion, blood pool, static) is very sensitive and positive in

24 hours and shows a well-defined focus of tracer uptake in all phases. It is useful in looking at multifocal sites of osteomyelitis. The uptake on the three-phase bone scans is related to blood flow and osteoblastic activity. Gallium scans can be used to confirm the diagnosis of osteomyelitis. Osteomyelitis is suggested if there is concordant uptake of gallium and diphosphonate. ^{111}In- or ^{99m}Tc-labelled leukocytes are very specific in localising infections. Ultrasonography can show a hypoechoic collection close to the bone, earlier than radiological detection. MRI is also a very sensitive tool. Osteomyelitis is seen as low signal in T1 and high signal in T2. MRI is useful in assessing the extent of osteomyelitis and subperiosteal abscess. The inflammatory component enhances on contrast whereas necrotic pus does not. CT can also detect osteomyelitis earlier than an X-ray but is typically used in chronic osteomyelitis.

Case 4.4: Answers

1. The X-ray of the leg, shows many, well-defined, round areas of sclerosis. The joint space appears normal. There is no periosteal reaction, soft-tissue lesion or bony destruction.

2. Osteopoikilosis.

3. Osteopoikilosis is an autosomal dominant disorder, which is more common in males and characterised by the presence of multiple, compact, bone islands. The lesions are mostly seen in metaphysis and epiphysis. They are seen as multiple oval or lenticular bone islands, which are sclerotic (2–10 mm), with their long axes parallel to the long axis of the bone. The most commonly involved bones are the glenoid, acetabulum, wrist, ankle and pelvis. It is rare in the skull, ribs, vertebra and mandible. There is no increased uptake on a bone scan.

4. Differential diagnoses:

   Melorheostosis: diaphyseal, waxy periosteal reaction along the cortex

   Epiphyseal dysplasia: affects epiphysis, metaphysis spared

   Osteopathia striata: linear stripes.

5. Osteopoikilosis is associated with dermatofibrosis lenticularis disseminata.

Case 4.5: Answers

1. The X-ray of the hands shows diffuse sclerosis and appearance of bone within bone. This appearance is also seen in the pelvis.

2. Osteopetrosis.

3 Differential diagnoses of bone-within-bone appearance: normal variant – in thoracic and lumbar vertebrae in children; growth recovery lines; osteopetrosis; Caffey's disease; sickle cell disease; thalassaemia; congenital syphilis; Paget's disease; acromegaly; reflex dystrophy; lead, bismuth and thorium; leukaemia, TB, rickets, scurvy, vitamin D toxicity.

4. Osteopetrosis (Albers–Schonbert disease, marble bone disease) is characterised by defective osteoclast function and bone resorption, resulting in sclerotic and brittle bone. There are two types: a **lethal infantile autosomal recessive type** and a benign **adult autosomal dominant type**. The infantile type presents with failure to thrive, anaemia, caries, cranial nerve compression, hepatosplenomegaly and lymphadenopathy. There is a dense skeleton with metaphyseal splaying and fractures. Infants are stillborn or die in early life as a result of infection, haemorrhage or leukaemia.

5. The autosomal dominant type can present with diffuse sclerosis, cortical thickening and medullary narrowing. In the benign type, the characteristic appearance is bone within bone. Alternating sclerosing and lucent lines are seen in long bones. Rugger jersey spine with sclerotic and lucent areas is seen, and also metaphyseal striations, skull base sclerosis, obliteration of sinuses, recurrent fractures and the Erlenmeyer flask deformity. The life expectancy is normal. Complications are fractures, marrow narrowing with extramedullary haematopoiesis and leukaemia. Differential diagnoses for the overall appearance are pyknodysostosis, melorheostosis, heavy metal poisoning, hypervitaminosis D and fibrous dysplasia.

Case 4.6: Answers

1. The plain X-ray shows a spiral fracture in the distal tibial metaphysis. There is also a subtle fracture in the medial aspect of the metaphysis of the distal femur.

2. Non-accidental injury (NAI) with corner sign.

3. Metaphyseal irregularity and fracture can be seen as a result of trauma, infection, metastatic neuroblastoma, leukaemia, congenital syphilis and scurvy.

4. NAI is the third most common cause of death in children after SIDS and accidents. Usually the children are brought to hospital with a history of trauma. Multiple injuries are seen in different stages of healing. Usually they are seen before the age of 2. The usual sites of fractures are the ribs, costochondral junction, acromion, skull, vertebra, tibia and metacarpals. There are multiple fractures in different stages of healing, with exuberant callus formation. An avulsion fracture at ligamentous insertion is seen without periosteal reaction. Epiphyses are separated. Metaphysis shows irregularity, fragments, corner/bucket-handle fracture, which results from avulsion of arcuate metaphyseal fragment overlying epiphyseal cartilage because of sudden twisting of an extremity, with periosteum pulled from the diaphysis but attached to the metaphysis. Spiral fracture of the diaphysis can be seen and also extensive periosteal reaction.

5. **Fractures pathognomonic of NAI**:

Rib fractures, costochondral junction fractures, especially first rib fractures and posterior fractures

Metaphyseal fractures, bucket-handle type

Fractures of different ages.

Fractures highly suggestive of NAI:

Scapula, outer third of clavicle, vertebral (dorsolumbar, C2–3), digital injuries

Diaphyseal fractures.

Case 4.7: Answers

1. The X-ray of the spine shows normal alignment, but there is discal calcification and narrowing of the disc spaces.

2. Ochronosis.

3. The characteristic finding is intervertebral discal calcification. Other features of ochronosis are joint space narrowing at multiple levels, with subchondral sclerosis and cyst formation, destruction of subchondral bone, soft-tissue swelling and loose bodies.

4. Discal calcification is also seen in trauma, infection, degenerative, spinal fusion, ochronosis, CPPD (calcium pyrophosphate deposition), Wilson's disease, haemochromatosis, homocystinuria, hyperparathyroidism, gout, idiopathic skeletal hyperostosis, ankylosing spondylitis, amyloidosis and acromegaly.

5. Ochronosis is a genetic disorder resulting from lack of homogentisic acid oxidase. This results in the accumulation of homogentisic acid in the cartilage, which causes the characteristic bluish-black pigmentation. The affected tissues become brittle with time, resulting in chronic inflammation, degeneration and osteoarthritis. It is inherited in an autosomal recessive fashion and often diagnosed at birth, by discoloration of diapers or dark urine staining. Pigmented patches may develop in the sclerae in the second or third decades. Changes in the ear cartilage are seen in the fourth decade. The skin changes are seen in the eyelids, forehead, cheeks, axillae, genitalia, nail beds, eardrum and mouth. Arthritis develops in the third and fourth decades. Heart valve dysfunction can result from pigment deposition in the heart. Elevated levels of homogentisic acid are seen in the blood, urine and other tissues. A dermatological biopsy can be acquired. There is no specific treatment. A diet high in vitamin C or nitisinone is tried, which inhibits 4-hydroxyphenylpyruvate dioxygenase. Arthropathy is treated with physiotherapy, analgesia, rest and joint replacement. Patients can expect a normal life span, but complications such as arthritis, and cardiovascular and skin changes will occur.

Case 4.8: Answers

1. The X-ray of the right shoulder shows a well-defined, central, lucent lesion in the proximal metaphysis of the right humerus. There is extension to the joint space. No soft-tissue component is seen.

2. Simple bone cyst.

3. Simple bone cyst is a benign fluid-filled lesion of unknown aetiology. Venous obstruction and blockage of interstitial fluid drainage, in rapidly growing and remodelling cancellous bone, are a possible mechanism. Pathologically the cyst is lined by membrane and filled with clear yellow fluid. It is seen between age 10 and 20 years. Clinical features include pain and fractures.

4. Simple bone cysts are found in tubular bones in 95% of patients. The most common location is the proximal metaphysis of the humerus or femur. It can also be seen in other flat bones. The cysts are usually centrally located in the proximal metaphysis. A diaphyseal location is seen in only 4–12% of patients. Involvement of the epiphysis is rare. It is seen as a simple, expansile lesion, with a fluid-filled cavity. The long axis of the lesion is parallel to the long axis of the bone. Loculations are seen only rarely. Expansion of the bone causes cortical thinning. A fallen fragment sign is seen secondary to pathological fracture. The fractured fragment migrates to the dependent portion of the cyst. This sign is pathognomonic of a simple bone cyst. A periosteal reaction is seen when there is fracture. A CT scan is not necessary, but, if done, shows a fluid-filled bone lesion. On MRI, the lesion is of low signal intensity in T1-weighted images and high signal intensity in T2-weighted images.

5. Differential diagnoses include aneurysmal bone cyst (multiloculated, expansile, eccentric), giant cell tumour (seen after epiphyseal fusion, narrow transition point, may be locally aggressive, may erode into joint), subarticular geode, Brodie's abscess, benign fibrous histiocytoma, chondroblastoma, haemophilic pseudotumour, expansile neuroblastoma metastasis, hydatid cyst and fibrous dysplasia. The cysts usually enlarge during periods of skeletal activity and then become inactive or latent when growth ceases. Simple bone cysts can be treated with curettage and bone grafting, intramedullary nailing, cryotherapy, methylprednisolone injection or injection of bone marrow. The aim of treatment is to prevent pathological fracture, promote cyst healing and avoid cyst recurrence or re-fracture.

Case 4.9: Answers

1. The two views are an AP view and a frog lateral view of the pelvis. The right femoral epiphysis appears smaller. There is medial displacement of the epiphysis, which can be confirmed by drawing a line tangentially along the lateral margin of the metaphysis that does not intersect the epiphysis. The femoral neck shaft angle is also reduced.

2. Slipped upper capital epiphysis (SUFE).

3. SUFE is an orthopaedic emergency, which is caused by atraumatic fracture through the hypertrophic zone of the physeal plate and results in slippage of the epiphysis posteriorly and medially The incidence is 1/100 000; it is common in males and is typically seen in adolescents (boys aged 10–16, girls 12–14). Growth spurt, hormones, renal osteodystrophy, irradiation, growth hormone therapy and a Salter–Harris type I epiphyseal injury are all aetiologies. Pathologically there is widening of the physeal plate during the growth spurt, which when associated with a change in orientation of the physis from horizontal to oblique increases the shear force. It is more common in overweight, adolescent boys.

4. It is usually unilateral and bilateral in 25%. In the earliest stages, there is irregularity and blurring of the physis and demineralisation of the neck metaphysis. The characteristic findings are displacement of the epiphysis posteriorly and medially. This is assessed by drawing the Klein line – drawn tangentially along the superior edge of the femoral neck. Normally this line intersects some part of the femoral head but, if there is slip, the line will not intersect the femoral head. The neck shaft angle is decreased with alignment of the growth plate being more vertical than normal. The epiphysis appears smaller as a result of a posterior slip. Sclerosis and irregularity of the wide physis are seen in the chronic phases. When healing starts, there is an area of increased opacity in the proximal metaphysis (blanching). CT and MRI can detect early slippages, but are rarely needed. A lateral view demonstrates the slippage earliest, because the slip is posterior.

5. Grading is based on the femoral head position. In **mild** grade the displacement is less than a third of the metaphyseal diameter; in **moderate** grade it is a third to two-thirds of the femoral diameter; and in **severe** grade it is more than two-thirds of the metaphyseal diameter.

The prognosis depends on the severity at the time of presentation. Common differential diagnoses are Perthes' disease, Osgood–Schlatter disease, muscle strain and flat feet.

6. Wires, pins and screws are used to stabilise the hips, by crossing the physis and fixing the epiphysis, to prevent further damage to penetrating vessels by stabilisation of the fracture. The physis closes after treatment. Osteotomy may be done for deformities. Complications are acute chondrolysis (acute cartilage necrosis, more common in African–Caribbean children), avascular necrosis of the femoral head (in advanced slips, delayed surgery, anterior pin placement, large number of pins, subcapital osteotomy), pistol grip deformity, degenerative changes and limb length discrepancy.

Case 4.10: Answers

1. There is a detached fragment of bone with well-defined lucency seen in the lateral aspect of the medial femoral condyle.

2. MRI shows a defect in the medial femoral condyle. The cartilage is absent and there is high signal within the bone marrow.

3. Osteochondral defect (osteochondrosis dissecans) of the medial femoral condyle.

4. Osteochondral defect is fragmentation of a part of an articular surface. It is a fatigue fracture caused by shearing, rotatory/tangentially aligned impaction forces, resulting in a defect in the subchondral region with partial or complete separation of the bone fragment.

5. It is commonly seen in adolescents and is more common in boys. Clinically it may be asymptomatic or present with pain, clicking, locking, crepitus, swelling and pain aggravated by movement. In the knee, the characteristic location is the posterolateral aspect of the medial femoral condyle close to the fossa intercondylaris. Rarely it is seen in the posterior aspect of the lateral femoral condyle. It is bilateral in 25%. The defect can be cartilaginous or osteocartilaginous. On an X-ray, the line is seen parallel to the articular surface. The defect is not seen if it is purely cartilaginous. An osteochondral defect can be detached and seen in the posterior aspect of the knee joint. MRI can be used to locate the osteochondral defect, grade it and find any loose fragment. The following is the classification:

I: depressed osteochondral fracture

II: osteochondral fragment attached by osseus ridge

III: detached, non-displaced fragment

IV: displaced fragment.

6. Differential diagnoses are osteochondral fracture, osteochondromatosis, spontaneous osteonecrosis of the knee (SONK), neuropathic joints and loose bodies after degeneration. Prognosis is good for skeletally immature patients as healing is good. Non-detached fragments, in those aged < 12 years, are managed conservatively, with a cast for 6 weeks and a crutch, and a gentle range of movements, which promotes cartilage healing. Detached fragments are removed under arthroscopy.

Case 4.11: Answers

1. The acetabular angle is > 30° on the left side. The unossified femoral head is situated in the superolateral quadrant of the Perkins lines. The Shenton line is broken. The right side is normal.

2. This is high-resolution ultrasonography of the left hip, showing an α angle of 50°, between the baseline and roofline. The femoral head is situated abnormally outside the acetabulum.

3. Developmental dysplasia of the hip (DDH).

4. The plain X-ray – **acetabular angle** – is measured between the Hilgenreiner line (horizontal line between the two triradiate cartilages) and a line connecting the superolateral and inferomedial margins of the acetabular roof. The normal acetabular angle is < 3°; in DDH, it is > 30°. **Quadrants**: the hip is divided into four quadrants by the Hilgenreiner line and the Perkins line, which is drawn at the outer acetabular margin, perpendicular to the Hilgenreiner line. Normal femoral head is centred in the inferomedial quadrant. The **Shenton line** is a smooth unbroken arc that bridges the medial femoral metaphysis and the inferior edge of the superior pubic ramus. This line is disrupted in DDH. Plain radiographs of

the pelvis are most helpful when significant ossification of the capital femoral epiphyses has occurred and when adequate ultrasonic evaluation cannot be performed

5. Ultrasonography of the hip is performed with a high-resolution linear array transducer, with the infant in the lateral decubitus position – the hip in a 90° flexed position and the knee flexed 90°. The unossified cartilaginous femoral head appears as a speckled ball in the acetabular fossa. To quantify acetabular maturity, α and β angles are determined by the application of three lines drawn in the standard coronal plane. The baseline passes through the plane of the ileum, where it connects to the osseous acetabular convexity. The inclination line passes from the lateral end of the acetabulum to the labrum, parallel to the cartilaginous roof. The roofline passes along the plane of the bony acetabular convexity. The α angle is the angle between the baseline and roofline and normally measures ≥ 60°. Angles of 50–60° may be physiologically typical in the immediate neonatal period, but hips with these angles are considered immature and require clinical and ultrasound follow-up. Angles < 50° are always considered abnormal and require treatment. The β angle is measured between the baseline and the inclination line. An angle < 55° is considered normal. The smaller the angle, the less the cartilaginous coverage and the better the bony acetabular coverage of the femoral head.

6. DDH is the result of a disruption in the normal relationship between the acetabulum and the femoral head. Without adequate contact between them, neither develops normally Complications are persistent dysplasia, recurrent dislocation and avascular necrosis of the femoral head.

Case 4.12: Answers

1. The X-ray of the left arm shows expansion of the shaft of the left humerus, with marked cortical thickening. There is a multilamellated periosteal reaction, and a focal sclerotic area within the lucency in the midshaft of the humerus.

2. Chronic osteomyelitis of the left humerus.

3. Chronic osteomyelitis is a chronic, severe, persistent infection of bone and bone marrow. It can appear de novo or follow acute and subacute osteomyelitis. It can result from inadequately treated acute osteomyelitis,

haematogenous spread or trauma, iatrogenic or compound fractures, infection with TB or syphilis, or contiguous spread. *Staphylococcus aureus* is the most common organism. Infection leads to increased intramedullary pressure by exudates, as in vascular thrombosis, which results in necrotic bone (sequestra); this is surrounded by sclerotic avascular bone. Haversian canals are blocked by scar tissue. New bone formation is called involucrum and multiple openings appear in this involucrum, through which exudates from sequestrum drain through the sinuses. A periosteal reaction circumscribes the sequestrum.

4. In chronic osteomyelitis, the bone is thickened, irregular and sclerotic with radiolucencies. Periosteal reaction and soft-tissue swelling are seen. Chronic draining sinuses are seen. A CT scan can also be used to define the extent of disease. MRI is very useful in assessing the extent of bone marrow involvement, sinuses and soft-tissue abscesses, which show contrast enhancement. MRI shows thick bones; sequestrum is hypointense in all sequences and shows no enhancement. Granulation tissue is hypointense in T1, hyperintense in T2 and shows contrast enhancement. Brodie's abscess shows a double line as a result of the high signal of granulation tissue surrounded by low-signal sclerotic bone in T2-weighted MRI. Differential diagnoses are osteosarcoma, Ewing's sarcoma, Caffey's disease and hypervitaminosis A, but none of these has the characteristic constellation of findings.

5. Variants of chronic osteomyelitis are chronic sclerosing osteomyelitis of Garre, chronic recurrent multifocal osteomyelitis, Brodie's abscess, tuberculous osteomyelitis and SAPHO syndrome (**s**ynovitis, **a**cne, **p**ustulosis, **h**yperostosis, **o**steitis). In Brodie's abscess, the disease is usually in metaphysis and is seen as a central lucency surrounded by reactive sclerosis, periosteal reaction and soft-tissue swelling. Complications are soft-tissue abscess, fistula, fracture, extension to joint, growth disturbance and deformity. Secondary amyloidosis and epidermoid carcinoma are long-term complications.

Case 4.13: Answers

1. The X-ray of the right arm shows a well-defined lucent lesion in the diaphysis of the proximal tibia with a surrounding rim of sclerosis (rind sign). There is also pathological fracture, but there is no periosteal reaction or soft-tissue extension.

2. The radiological findings are consistent with fibrous dysplasia. The clinical diagnosis is McCune–Albright syndrome, which includes polyostotic fibrous dysplasia, precocious puberty and pigmentation.

3. Fibrous dysplasia is a skeletal developmental anomaly of the bone-forming mesenchyme, with a defect in osteoblastic differentiation and maturation. The medullary bone is replaced by fibrous tissue, which has the characteristic ground-glass appearance on a plain X-ray. Clinically there are four forms: **monostotic** (70%), **polyostotic**, **craniofacial** and **cherubism**. It is commonly seen between age 3 and 15. The monostotic form is more common in the ribs, femur, tibia or craniofacial bones. The polyostotic form is more common in the femur, tibia, pelvis, ribs and craniofacial bones. Fibrous dysplasia may be associated with endocrinopathies in 2–3% of cases (precocious puberty in girls, hyperthyroidism, hyperparathyroidism, acromegaly, diabetes mellitus and Cushing syndrome). Elevated alkaline phosphatase (ALP) is seen. Clinical features are pain, tenderness, deformity, scoliosis, endocrine changes and café-au-lait spots.

4. The usual appearance of fibrous dysplasia is a lucent lesion in the diaphysis or metaphysis, with endosteal scalloping, with or without bone expansion, and the absence of periosteal reaction. Usually, the matrix of the lucency is smooth and relatively homogeneous (ground glass). Irregular areas of sclerosis may be present with or without calcification. The lucent lesion has a thick sclerotic border and is called the rind sign. The lesion may extend into the epiphysis only after fusion. The dysplastic bone may undergo calcification and endochondral bone formation. In the skull, the lesion is convex and expands the outer table. The tables are intact but thinned. A CT scan shows a lucent lesion with attenuation values of 70–130 HU. On MRI, the lesion has low-to-intermediate signal in T1 and high signal in T2. Fluid–fluid levels are seen.

5. Differential diagnoses of a well-corticated lucent lesion in a child's metaphysis include simple bone cyst, enchondroma, fibrous cortical defect/non-ossifying fibroma, giant cell tumour, haemangioma, primary hyperparathyroidism, neurofibromatosis and Paget's disease (older patients).

6. The complications of fibrous dysplasia are fracture, deformities including severe coxa vara (shepherd's crook deformity), premature fusion of ossification centres with dwarfism, leg length discrepancy, hypophosphataemic rickets and osteomalacia. Malignant conversion is seen in 1% (osteosarcoma, fibrosarcoma and chondrosarcoma).

Case 4.14: Answers

1. The X-ray shows upward displacement of the left scapula and an abnormal bony structure connecting the scapula to the cervical spine.

2. Sprengel's shoulder.

3. Sprengel's shoulder refers to failure of descent of the scapula, secondary to fibrosis or an omovertebral connection. The scapula normally differentiates opposite C4, C5 and C6 at 5 weeks and descends to the thorax by the third intrauterine month. Interruption in this migration occurs during weeks 9–12 and is associated with arrest in the development of bone, muscle and cartilage. It is associated with many malformations and syndromes – the higher the scapula, the less the glenoid rotation. The scapuloclavicular space is narrow, which may result in brachial plexus compression. A well-known association is an omovertebral bone (a third), and this bone (cartilage, fibrous or bone) extends from the superomedial border of the scapula to the spinous process/lamina/transverse process of C4–7. It is rhomboid or trapezoid in shape and lies in a fascial sheath. A joint can form between the scapula and omovertebral bone. It can be a solid osseus bridge, and is best seen in a lateral or oblique view of the cervical spine. It is usually unilateral and always associated with a fixed elevated scapula. Periscapular muscles are fibrotic and contracted, trapezius being the most common. A lateral view of the spine should be obtained to rule out anomalies. Scapular displacement can be measured by drawing three lines:

Line 1: from midpoint of acromioclavicular joint to midpoint of scapuloclavicular joint

Line 2: from midpoint of acromioclavicular joint to inferior angle of scapula

Line 3: along the spinous processes of the vertebrae.

The superior scapular angle is between lines 1 and 2, and the inferior scapular angle between lines 2 and 3.

4. The scapula is elevated 2–10 cm, adducted, and the inferior pole medially rotated. It is hypoplastic. The length of the vertebral border is decreased, scapulothoracic movements of the shoulder joint are limited, omovertebral bone limits abduction and the left side is more commonly affected.

5. Sprengel's deformity is associated with Klippel–Feil syndrome, Poland syndrome, VATER, Grieg syndrome, velocardiofacial syndrome, Goldenhar syndrome and floating harbour syndrome.

Case 4.15: Answers

1. The chest X-ray shows a normal appearance of the heart and lungs. However, the clavicles are not seen.

2. The X-ray of the pelvis shows separation of the pubic bones (pubic diastasis). The X-ray of the skull shows multiple small wormian bones at the junction of the lambdoid and coronal sutures.

3. Cleidocranial dysostosis

4. Cleidocranial dysostosis is a skeletal dysplasia that is transmitted in an autosomal dominant pattern and caused by a mutation in the gene for the transcription factor CBFA1 (core-binding factor α subunit 1), which is located on chromosome 6.

5. Cleidocranial dysostosis is characterised by a defect in ossification of the enchondral and intramembranous bones. Multiple wormian bones are seen in the skull. The clavicle is absent, partially absent or unfused. Failure of midline ossification manifests as delayed closure of symphysis pubis, fontanelles, mandible, neural arches, sternum and vertebral bodies.

6. Wormian bones are intrasutural bones seen in the skull, most commonly in the lambdoid suture. It is a normal finding until age 1 year. The other causes are pyknodysostosis, osteogenesis imperfecta, rickets, kinky hair syndrome (Menkes), hypothyroidism, otopalatodigital syndrome, pachydermoperiostitis and Down syndrome. The normal gap in pubic symphysis is 4–5 mm. Pubic diastasis is caused by trauma, infection, osteitis pubis, osteomyelitis, bladder exstrophy, epispadias, cleidocranial dysostosis, pyknodysostosis, pregnancy, rheumatoid , hyperparathyroidism, Reiter syndrome and metastasis. Differential diagnoses for an irregular clavicle are trauma, infection, pyknodysostosis, rheumatoid arthritis, hyperparathyroidism, post-traumatic osteolysis, metastasis and myeloma.

Case 4.16: Answers

1. There is atrophy of the fingertips and autoamputation of the phalangeal tufts, resulting in defects in the distal portion of the fingers in both hands symmetrically.

2. Acro-osteolysis caused by amniotic band syndrome

3. The appearances are pathognomonic in children. Differential diagnoses in older children and adults include trauma, surgery, insensitivity to pain (Lesch–Nyhan syndrome), diabetes mellitus, frostbite and post-meningococcaemic gangrene. Other causes are psoriasis, hyperparathyroidism, frostbite, sarcoidosis, leprosy, occupational exposure (polyvinyl chloride), post-traumatic and congenital (syndromes of Hajdu and Cheney).

4. Amniotic or constricting band syndrome (ABS), or Streeter's dysplasia, is progressive intrauterine amputation of the fingers or limbs associated with a wide spectrum of congenital anomalies involving the trunk and craniofacial region. Incidence is 1 in 15 000 live births. Most amputations occur in the upper limb (90%). In the hand, digital amputations are most common in the index, middle and ring fingers, whereas, in the foot, amputations of the hallux are most often noted. Mild band pressure causes just indentations at the base of the phalanx, usually distal to the metacarpophalangeal (MCP) joints. Progressive constriction is the result of the maceration of the indentation and subsequent healing by scar tissue formation. If the compression from the band is severe, lymphatic and vascular compromise may ensue, and the child presents at birth with a swollen engorged digit or limb that may require immediate surgical release. Theories of formation:

Intrinsic theory: disruptive event occurs during blastogenesis, leading to an intrinsic germ plasm defect, which causes the soft tissue to slough. External healing of the slough leads to the constricting rings and the resultant localised developmental defects.

Extrinsic theory: intrauterine trauma leads to premature rupture of the membranes, and strands of residual membranes could encircle the digits or might even be swallowed.

The congenital (intrauterine) band is a product of rupture of the amnion and produces compression and chronic ischaemia of the affected limb. Associated anomalies are orbital defects (ocular, lids, lacrimal), waist constriction, clubfoot, cleft palate and lips, encephalocele, cleft lip/palate, renal/cardiac anomalies, hemihypertrophy, tibial pseudarthrosis/bowing, leg length discrepancy, gastro-/thoracoschisis and extrathoracic heart.

5. The management depends on the clinical findings at birth, and the prognosis on the severity of the abnormalities and involvement of internal organs. Urgent surgical treatment is necessary for patients with vascular compromise. Surgery is also indicated in syndactyly or acrosyndactyly that compromises hand function. Early intervention for severe constriction bands after birth includes band excision with 1–2 mm normal skin to avoid recurrence. This is performed on a maximum of 65%, by Z-plasty for lesser constrictions and V-Y-plasty or W-plasty for tighter bands. A staged correction ensures the adequacy of vascularity to the residual limb or digit. In addition, debulking of the fibrofatty soft tissues, followed by subcutaneous tissue advancement as described (Upton), may further improve the cosmetic appearance of the digits after band release.

Case 4.17: Answers

1. The plain X-ray of the whole body shows H-shaped abnormal vertebrae, failure to increase the interpedunculate distance in the lower lumbar vertebrae, hypoplastic iliac bones, short iliac bones, narrow sacrosciatic notch, short and bowed peripheral bones with telephone-handle appearance, metaphyseal projections and a narrow chest with a large head.

2. Thanatophoric dysplasia. This is a lethal sporadic skeletal dysplasia that is autosomal dominant. It is characterised by severe rhizomelic dwarfism, and is the second most common lethal bone dysplasia after osteogenesis imperfecta.

3. **Chest**: narrow, short horizontal ribs not extending beyond the anterior axillary line, short curved telephone-handle humeri, small scapula, normal clavicles, H-/U-shaped vertebrae

   Head: large head, short base, frontal bossing, trilobed cloverleaf skull

   Spine: platyspondyly, H-/U-shaped vertebrae, reduction of interpedunculate distance of the lower lumbar vertebrae

   Pelvis: hypoplastic iliac bones, flat acetabulum, narrow sacrosciatic notch, short pubic bones

Extremities: small and bowed bones, metaphyseal flaring producing telephone handle appearance, metaphyseal thorn-like projections, polydactyly.

4. Achondroplasia, achondrogenesis, Ellis–van Creveld syndrome (extra digit, acromesomelic short limbs), Jeune syndrome (less marked bone shortening, sparing of vertebrae) and short rib polydactyly syndromes are considered in the differential diagnosis of thanatophoric dysplasia.

5. Most of these children are stillborn or present with respiratory distress, hypotonia, protuberant abdomen and extended arms, with externally rotated, abducted thighs. Most of these cases are fatal within a few hours or days of birth as a result of respiratory failure.

Case 4.18: Answers

1. The plain X-ray of the spine shows rugger jersey spine, with areas of sclerosis and luceny. The X-ray of the hands shows subperiosteal bone resorption in the lateral aspect of the middle phalanges. There is also acro-osteolysis, more prominent in the proximal phalanges of the first to third digits.

2. Secondary hyperparathyroidism.

3. Secondary hyperparathyroidism results from a compensatory hyperplasia of the parathyroid glands in response to hypocalcaemia caused by chronic renal failure and other metabolic abnormalities. The common causes are renal osteodystrophy, calcium deprivation, hypovitaminosis D, pregnancy, maternal hypoparathyroidism and hyperphosphataemia. The low-to-normal calcium levels result in high parathyroid hormone (PTH) levels and a calcium phosphate level that exceeds the solubility product.

4. Radiological features are diffuse sclerosis of bones (osteoblastic activity of PTH or calcitonin, more common in axial skeleton, pelvis, ribs, clavicles, metaphysis, epiphysis), subperiosteal bone resorption (pathognomonic – lacy irregularity of cortical marking, most common in the radial aspect of the middle phalanx of the second and third fingers, and also in the medial tibial plateau, medial femoral neck, medial humerus neck, distal ulna, rib margins, base of terminal tuft), rugger jersey spine with sclerotic

and lucent areas, soft-tissue calcification, periosteal new bone formation and diffuse osteopenia. Brown tumours are uncommon in secondary hyperparathyroidism. A bone scan shows a characteristic appearance of a superscan, with high axial uptake and no uptake in the kidneys.

5. Sequelae of secondary hyperparathyroidism are deformities, SUFE, basilar impression of skull, wedge vertebrae, scoliosis, renal stones, nephrocalcinosis, peptic ulcer, calcific pancreatitis, soft-tissue calcification, joint erosions and fractures.

Case 4.19: Answers

1. The X-ray shows discontinuity in the midportion of the right clavicle. There is no lytic lesion. The defect is smoothly corticated and there is no periosteal reaction or soft-tissue swelling. The acromioclavicular and glenohumeral joints are normal.

2. There is deformity of the midtibia and fibula with an abnormal joint.

3. Congenital pseudarthrosis of clavicle and pseudarthrosis of tibia and fibula.

4. Pseudarthrosis can be caused by osteogenesis imperfecta, neurofibromatosis 1, osteomalacia/rickets and fibrous dysplasia.

5. Congenital failure of the clavicle to form is rare. Congenital pseudarthrosis of the midportion of the clavicle occurs when an environmental insult or anatomical or mechanical event disrupts diaphyseal membranous ossification, resulting in failure of fusion of the two primary ossification centres of the clavicle. The two portions of the clavicle produced are connected by a fibrous bridge contiguous with the periosteum and a synovial membrane develops between the two. It always occurs on the right side, except in situs inversus, suggesting that vascular anlage of the subclavian artery, which crosses the first rib just below the pseudarthrosis site, may be involved in the aetiology. Bilateral cases are associated with syndromes. Cervical rib is associated in 15%. A painless mass over the right clavicle is the most common finding that prompts parents to seek consultation with a doctor. In the typical presentation, the larger sternal side is tilted anteriorly and superiorly, and the smaller acromial portion curves gently to meet the pseudarthrosis. The mass is usually painless, the range of motion full and function normal. On X-rays, pseudarthrosis of the midclavicle on the right is easily visualised and has a characteristic pattern with anterior and superior tilting of the sternal half and a smaller acromial portion. MRI may be used to determine the extent of the fibrous union, the location of the great vessels and the space available within the thoracic outlet.

6. Mere observation may be appropriate. No non-surgical techniques achieve union. Surgical resection or osteosynthesis is indicated for cosmetic reasons and pain.

Case 4.20: Answers

1. The X-ray of the hand shows a short fourth metacarpal. The metacarpal sign is positive.

2. Turner syndrome.

3. **Positive metacarpal sign**: a tangential line through the head of the fourth and fifth metacarpals intersects the head of the third metacarpal. This indicates a short fourth metacarpal. **Differential diagnoses**: Turner syndrome, Klinefelter syndrome, pseudohypoparathyroidism, pseudo-pseudohypoparathyroidism, multiple epiphyseal dysplasia, enchondromatosis, diaphyseal aclasis, sickle cell disease, juvenile rheumatoid arthritis and trauma.

4. Turner syndrome is a chromosomal anomaly caused by non-disjunction of the sex chromosomes, with a 45 X phenotype. Partial monosomy can be seen. Affected girls have short stature, with growth retardation, webbed neck, shield-shaped chest, low hairline, learning disability, high palate and primary amenorrhoea. It is associated with coarctation, aortic stenosis and horseshoe kidney.

5. Radiological features are:

Hands: positive metacarpal sign, narrowing of scaphoid triquestrum lunate angle, short second and fifth phalanges, drumstick distal phalanges, insetting of epiphysis into metaphysis, Madelung's deformity, cubitus valgus and osteopenia

Knee: tibia vara, exostosis from the medial aspect of proximal tibial metaphysis

Axial: hypoplastic odontoid, squared lumbar vertebrae, osteopenic vertebrae, small iliac wings

Skull: basilar impression, parietal thinning

General: growth arrest, delayed epiphyseal fusion, osteoporosis.

Case 4.21: Answers

1. The X-ray of the spine shows scoliosis and middle beaking of the vertebrae. The X-ray of the hand shows widening of the proximal end of the metacarpals and phalanges, and proximal pointing of the metacarpals.

2. Morquio syndrome – a subtype of the mucopolysaccharidoses.

3. The mucopolysaccharidoses are a group of lysosomal storage disorders caused by deficiency of lysosomal enzymes. Types of mucopolysaccharidoses:

Type	Eponymous syndrome	Inheritance	Enzyme
IH	Hurler	AR (autosomal recessive)	α-l-Iduronidase
II	Hunter	XR (X-linked recessive)	Iduronate sulphatase
III	San Filippo	AR	Heparan sulphatase, N-acetyl-α-d-glucosaminase, α-glucosamine-6-sulphate, N-acetylglucosamine-6-sulphate sulphatase
IV	Morquio	AR	N-Acetylgalactosamine-6-sulphate sulphatase
V-IS	Scheie	AR	α-l-Iduronidase
VI	Maroteux–Lamy	AR	Arylsulphatase B
VII	Sly	AR	β-Glucuronidase

4. **Dysostosis multiplex** refers to a constellation of radiological findings in mucopolysaccharidoses:

Large skull, thick calvaria, frontal and parietal hyperostosis

Hypertelorism

J-shaped sella turcica

Wedge-shaped vertebrae: in Morquio syndrome platyspondyly at multiple levels, middle vertebral beaking

Anterior hypoplasia of lumbar vertebrae and kyphosis

Thoracolumbar kyphosis.

Poorly formed pelvis with small femoral hands and coxa valga

Hip subluxation, genu valgum

Enlarged diaphysis of long bones, irregular wide metaphysis, tapering distal portions

Irregular carpal bones

Wide metacarpals, brachydactyly, proximal pointing

Short wide and trapezoid-shaped phalanges.

5. In **Hurler syndrome**, the vertebral beaking is seen inferiorly. In Morquio syndrome, beaking is situated centrally. **Spondyloepiphyseal dysplasia** is another differential diagnosis, with smaller acetabular angle and varus femora deformities. Treatment consists of enzyme replacement therapy and bone marrow transplantation.

Case 4.22: Answers

1. There is expansion of the distal metaphysis of the femur. There is no lytic or sclerotic lesion in the bone. MRI shows similar change without signal abnormality.

2. Erlenmeyer flask deformity in Gaucher's disease.

3. Erlenmeyer flask deformity is characterised by expansion of the distal end of long bones.

4. Causes of Erlenmeyer flask deformity: Gaucher's disease, Niemann–Pick disease, anaemia, thalassaemia, sickle cell disease, osteopetrosis, rickets, metaphyseal dysplasia, fibrous dysplasia, hypophosphatasia, achondroplasia, Down syndrome and rheumatoid arthritis.

5. Gaucher's disease is an autosomal recessive disease caused by deficiency of β-glucocerebrosidase resulting in accumulation of glucocerebroside in the reticuloendothelial system. There are many types: adult/chronic neuropathic form, rapidly fatal infantile/acute neuropathic form and juvenile/subacute neuropathic forms. Skeletal changes in Gaucher's disease are seen predominantly in long tubular bones (especially the distal end of the femur), axial skeleton, hip, shoulder and pelvis. Skeletal changes are seen in 75%. The changes are bilateral and symmetrical. The characteristic finding is Erlenmeyer flask deformity. Other features are diffuse osteopenia, lytic lesions, periosteal reaction, avascular necrosis, bone infarction and H-shaped vertebrae. Other radiological findings are hepatosplenomegaly, lymphadenoapthy, multiple hypodense lesions in the spleen and reticulonodular infiltrates in the lung base. Complications are pathological fractures, avascular necrosis, osteomyelitis, myelosclerosis and pulmonary infections. Clinically, there is hepatosplenomegaly, impaired liver function, elevated acid phosphatase, pancytopenia caused by hypersplenism, ascites, haemochromatosis and dull bone pain.

Case 4.23: Answers

1. The plain X-ray shows a bilateral diffuse increase in bone density with patchy areas of lucencies seen within the metaphysis.

2. Leukaemia.

3. Differential diagnoses for metaphyseal lucencies are normal variant, growth lines, syphilis, neuroblastoma, rickets, scurvy. The most common differential diagnoses are neuroblastoma metastasis, eosinophilic granuloma and metastases.

4. Leukaemia is the most common malignancy in children (33%). Most cases are acute lymphocytic leukaemia. Clinical features are low-grade fever, fatigue, pain, bruising, joint pains, hepatosplenomegaly and lymphadenopathy. Lab examination shows high ESR and anaemia. Peripheral smear confirms leukaemia.

5. Bone symptoms are seen in 50–90%. There are various presentations:

Leukaemic lines: metaphyseal lucencies caused by leukaemic infiltration at sites of rapid growth, seen in the proximal tibia, distal femur, proximal humerus, distal radius, ulna and vertebrae

Diffuse osteopenia with coarse trabeculations

Bilateral periosteal reaction

Metaphyseal sclerosis

Focal lytic lesions with moth-eaten appearance, especially distal to the knee.

Case 4.24: Answers

1. The X-ray of the ankle shows an increased distance between the shaft and epiphyseal centre with cupping and fraying of the metaphysis.

2. Rickets.

3. Rickets is a metabolic abnormality affecting endochondral bone growth, in which the zone of preparatory calcification does not form, with heaping of maturing cartilage cells and failure of osteoid mineralisation in the shaft with elevated periosteum.

4. Causes of rickets:

Primary vitamin D deficiency

Malabsorption: gastrectomy, enteropathy, enteritis, biliary obstruction, biliary cirrhosis, pancreatitis

Primary hypophosphataemia

Hypophosphatasia, pseudohypophosphatasia

Fibrogenesis imperfecta osseum

Axial osteomalacia

Hypoparathyroidism, hyperparathyroidism, thyrotoxicosis, Paget's disease, fluorides, neurofibromatosis, osteopetrosis, malignancy, macroglobulinaemia, ureterosigmoidostomy.

5. Radiological features: rickets is commonly seen in the metaphysis of long bones such as the wrists, ankles and knees. An X-ray shows delayed formation of poorly mineralised epiphysis and the epiphyseal plates are wide and irregular. Increased distance is seen between the end of the shaft and the epiphysis. Cupping and fraying of the metaphysis, metaphyseal spurs, coarse trabeculation, periosteal reaction, deformities such as bowed legs, and bowing of the diaphysis and frontal bossing are other features. Children present with irritability, bone pain, tenderness, craniotabes, rachitic rosary, bowed legs, delayed dentition, and swelling of the wrists and ankles. Differential diagnoses are metaphyseal dysplasia and healing scurvy

Case 4.25: Answers

1. The X-ray shows subtle narrowing of the disc space between L4 and L5 with irregular endplates. T1-weighted MRI shows reduction of the disc space at the L4–5 level, with irregular endplates. There is an abnormally low signal in L4 and L5 vertebrae. T2-weighted images show high signal in the corresponding vertebrae. High signal is also seen in the disc.

2. Discitis.

3. Discitis is infection of the intervertebral disc. *Staphylococcus aureus* is the most commonly identified organism. In 70% of children, the causative organism is not identified and can be streptococci, enterococci, *E. coli, Salmonella, Pseudomonas* and *Klebsiella* spp., TB, brucellosis, fungi and parasitic diseases. The infection usually spreads haematogenously. L2–3 and L3–4 are the discs commonly involved. Children classically present with fever, back pain, irritability and refusal to walk. In children, the discs are well vascularised, the vessels becoming obliterated by age 13. As a result, isolated discitis occurs in childhood, but by adulthood infection starts in the vertebral body and spreads to the disc.

4. The plain X-ray is normal in the acute phase, but after 2–8 weeks shows narrowing of the disc space and erosion of the endplates of adjacent vertebrae. A bone scan shows high uptake in the affected region. MRI is the imaging method of choice with the highest sensitivity. The MR features are disc space narrowing, high signal in T2-weighted images and marrow oedema in adjacent vertebrae. Disc enhancement is seen, and often extension into adjacent soft tissues. The soft-tissue abscess can extend

anteriorly or posteriorly into the spinal canal, causing cord compression. In chronic infection, collapse of the vertebral body and deformity are seen. Blood culture is used to decide on treatment. CT-guided biopsy can be done if complications develop. The causative organism can be identified.

5. Intravenous antibiotics are given. Immediate surgery is performed if there is spinal cord compression. Deformities are treated by fusion of spinal segments.

Case 4.26: Answers

1. Lateral view of the spine shows kyphosis, decreased disc space and anterior wedging of multiple lower thoracic vertebrae. Sagittal MRI confirms this, showing kyphosis, anterior wedging, irregular end plates and disc space narrowing.

2. Scheuermann's disease.

3. Scheuermann's disease (juvenile kyphosis) is osteochondrosis of the secondary ossification centre of the vertebral bodies. Trauma might be a causative factor. It commonly affects the lower dorsal and upper lumbar vertebrae. It affects multiple bodies or the entire spine. It commonly presents between age 13 and 16, and is more common in boys. The affected children are taller and have rapid skeletal growth. They present with deformity, poor posture, dull aching and intermittent backache. Tenderness above and below the level of kyphosis, decreased flexibility of the spine and deformity are clinical features.

4. The X-ray and MRI show:

Kyphosis > 40°, loss or lordosis, scoliosis

Anterior wedging > 5° in three or more consecutive vertebrae

Increased AP diameter

Irregular endplates: flattened area in the anterosuperior aspect as a result of avulsion of the ring apophysis caused by migration of nucleus pulposus through the weak point between ring apophyses

Schmorl's nodes: herniation of nucleus pulposus into the vertebral body, producing depression in the posterior vertebral body

Slight narrowing of the disc space.

Calcifications are uncommon.

5. Differential diagnoses:

Osteochondrodystrophy: earlier presentation, changes in appendicular skeleton

Developmental notching of anterior vertebrae: no wedging, no Schmorl's nodes

Other causes of Schmorl's nodes: Wilson's disease, ochronosis, sickle cell disease, spinal stenosis

Congenital and other causes of kyphosis.

6. This mild non-progressive disease is treated by reducing weight bearing and strenuous activity. Severe disease is managed though use of casting, a brace and rest. Surgery is done only when there is severe deformity or severe pain.

Case 4.27: Answers

1. The X-ray of the left leg shows extensive sclerosis, cortical thickening and periosteal reaction. There is no soft-tissue swelling or fracture.

2. Osteoid osteoma.

3. Osteoid osteoma is a benign tumour of osteoid and woven bone, measuring < 1.5 cm (> 1.5 cm – osteoblastoma). It is common in the second and third decades. Clinically, osteoid osteomas present with pain, which is worse in the night and relieved by salicylates.

4. Osteoid osteoma is seen in the metaphysis or diaphysis of long bones or posterior elements of the spine or flat bones. In the bones the usual location is in the cortex. Occasionally it is seen in cancellous bone or subperiosteally. The characteristic lesion is a round or oval radiolucent nidus (< 1.5 cm), with a surrounding rim of sclerosis and central calcification. In the spine, there is painful scoliosis concave to the lesion. When the lesion is intra-articular, effusion, cartilage loss and degenerative changes are seen. Disuse osteoporosis can be seen. The CT scan shows nidus surrounded by sclerosis and variable amounts of mineralisation. MRI shows nidus isointense in T1 and low in T2 with perinidal oedema. An angiogram shows vascular nidus.

5. Differential diagnoses: stress fracture, Brodie's abscess, sclerosing osteomyelitis, syphilis, osteoblastoma, bone island, Ewing's sarcoma metastases, lymphoma and subperiosteal ABC (Aneurysmal bone cyst).

6. The nidus can be removed surgically or by radiofrequency (RF) ablation under CT guidance. The tumour can be percutaneously ablated by using RF, ethanol, laser or thermocoagulation therapy under CT guidance. In spinal tumours, complete ablation or resection of the tumour is desirable but not always feasible. Percutaneous RF ablation is performed under CT guidance by using general or spinal anaesthesia. After localisation of the nidus with 1- to 3-mm CT sections, an osseous access is established and ablation performed at 90°C for 4–5 min by using a rigid RF electrode. The procedure is successful when the electrode is heated to the desired temperature within the nidus.

Case 4.28: Answers

1. The X-ray of the spine shows an expansile, dense lesion, seen in the left transverse process of the L4 lumbar vertebra. The CT scan shows the lesion more exquisitely. There is an expansile lesion with areas of calcification and extensive sclerosis, in the left transverse process of the L4 vertebra. There is no soft-tissue mass in the paraspinal region. There is no mass in the spinal canal.

2. Osteoblastoma. This is a benign tumour with osteoid, osteoclast, connective tissue stroma and interconnecting trabecular bone, > 1.5 cm (osteoid osteoma < 1.5 cm). Patients present with dull pain, worse at night, responding to salicylates, and swelling, tenderness, decreased range of movements, painful scoliosis, muscle weakness, paraesthesiae, paraparesis and paraplegia.

3. Osteoblastoma is common in the spine. It can be seen in the long bones, and small bones of the hand and skull. It is located in the diaphysis or metaphysis. On an X-ray, there is a radiolucent nidus > 2 cm, with well-demarcated margins, matrix calcification and reactive sclerosis. Another appearance is an expansile lesion with cortical expansion, lucent or

ossified matrix, a soft-tissue component and thick periosteal reaction. Scoliosis and osteoporosis are seen. A CT scan shows matrix calcification, soft-tissue, periosteal reaction and bone remodelling. A bone scan shows increased uptake and an angiogram tumour blush.

4. Differential diagnoses: when a well-defined, expansile lesion occurs in the spine, osteoblastoma is the most common diagnosis. Matrix calcification is seen in 50% of patients. Other differential diagnoses are: osteoid osteoma – dense calcification, nidus < 1.5 cm, periosteal new bone; chondroblastoma; osteosarcoma – periosteal new bone; chondrosarcoma – soft tissue; giant cell tumour – no calcification, epiphysis; aneurysmal bone cyst; osteomyelitis; haemangioma; lipoma; epidermoid; fibrous dysplasia; metastasis; and Ewing's sarcoma.

5. Complications are fracture, continued growth and recurrence (20%). Osteoblastomas can be difficult to treat. Usually they are diagnosed by excision biopsy and treated with curettage and grafting. En-bloc resection can also be performed. Larger lesions may require internal fixation. Irradiation is another therapeutic option. Rates of recurrence are lower with wide surgical excision, but the location of the lesion does not always allow for this option. Cementation in conjunction with excision may be helpful in extending the surgical margin.

Case 4.29: Answers

1. The X-ray of the right leg shows a well-defined, expansile, multiloculated, lytic lesion arising from the proximal metaphysis of the tibia, causing cortical thinning. No periosteal reaction or soft-tissue component is identified. The knee joint appears normal.

2. This is a T2-weighted MR image of the same patient. The lesion appears expansile, with a high signal intensity.

3. Aneurysmal bone cyst. This is an expansile osteolytic lesion with a thin wall, containing blood-filled cystic cavities. It is seen between age 5 and 20 years. An aneurysmal bone cyst can arise secondary to pre-existing bone tumours in 30% of cases, such as chondroblastoma, fibrous dysplasia, giant cell tumour and osteoblastoma.

4. Common locations are in metaphyses of long tubular bones, posterior elements of the spine and the pelvis. Pain, swelling and limitation of joint movements are some of the clinical features. It is usually seen in the metaphysis as an expansile, multiloculated (soap bubble) eccentric lesion, with thin intact cortex, respecting the epiphyseal plate, with no periosteal reaction (unless fractured). Fluid–fluid levels are seen in cystic components. Large lesions can be aggressive resembling lytic metastasis. MRI shows a low-to-intermediate signal in T1 and heterogeneous low-to-intermediate signal in T2. High signal in T1 can be seen in acute haemorrhage. A fluid–fluid level is a characteristic finding on MRI and CT. A bone scan shows high uptake in the margin.

5. Fractures can be seen. Periosteal reaction develops if there is a fracture. Differential diagnoses include simple bone cyst (unicameral, located centrally), giant cell tumour (seen after epiphyseal fusion, narrow transition point, maybe locally aggressive, may erode into joint), subarticular geode, Brodie's abscess, benign fibrous histiocytoma, chondroblastoma, haemophilic pseudotumour and expansile neuroblastoma metastasis. Differential diagnosis of fluid–fluid level in bone lesion on MRI is ABC (Aneurysmal bone cyst), SBC (Simple bone cyst), chondroblastoma, giant cell tumour, telangiectactic osteosarcoma and fibrous dysplasia.

Case 4.30: Answers

1. This is the X-ray of the left hand.

2. The X-ray of the left hand is used for assessing bone age.

3. The X-ray of the left hand is taken and then it is compared with standard X-rays of left hands in *The Atlas* by Greulich and Pyle . *The Atlas* has normal pictures of bone development of an average person of known chronological age. Separate pictures are available for males and females. Another method is to use the atlas of Tanner and Whitehouse, where indices are used.

4. The left hand is the non-dominant hand in most individuals. In left-handed individuals, a right hand X-ray is used.

5. Causes of **delayed bone age** are:

Constitutional

Metabolic: hypothyroidism, hypogonadism, hypopituitarism, diabetes mellitus, Cushing syndrome, rickets

Systemic disease: heart disease, renal diseases, gastrointestinal disease, anaemia, bone marrow transplant recipient

Syndromes: Down, Noonan, Edward, Patau, Cornelia de Lange and Lesch–Nyhan syndromes, cleidocranial dysplasia, metatrophic dwarfism

Causes of advanced bone age: precocious puberty, congenital adrenal hyperplasia, adrenarche, and Soto, Marshall–Smith and Beckwith–Wiedemann syndromes.

Case 4.31: Answers

1. The X-ray the right leg shows extensive intramedullary sclerosis in the proximal tibial metaphysis. There is sunburst periosteal reaction and severe soft-tissue swelling, with Codman's triangle.

2. Osteosarcoma of the right femur.

3. Osteosarcoma is a malignant tumour that arises from undifferentiated mesenchyme, which forms neoplastic immature bone. It has a bimodal age distribution of 10–25 and > 60 years. Clinical features are sudden onset of pain, swelling, redness, fever, elevation of ALP and diabetes mellitus (paraneoplastic syndrome). It is usually seen in the long bones in the metaphysis. Complications are pathological fracture and radiation-induced osteosarcoma. Metastasis, soft-tissue mass > 20 cm, pathological fractures and skip lesions are bad prognostic indicators. Treatment is by chemotherapy followed by wide surgical resection.

4. Osteosarcoma is commonly seen in leg bones, with 50–55% seen around the knee joint. It is located within the metaphysis and can extend into other areas. It is very aggressive, with ill-defined tumour margins. The lesion shows extensive areas of new bone formation or lytic areas of a moth-eaten or permeative pattern of bone destruction. Periosteal reaction is a sunburst (tumour extending through the periosteum), hair-on-end, onion-peel type. Codman's triangle is seen (the interface between a growing bone tumour and normal bone, appearing as an incomplete triangle formed by the elevated periosteum). Soft-tissue mass with new bone formation is seen. A bone scan shows high uptake. A CT scan can demonstrate the new bone formation. MRI shows the extent of marrow involvement, soft-tissue involvement and joints, and demonstrates areas of viable tumour that are suitable for biopsy. A chest X-ray is done for detecting metastasis. Lung metastasis can be ossified or cavitatory and can produce pneumothorax. Skeletal metastasis is uncommon. Acute osteomyelitis, sclerosing chronic osteomyelitis and Charcot's joint are the differential diagnoses. Acute osteomyelitis has a similar clinical presentation as osteosarcoma, but extensive new bone formation is not seen.

5. Variants of ostesarcoma:

Parosteal osteosarcoma: outer layer of periosteum, slow growing, fulminating course once it reaches medulla

Periosteal osteosarcoma: deep layer of periosteum

Secondary type: from Paget's disease, irradiation, osteonecrosis, fibrous dysplasia, osteogenesis imperfecta, chronic osteomyelitis, retinoblastoma

Telangiectactic: aneurysmal expansion of bone

Osteosarcomatosis: multifocal

Low-grade intraosseus

High-grade surface

Extraskeletal osteosarcoma.

Case 4.32: Answers

1. There is a calcified lesion arising from the lower cervical vertebrae. The lateral view shows an exophytic bony lesion with cartilaginous type of calcification protruding into the posterior soft tissue of neck.

2. Osteochondroma.

3. Osteochondroma (exostosis) is the most common benign tumour of the bone and the most common benign cartilage-containing tumour. It is a developmental anomaly that is caused by herniation of a fragment of physeal cartilage through the periosteal cuff surrounding the growth plate which continues its ossification. Theories of formation include microtrauma and radiotherapy. Multiple osteochondromas are seen in hereditary multiple exostoses (HMEs), which is an autosomal dominant disorder. Multiple epiphyseal dysplasia and dysplasia epiphysealis hemimelica (DEH), or Trevor's disease, are also autosomal dominant conditions in which multiple exostoses are seen. Most of the osteochondromas present as slow-growing, painless masses. Symptoms are more common when complications develop.

4. Osteochondromas are common in the metaphysis at sites of tendon and ligamentous attachments. It is common in the distal femur, proximal femur, tibia and fibula. X-rays show a metaphyseal lesion with a cortex and medulla that continue with the cortex and medulla of the native bone. There is a hyaline cartilaginous cap, which is seen only if there is calcification. Osteochondromas point away from their point of attachment towards the diaphysis. The metaphysis may be widened. CT demonstrates the lesion better and the cartilage cap is seen as a hypodense area if it is non-calcified. The thickness of the cap depends on the age. It can be up to 3 cm in children and adolescents, and measures 6–8 mm in skeletally mature individuals. A thick cap, > 1 cm in adults, is suspicious for malignant transformation. The presence of a soft-tissue mass is another feature suspicious of malignancy. MRI is useful in characterising the lesion. The cartilage cap is hyperintense in T2 and intermediate in T1. Calcification is hypotense. Septal calcification can be seen. In the chest, osteochondromas arise from the costochondral junction and can cause pneumothorax. Osteochondromas in the pelvis can have a soft-tissue component.

5. Other conditions that produce metaphyseal spurs are hyperparathyroidism, hypophosphatasia, Menkes' disease and short rib polydactyly syndromes. Conditions that produce bony excrescences are osteoma, osteophyte, enthesiophyte, heterotopic ossification, Turner syndrome, tuberous sclerosis, trauma, chondroectodermal dysplasia, bizarre parosteal osteochondromatous proliferation, fetal alcohol syndrome, acrodysostosis and anatomical variants. Chondrosarcomas and parosteal sarcomas are the important differential diagnoses.

6. Osteochondroma stops growing when the epiphyseal centre fuses. Treatment is by surgical excision. Deformities, fractures, vascular complications (thrombosis, occlusion, pseudoaneurysm), neurological complications, reactive bursitis and malignant transformation (1%) are the complications. Malignant transformation is usually to chondrosarcoma/osteosarcoma. Increasing pain, cartilage cap > 1.5 cm, irregular margins and soft-tissue mass are signs of malignant transformation.

Case 4.33: Answers

1. The X-ray of the pelvis appears normal.

2. This is a high-resolution ultrasound scan of the hip, obtained in the longitudinal position. There is a convex dark collection of fluid anterior to the femur.

3. Hip effusion.

4. Ultrasonography of the hip is a very sensitive and accurate method for evaluating hip effusion. There are various causes of hip pain in children, including SUFE, Perthes' disease, septic arthritis, toxic synovitis, juvenile rheumatoid arthritis and fracture. Hip effusion is seen in many conditions, especially in septic arthritis. X-ray is the first step, but it is not sensitive. It might show displacement of fat stripes when the effusion is huge. If the X-ray is normal, ultrasonography of the hip should be done to evaluate the effusion and see if it is septic. The patient lies down in a supine position. The ultrasound probe is oriented longitudinally along the length of the femur. The area of focus is the joint space, under the proximal metaphysis of the shaft of the femur. Normally this area shows the capsule as a dark band, which is flat or concave. If this band is prominent, with convexity > 6 mm, it indicates effusion. If in doubt, this appearance can be compared with the opposite side to exclude effusion.

5. When the patient shows hip effusion and there are signs of sepsis, an ultrasound-guided aspiration of the effusion should be done. This is performed under local anaesthesia and the needle is advanced under ultrasound guidance, into the area of the maximum fluid collection, and aspirated. Gram staining will confirm septic arthritis in 30–50% of cases. The WBC count is elevated, with > 90% neutrophils, and an aspirate glucose concentration < 40 mg/dl or significantly less than the serum level. Gram staining and culture can be done and appropriate antibiotics determined on the basis of culture and sensitivity.

Case 4.34: Answers

1. The plain X-ray shows collapse of the right femoral head with dense sclerosis. The joint space is normal. The second film is a frog lateral view, which shows the collapse of the head again.

2. Legg–Calve–Perthes disease

3. Perthes' disease refers to idiopathic avascular necrosis of the capital femoral epiphysis. Classically, it seen in children between age 3 and 12 years with peak incidence between 4 and 6 years, as a result of changing blood supply to the femoral head in this age group. It usually starts in the anterolateral aspect of the femoral head because of compression of the posterosuperior epiphyseal branch of the medial circumflex artery. It is more common in boys and is usually unilateral. It is bilateral in 15%. It presents with insidious hip pain and limp in a systemically well child.

4. Early X-rays are normal or show a subtle widening of joint space as a result of effusion or thickening of the cartilage. With time, there is increased density, subchondral lucency caused by fracture, increasing sclerosis and fragmentation with femoral neck cysts. Unlike septic arthritis, there is no destruction of articular cartilage. Remodelling and reossification occurs over 18–24 months. Deformities include coxa plana (flattening), coxa vara and coxa magna (enlargement). Treatment is with varus derotational femoral osteomy or iliac osteotomy. MRI is the most sensitive method to detect early and intermediate stages. In the early stages, irregular linear changes of low signal intensity are seen in the bone marrow. Low signal on T1 and high signal on T2 is called an asterisk sign. Presence of a dark, sclerotic rim is called a double-line sign. An X-ray, CT and MRI are all useful in the late remodelling phase.

Caterall grading:

– stage I: histological and clinical diagnosis without radiological findings

– stage II: sclerosis with or without cystic changes with preservation of the contour and surface of the femoral head

– stage III: loss of structural integrity of the femoral head

– stage IV: loss of structural integrity of the acetabulum in addition.

5. Differential diagnoses for unilateral disease: septic hip, toxic synovitis, slipped femoral capital epiphysis, metaphyseal dysplasia, spondyloepiphyseal dysplasia, eosinophilic granuloma, haemophilia, overtreated developmental dysplasia and lymphoma. Differential diagnoses for bilateral disease: hypothyroidism, multiple epiphyseal dysplasia, spondyloepiphyseal dysplasia and sickle cell disease.

6. Prognosis depends on extent, age and sex of child. It is poor in children > 9 years, worse for girls (reduced remaining growth potential) and when it involves the entire femoral epiphysis. Deformities and secondary degeneration are the complications.

Case 4.35: Answers

1. The X-ray of the spine shows narrowing of the interpedun cular distance in the lumbar spine. The iliac wings are short and square. There is shortening of the long bones in the leg with a short and broad femoral neck. In the hands, the bones are short and pointed.

2. Achondroplasia.

3. Achondroplasia is an autosomal dominant disease that results in rhizomelic (proximal limb) dwarfism. It is the most common cause of short-limbed disproportionate dwarfism. The affected patients have short toes and fingers, a large head with a prominent forehead, small midface with flattened nasal bridge, spinal kyphosis and lordosis, genus varus (bow leg) or genu valgus (knock knee). Delayed motor development is seen with the standing height below the third percentile. The autosomal dominant mutation is seen in the fibroblast growth factor receptor gene 3, which results in abnormal cartilage formation.

4. Radiological findings include a large skull with narrow foramen magnum and small skull base. The primary radiological criteria for diagnosis are: decrease in interpeduncular distance in the lumbar spine (in normal people, the interpeduncular distance progressively increases downwards), short square iliac wings, short and broad neck of femur, shortening of long tubular bones and brachydactyly. Secondary features include anteroposterior shortening of lumbar pedicles, dorsal concavity of lumbar vertebrae, long distal fibula, short distal ulna and long ulnar styloid. A

CT scan can be used to assess the spinal deformities. MRI is very useful in assessing cervicomedullary compression, and can also show myelomalacia, intramedullary cyst, angulation at the craniocervical junction and spinal stenosis. MRI of the brain shows hydrocephalus and other abnormalities. Phase contrast CSF flow studies can be used to assess flow across the aqueduct and quantify hydrocephalus. Prenatal ultrasonography can identify short-limbed dwarfism.

5. Complications include recurrent otitis media (poor drainage of eustachian tubes as a result of midface hypoplasia, hypertrophied tonsils and temporal bone abnormalities), complications resulting from cervicomedullary compression (hypotonia, respiratory insufficiency, apnoea, cyanotic episodes, feeding problems, quadriparesis, sudden death), hydrocephalus, obstructive and restrictive respiratory complications, spinal deformities, obesity, spinal canal stenosis (low backache, neurogenic claudication, paraesthesia, paraparesis, incontinence), lower extremity radiculopathy (caused by nerve root compression or cauda equina syndrome), genu varum and cardiovascular complications. Under 25 years, CNS and respiratory complications are the common cause of death. Over 25 years, death results from cardiovascular causes. Recombinant growth hormone and limb-lengthening procedures are used to address dwarfism. Orthopaedic procedures are done for correction of spinal deformities, spinal stenosis, foramen magnum narrowing and genu valgum/varum. Ventriculoperitoneal shunts are placed in severe hydrocephalus with macrocephaly.

Case 4.36: Answers

1. The X-ray shows a rib arising from the seventh cervical vertebra on both sides.

2. Cervical rib with thoracic outlet syndrome.

3. Cervical rib is seen in 0.2–2.0% of the population and is common in females. It is usually asymptomatic, but can produce thoracic outlet syndrome.

4. The rib can be a complete or incomplete type, bony or fibrous, unilateral or bilateral. Radiologically the differential diagnosis includes a hypertrophied transverse process of the C7 or a hypoplastic first thoracic rib. The rib may fuse with the first rib anteriorly and the adjacent transverse process is angulated inferiorly. It can be associated with Klippel–Feil syndrome. Other investigations such as a venogram, arteriogram or duplex ultrasonography may be required to assess for vascular compression.

5. Usually cervical ribs are asymptomatic, but they can produce thoracic outlet syndrome as a result of elevation of the floor or scalene triangle with a decrease of costoclavicular space. Of those with thoracic outlet syndrome 10–20% have cervical rib; 5–10% of those with complete cervical rib have symptoms. Thoracic outlet syndrome presents with neurological, venous or arterial symptoms. Neurological symptoms involve the nerve roots C8, T1 or the upper three nerve roots, C5, C6 and C7. Pain is present in the medial aspect of the arm, forearm, ring and small digits, and there are paraesthesiae, loss of dexterity, cold intolerance and headache. Claudication with arm activity is the vascular complication. The elevated arm stress test is the most reliable test. The patient sits with the arms abducted 90° from the thorax and elbows flexed 90°. Then the patient opens and closes the hands for 3 min. Those with the syndrome have reproduction of symptoms in these 3 min. Tenderness, sensory loss, weakness, oedema, cyanosis, pallor, pulselessness and low blood pressures are other clinical features. A cervical rib is found in most arterial cases, and it is resected if it is found to cause thoracic outlet syndrome.

Case 4.37: Answers

1. The X-ray of the spine shows a dorsolumbar scoliosis concave to the right side. There are multiple abnormal, split vertebrae in the spine.

2. The coronal CT scan and three-dimensional coronal CT scan sections show a vertically split midthoracic vertebra.

3. Butterfly vertebra. This is one of the types of segmentation anomalies of the spine. A normal spine has two centres of ossification for the bodies, a dorsal and ventral, which are formed in weeks 9–12.

4. Types of segmentation anomalies of vertebral bodies:

   Butterfly vertebra: failure of fusion of the lateral halves of vertebral bodies, as a result of the persistence of notochordal tissue.

The vertebrae are widened. The AP view shows a split vertebra with a butterfly configuration. It is associated with spina bifida, meningocele, diastomatomyelia, the foregut and cardiac anomalies.

Block vertebra: congenital fusion of vertebrae, common in lumbar or cervical region, in which the height of the fused vertebrae is the sum of the individual vertebrae and discs. There is a waist at the level of the disc space. Differential diagnoses: acquired fusion of infection and ankylosing spondylitis.

Klippel–Feil syndrome: block vertebrae, Sprengel's shoulder.

Hypoplastic vertebrae.

Asomia: absence of vertebral bodies; posterior elements can be seen.

Hemivertebrae: unilateral wedge vertebra (right and left hemivertebrae), dorsal hemivertebrae, ventral hemivertebra.

Coronal cleft: failure of fusion of anterior and posterior ossification centres, best seen in lateral view; seen in preterm males, chondrodysplasia punctata.

---

5. The most common differential diagnosis is a fracture. The presence of a smooth corticated margin in the absence of a history of trauma favours a segmentation anomaly. The disease is longstanding.

---

6. They are usually asymptomatic and require no treatment. Severe cases of deformity and pain require surgical stabilisation.

Case 4.38: Answers

1. The X-ray of the right hand shows multiple lucent lesions with calcifications involving most of the phalanges and some of the metacarpals. There are multiple areas of calcification in the soft tissue between the joints. There is a large soft-tissue swelling in the ulnar aspect of the joint.

---

2. Mafucci syndrome: multiple enchondromas with haemangioma.

---

3. Enchondromas are benign cartilaginous tumours in the medullary cavity. They are caused by derangement of cartilaginous growth, which results in migration of cartilaginous rests from the epiphyseal plate to the medullary cavity in the metaphysis, where they proliferate. It is usually unilateral and monomelic and can be local, regional or generalised. Multiple enchondromas may occur in three distinct disorders:

Ollier's disease: non-hereditary, multiple enchondromas, unilateral

Maffucci syndrome: non-hereditary, multiple enchondromas and haemangioma

Metachondromatosis: multiple enchondromas and osteochondromas, autosomal dominant transmission.

---

4. Enchondromas are seen in the 20- to 40-year age group. They are very common in the small bones of the hands and feet, with most in the proximal phalanx. Other locations are the shoulder, pelvis and long bones. They are seen in the diaphysis of short tubular bones and the metaphysis of longer bones. On X-rays, enchondromas are seen as oval or round areas of geographical destruction with a lobulated contour. The characteristic feature is ring- and arc-type matrix mineralisation. The enchondromas are larger in Ollier's disease. There is shortening of bone as a result of an impaired epiphyseal fusion. Deformities and limb length discrepancy are seen. Metaphyseal expansion, thinning of cortex and endosteal scalloping are also seen. Haemangiomas in Maffucci syndrome produce phleboliths, which are seen as calcifications with central lucencies on X-rays. The osteochondromas in metachondromatosis point towards the joint, unlike the conventional osteochondromas. Cortical breakthrough, soft-tissue mass and deep endosteal scalloping (in long bones) indicate development of chondrosarcoma. CT and MRI are also helpful in diagnosis and differentiation from other lesions.

---

5. Bone infarct (serpiginous rind of sclerosis around the lesion) and exostoses (point away from joint); chondrosarcoma (low-grade chondrosarcoma difficult to differentiate from enchondroma; normal X-ray does not exclude chondrosarcoma).

---

6. Pathological fractures and malignant transformation are the main complications. The incidence of malignancy is 1–2% in solitary enchondromas. In Ollier's disease and Maffucci syndrome, the incidence is 25–50%. Malignancy is seen in the long bones and flat bones and is uncommon in the hands and feet. Osteosarcoma, chondrosarcoma and fibrosarcoma are the malignant tumours. In Mafucci syndrome, haemangiomas can also undergo sarcomatous transformation, and are associated with a granulosa cell tumour of the ovary. There is increased prevalence of ovarian carcinoma, pancreatic carcinoma, CNS glioma and gastrointestinal adenocarcinoma in Mafucci syndrome.

Case 4.39: Answers

1. The X-ray of the right leg shows a well-defined, oval, multiloculated lesion in the tibia with a sclerotic rim and endosteal scalloping. There is no periosteal reaction or soft-tissue swelling.

2. Non-ossifying fibroma.

3. Non-ossifying fibroma is a benign non-aggressive tumour that is composed of spindle-shaped fibroblasts, with a storiform whorled pattern and scattered giant cells, foam cells and collagen. It is seen between age 8 and 20 years. A fibrous cortical defect also has similar appearance, but it is seen in younger patients. Common sites are the femur, proximal and distal tibia, and knee. They are seen in metaphysis, close to the physeal plate.

4. Non-ossifying fibroma is usually seen around the knee joint, in the metaphysis, arising eccentrically within the medullary cavity, from the posterior wall of tubular bone. The X-ray shows a well-defined, oval/round, lucent lesion, with the long axis along the long axis of bone, with sclerotic rim, endosteal scalloping and cortical thinning. Large tumours are multilocular. The epiphysis is never affected. A bone scan shows mild uptake. MRI shows a hypointense lesion in T1 and T2. If there are lot of histiocytes, it is hypointense in T1 and hyperintense in T2. Contrast enhancement is seen. Complications are fractures and hypophosphataemic rickets.

5. Jaffe–Campanacci syndrome consists of non-ossifying fibromas, learning disability, hypogonadism, CVS defects and café-au-lait spots. No specific treatment is required for non-ossifying fibromas and fibrous cortical defects. The latter persist without complications and eventually become non-ossifying fibromas. Large asymptomatic non-ossifying fibromas can be treated with curettage and bone grafting.

6. Differential diagnoses for non-ossifying fibromas (NOFs – > 3 cm, eccentric, intramedullary abutting cortex, superficial scalloping pattern in cortex, can continue into adulthood) are fibrous cortical defects, which are similar to non-ossifying fibroma but smaller (< 3 cm), and asymptomatic, eccentrically located, metaphyseal, cortical defects, which disappear spontaneously. A common location is the posteromedial aspect of the distal femoral cortex along the medial supracondylar ridge

just proximal to the adductor tubercle. Other differential diagnoses are adamantinoma (older age group, tibia), chondromyxoid fibroma (cortical bulge), fibrous dysplasia, aneurysmal bone cyst, intraosseus ganglion and giant cell tumour.

Case 4.40: Answers

1. AP and oblique X-rays of the hand show an oblique lucency running through the metaphysis of the proximal phalanx, extending into the growth plate, resulting in a triangular fragment.

2. Salter Harris Type II fracture of the phalanx. This is the most common type of Salter Harris fractures, accounting for 75% of cases.

3. The cartilaginous growth plate of the paediatric skeleton separates metaphysis and epiphysis. The germinal layer for the growth plate is contiguous with the epiphysis and is supplied by epiphyseal vessels. Injuries to the growth plate heal rapidly except when the epiphyseal blood supply or germinal layer has been damaged. Of the layers of growth plate, the resting cartilage, proliferating cartilage and zone of provisional calcification have a strong matrix that resists shearing force. The zone of hypertrophying cartilage is the weakest one and vulnerable to shearing injuries. The cartilaginous growth plate is weaker in children than the capsule and ligaments, so any force that produces sprain or dislocation in adults causes growth plate injury in children.

4. **Salter–Harris** classification of epiphyseal injuries:

   Type 1: slip of epiphysis

   Type 2: fracture line through physis and metaphysis, separating a triangular metaphyseal fragment

   Type 3: fracture in epiphysis extending to the physis

   Type 4: fracture involving metaphysis, physis and epiphysis

   Type 5: crush injury of physis

   Rang–Ogdens additions:

   Type 6: injury to perichondrial structures

   Type 7: isolated injury to epiphyseal plate

Type 8: isolated injury to the metaphysis, with potential injury related to endochondral ossification

Type 9: periosteal injury interfering with membranous growth.

5. Type 2 epiphyseal injuries need closed reduction and immobilisation to avoid damage to the cartilage that might hinder growth or produce deformity, depending on the extent of involvement. Damage to either the epiphyseal or the metaphyseal vascular supply disrupts bone growth, but the damage to the cartilage layer may not be significant if the surfaces are reapposed and vascular supply is not permanently interrupted.

Case 4.41: Answers

1. The X-ray of the forearm and wrist shows ulnar angulation of the distal radius. The radius appears foreshortened and there appears to be premature fusion of the ulnar aspect of the radial epiphysis.

2. Madelung's deformity.

3. Madelung's deformity of the wrist is characterised by a growth disturbance in the volar and ulnar aspect of distal radial physis, which results in a volar and ulnar tilted distal radial articular surface, volar translation of the hand and wrist, and a dorsally prominent distal ulna.

4. Madelung's deformity can be primary/idiopathic or secondary to Turner syndrome, Hurler syndrome, Leri–Weil syndrome of dyschondrosteosis, osteochondromatosis, Ollier's disease, achondroplasia, multiple epiphyseal dysplasia, trauma, infection, sickle cell disease and rickets. It can be transmitted in an autosomal dominant inheritance in a third. It is bilateral in 50% and more common in girls. Although it is congenital, clinically it does not manifest until late childhood or early adolescence. Insidious onset of pain in one wrist and then the other, increasing prominence of the dorsal ulnar head and bowing of the distal radius are common features. The wrist appears subluxed as a result of the presence of normal distal ulna. It is bilateral in two-thirds. Extension and supination are limited at the wrist.

5. The features of Madelung's deformity are ulnar angulation of the distal radius, decreased carpal angle, dorsal subluxation of the ulna, lateral and dorsal curvature of the radius, widened interosseous space, true shortening of the

total length of the radius, premature fusion of the ulnar half of the distal-radial physis, focal osteopenia in the area of the ulnar portion of the distal radius, exostosis at the distal-ulnar border of the radius, triangularisation of the distal-radial epiphysis, ulnar and palmar facing the distal-radial articular surface, relative dorsal subluxation of the ulna, increased radiodensity of the ulnar head and carpal wedging with the lunate at the apex of the wedge. An arched curvature of the carpal bones in direct continuation of the dorsal bowing of the radius is seen on the lateral radiograph. In some cases, there is atrophy of the radial head and hypertrophy of the capitellum. Pain usually subsides at maturity, but there is recurrence of pain when the deformity is stabilised and joint surfaces become incongruent. Ulnar shortening or radial osteotomy is done in severe cases.

Case 4.42: Answers

1. The plain film of the hip shows coxa valga (increased femoral neck-shaft angle), with subluxation and increased femoral anteversion. The bones are osteopenic and gracile. There is reduction of the soft tissue.

2. Neuropathic changes in the bones.

3. Cerebral palsy. This is a CNS disorder with motor impairment. Spastic diplegia is the most common presentation. Preterm delivery, low birthweight, asphyxia, infection, placental infarction and occlusion of cerebral vessels are causes of cerebral palsy. Loss of supraspinal inhibition leads to spasticity, motor weakness, impaired sensory perception, and muscle and joint contractures. The most commonly affected muscles are paraspinal muscles, hip flexors, hip adductors, hamstrings, gastrocnemius and soleus.

4. In the spine, thoracic kyphosis, lumbar lordosis, spondylolisthesis, spondylolysis, scoliosis and pelvic obliquity are seen. In the hips, progressive hip flexion and adduction lead to:

Scissor gait: bilateral adduction hip deformity

Windswept deformity: adduction contracture of one hip and abduction contracture of other hip

Increased femoral anteversion (angle between a line through the axis of femoral head and neck and a plane through femoral condyles; normal 8–15°)

Coxa valga, which is an increase in the femoral neck-shaft angle (angle between the midaxis of the shaft of a line along the midaxis of the femoral head and neck; normal 125–130°)

Subluxation – superolaterally

Dislocation

Deformed femoral head: medial or lateral flattening

Pseudoacetabulum along lateral margin of ileum.

In knee, flexion contracture, patella alta, patellar fragmentation and genu recurvatum are seen. In the foot, rocker-bottom deformity, equinovalgus, equinovarus and subluxation of the talonavicular joint are noted.

5. Treatment is prevention of adduction and flexion deformity and progression to subluxation. Stretching spastic agonist muscles and strengthening weaker antagonist muscles, abduction splinting, tenotomy, neurectomy and varus derotation osteotomy are all treatment options. Differential diagnosis includes San Filippo-type mucopoysaccharidosis.

Case 4.43: Answers

1. There is a transverse lucency along the proximal aspect of the fifth metatarsal bone; the other bones and joints are normal.

2. Fracture of the fifth metatarsal bone.

3. The fifth metatarsal bone is the most common site of mid-foot fractures. There are two types of fractures in this location:

Jones' fracture: transverse fracture at the base of the fifth metatarsal, 1.5–3 cm distal to the proximal tuberosity. This fracture is notorious for non-union and gets displaced with progressive weight bearing

Pseudo-Jones' fracture/tennis fracture: this is more common. Avulsion injury at the proximal tuberosity is caused by lateral ankle strain at the site of the peroneus brevis tendon.

4. Pseudo-Jones' fracture heals well with compression dressing and weight bearing is tolerated. Jones' fracture gets easily displaced by weight bearing and non-union is very common. Initial treatment is with immobilisation and non-weight bearing. Non-union requires internal fixation and bone grafting.

5. The most common diagnostic difficulty in this location is the presence of an apophysis. A secondary ossification centre is seen at the base of the fifth metatarsal (apophysis), which can be seen in girls aged 9–11 years and boys aged 11–14 years. This centre is always longitudinal and parallel to the base of the fifth metatarsal and should not be confused with a fracture, which is always transverse. In addition the apophysis is smooth and well corticated.

Case 4.44: Answers

1. AP X-ray shows compression of the distal aspect of the radius and ulna. In the lateral X-ray, there is buckling of the dorsal cortex of radius, with intact volar cortex. The distal fragment is angulated dorsally. There is also buckling of the distal ulna, but to a lesser extent.

2. Torus fracture of the distal radius and ulna.

3. A fall on outstretched hands is the common mechanism of torus fracture of the radius. Torus (protuberance in Latin) is unique to children, because of weakness of immature mineralisation of bone. When compressive force is placed on a tubular bone's long axis, the axial stress on the bone causes a buckling reaction, characterised by failure of cortex on the compression side, 2–3 cm proximal to the physis.

4. Torus fractures of the distal metaphysis of the radius and ulna are the most common fractures in the lower forearm in young children. The impact of indirect violence of a fall on an outstretched hand crumples the dorsal cortex, but the volar cortex is intact. The distal fragment is angulated dorsally. There is no deformity in torus fracture because the periosteum and cortex are intact on the opposite side of the bone. To summarise, in torus fracture the tension side (anterior) is intact. If the fracture is not on the compression side, the patient has a greenstick fracture, which will result in deformity. In a greenstick fracture, there is failure of the cortex on the tension side (convex side of angulation) with plastic deformation of the cortex on the concave side (compression side). A lateral view of the wrist is important for diagnosis.

5. Treatment consists of a short arm cast for 3 weeks to make the patient comfortable and prevent further injury. As a result of the compressive forces on the radius and the proximity of the radius and ulna, there is often involvement of the ulna, which will result in deformity of a thinner, longer ulna – greenstick fracture. There is pronation–supination carrying of the affected arm. Treatment is to reverse the torsional mechanism of injury, ie pronating the fracture with palmar angulation of the bone and supinating the dorsally angulated bone.

Case 4.45: Answers

1. The X-ray of the knee shows expansion of the epiphysis and metaphysis, with coarse trabeculations and widening of the intercondylar notch. The X-ray of the pelvis shows a large, expansile, lucent lesion in the right iliac bone, with no periosteal reaction or fracture.

2. Haemophilic joint with haemophilic pseudotumour in the pelvis.

3. Haemophilia is an X-linked disorder with deficiency of coagulation factor VIII. Haemophilic arthropathy is caused by repeated bleeding into a joint, which results in reactive pannus formation that erodes bone. It is seen in the first and second decades.

4. Haemophilic arthropathy is common in knee joints. Ankle joints, elbows and shoulders are also affected. The changes are bilateral. There is haemarthrosis, enlarged epiphysis (synovial hyperaemia), juxta-articular osteoporosis and widening of the intercondylar notch. Erosions, joint space narrowing, subchondral cysts and osteophytes are seen. In the knee, bulbous femoral condyles, widening of the intercondylar notch, flattening of condylar surfaces, genu valgum, slanted tibial plateaus, squared patella and contracted hamstrings are noted. MRI shows hypertrophied synovium, haemorrhage and erosions. Haemophilic pseudotumour is seen in the hip. It is a haemorrhagic cystic swelling in bone or muscle. It produces a multiloculated expansile lesion in flat bones, with bony destruction, soft-tissue extension and pathological fracture. MRI shows haemorrhage in varying stages. CT shows a mass with a high density and destruction.

5. Widening of the intercondylar notch is also caused by juvenile rheumatoid arthritis (JRA), haemophilia, gout, TB, synovial osteochondromatosis and synovial haemangioma. The combination of intercondylar notch widening and a widened epiphysis is seen only in haemophilia and JRA. An expansile lesion such as the pseudotumour can also be caused by giant cell tumour, aneurysmal bone cyst, plasmacytoma, hydatid cyst and a brown tumour of hyperparathyroidism.

Case 4.46: Answers

1. There is varus angulation of the tibia in the proximal metaphysis.

2. Blount's disease.

3. Blount's disease (tibia vara) is disordered ossification of the medial aspect of the proximal tibial physis, epiphysis and metaphysis, resulting in varus angulation and internal rotation of the tibia in the proximal metaphyseal region immediately below the knee. It is caused by biomechanical overload of the posteromedial proximal tibial physis as a result of static varus alignment and excessive body weight on the epiphysis, leading to growth suppression. Abnormal axial loading also results in a change in direction of the weight-bearing forces from the perpendicular to the oblique. The oblique angle tends to displace the tibial epiphysis in a lateral direction, overloading the posteromedial segment and inhibiting its growth Predisposing factors for the development of the condition include obesity and early walking. It is more common in African–Caribbean individuals.

4. There are three types: **early onset** (< 3 years), **juvenile** (4–10 years) and **adolescent** (> 11 years). Children with infantile tibia vara present with bowing and length discrepancy in the lower limbs. A non-tender bony protuberance can be palpated along the medial aspect of the proximal tibia; 80% of infantile and 50% of juvenile cases are bilateral.

5. A standing AP film of both legs shows bowing and an abnormal medial proximal tibial metaphysis. On a lateral X-ray, a posteriorly directed projection is seen at the proximal tibial metaphysis. The femoral–tibial angle helps confirm the varus position of the leg, but it can be misleading secondary to the rotation of the leg, which may be positional or result from a coexisting rotational abnormality. The metaphyseal–diaphyseal angle is obtained by measuring the angle formed between a line drawn parallel to the top of the proximal tibial metaphysis and another drawn perpendicular to the long axis of the shaft of the tibia. Angles > 20°

confirm true tibia vara in children, whereas angles of 15–20° may or may not indicate tibia vara. Another angle used is the tibial metaphyseal–metaphyseal angle. This angle is larger than the metaphyseal–diaphyseal angle in children with the most marked bowing and indicates distal tibial bowing in severe cases. There is a six-stage classification proposed by Langenskiold. Patients in stages 3–6 require surgical correction.

6. Differential diagnoses include physiological bowing, congenital bowing, rickets, Ollier's disease, trauma, osteomyelitis and metaphyseal chondrodysplasia. Physiological bowing involves both the tibia and the fibula and is a gradual curve. Congenital bowing occurs in the mid-tibia. Rickets affects other parts of the skeleton with biochemical abnormalities and loss of a zone of provisional calcification. Ollier's disease has multiple enchondromas in addition to the bowing. Metaphyseal dysplasia affects multiple metaphyses, with no biochemical abnormalities. Extreme physiological bowing may cause false-positive results.

Case 4.47: Answers

1. The anterior humeral line is seen intersecting anterior to the posterior third of the capitellum. The radiocapitellar line is not intersecting the centre of the capitellum. There is a fracture line seen in the distal humerus.

2. Supracondylar fracture of the humerus.

3. Fall on to outstretched hands with hyperextended elbows or with flexed elbows resulting in vertical stress is the mechanism for supracondylar fracture. This is the most common elbow fracture in children aged < 10 years. There are two broad types: **extension** (95%); **flexion** – **type I** is undisplaced, **type II** displaced with intact cortex and **type III** complete displacement.

4. A proper AP view of the elbow should be performed with the forearm in supination and the elbow in extension. Assess for the ossification centres. Look for the following things in the lateral view:

   Anterior fat pad displacement: anterior fat pad can be seen as a lucent area in the anterior aspect of the distal humerus, even in normal individuals. It is displaced anteriorly and superiorly when there is elbow effusion.

Posterior fat pad: posterior fat pad is over the olecranon fossa and is not normally seen. Visualisation of posterior fat pad indicates haemarthrosis secondary to intra-articular fracture.

Anterior humeral line: this line is drawn along the anterior surface of the distal humerus and in normal individuals intersects the middle third of the capitellum. In supracondylar fracture with posterior displacement of the fragments, the line intersects the anterior third of the capitellum or passes completely anterior to the capitellum.

Radiocapitellar line: a line drawn along the central axis of the radius should intersect the centre of the capitellum. If this line does not transect the middle of the capitellum, it indicates radial neck fracture or radial head dislocation.

Fracture lines: transverse fracture lines can be seen. The distal fragment is posteriorly displaced.

5. Suspected supracondylar fractures are initially splinted in 20° of elbow flexion pending evaluation. Closed reduction under anaesthesia is the definitive treatment. Percutaneous pin fixation is indicated for type II fractures and most type III fractures. Open reduction is indicated when closed reduction fails to achieve adequate alignment or with vascular injuries.

Case 4.48: Answers

1. The X-ray of the foot shows equinus deformity at the ankle joint and plantar flexion. There is also varus deformity in the hindfoot (medial deviation) and adduction at the level of metatarsal.

2. Congenital talipes equinovarus.

3. Congenital talipes equinovarus is characterised by hindfoot fixed plantar flexion (equinus) and varus (calcaneovarus) and forefoot varus. It is caused by interruption in the foot's development after 9 weeks' gestation. It is more common in boys and associated with early amniocentesis.

4. In a normal foot, the position of the talus is fixed. The calcaneum is in 10° valgus from midline. The talocalcaneal angle is between the long axis of the talus and the long axis of the calcaneum. The normal angle is 50° in newborns and 15-40° at 4 years. The line through the long axis of talus intersects the base of the first metatarsal. In talipes equinovarus, the talocalcaneal angle is reduced (< 25°) with talus and calcaneum approximating. The line through the talus passes lateral to the first metatarsal. The calcaneum is also plantar flexed, calcaneotibial angle > 90°. In the lateral view the fifth metatarsal is the most plantar.

5. Congenital talipes equinovarus is associated with arthrogryposis multiplex congenita, spina bifida, chrondrodysplasia punctata, neurofibromatosis and myelomeningocele. Treatment depends on the age at presentation and the severity of deformities. If the presentation is immediately after birth, Ponseti's method of serial manipulations and plaster casting is done. If there is no response and there are residual deformities, surgical correction of deformities is done. This involves surgical release of tendons/ligaments, tendon transfers or osteotomy/arthrodesis.

Case 4.49: Answers

1. MRI of the thighs shows bilateral diffuse increased signal intensity within the thigh muscles.

2. The clinical features and MRI findings are suggestive of dermatomyositis/ pyomyositis.

3. Blood test for muscle enzymes, EMG (electromyography) and muscle biopsy are required for confirmation. As dermatomyositis can be a paraneoplastic syndrome an X-ray of the chest is required to exclude bronchogenic neoplasm (which is rare in children). Gastroscopy, colonoscopy and barium studies may also be required.

4. Dermatomyositis is an idiopathic inflammatory myopathy with characteristic cutaneous findings. Diagnostic criteria are progressive proximal symmetrical weakness, elevated muscle enzymes, abnormal findings on EMG and muscle biopsy, and cutaneous disease. The characteristic feature is a heliotrope rash, which is a violaceous or dusky erythematous rash seen symmetrically in the periorbital region, and Gottron's papules, which are violaceous papules usually seen over the dorsum of the hand and extensor surfaces, but also in the feet, elbows or knees. Proximal muscle weakness is a characteristic feature. Muscle tenderness can be occasionally be seen. Calcinosis, myocarditis, pulmonary fibrosis, arthritis and dysphagia are other features resulting from multisystemic involvement. Creatine kinase is elevated, as are aldolase, LDH and antimyosin antibodies.

5. MRI is useful for confirming diagnosis and selecting a site for biopsy. On MRI, there is symmetrical high signal in proximal muscles. T1-weighted and STIR (fat suppression) images are acquired in the axial and coronal planes. A high signal in STIR indicates myositis and biopsy is done in areas showing maximum areas of inflammation. The muscle signal decreases after initiation of steroid therapy. Low signal in T1 and atrophy of muscles are seen in chronic involvement.

Case 4.50: Answers

1. The X-ray of the wrist shows diffuse osteopenia in all the bones. The X-ray of the right knee joint shows widened epiphysis and metaphysis and prominent intercondylar notch.

2. Juvenile rheumatoid arthritis.

3. JRA is seen in children under 16 years and is common in girls. There are many clinical types:

   Juvenile onset, adult type: 8–10 years, RA factor positive, poor prognosis, erosive changes and extensive periosteal reaction, protrusio acetabuli

   Polyarthritis of ankylosing spondylitis type: boys, 9–11 years, peripheral arthritis, fused bones, greater trochanter, heel spur, iridocyclitis

   Still's disease: systemic (fever, rash, lymphadenopathy, hepatosplenomegaly, pericarditis)/polyarticular/pauciarticular; common in caropometacarpal joints, girls, age 2–4 and 8-–11 years; periosteal reaction in phalanges, broad bones, early maturation and fusion.

4. Juvenile arthritis involves large joints such as the hips, knees, ankles, wrists and elbows. Periarticular soft-tissue swelling, late onset of bony changes, thinned cartilage, ballooned-out and widened epiphysis and metaphysis, juxta-articular osteoporosis, erosions, cyst-like lesions away from the joint line and ankylosis are the radiological features. In the cervical spine, there is decreased size of bodies, atlantoaxial subluxation, and fractures and ankylosis of the sacroiliac joint. In chest pleural and pericardial effusion, lung nodules are seen.

5. Differential diagnoses: **haemophilia** – expansion of joint space, wide epiphysis; septic arthritis – joint destruction, joint space narrowing.

Case 4.51: Answers

1. The X-ray of the skull shows dense bone with expansion of diploic space with hair-on-end appearance.

2. Thalassaemia.

3. Differential diagnoses for hair-on-end appearance: thalassaemia, sickle cell disease, hereditary spherocytosis, glucose-6-phosphate dehydrogenase deficiency, iron deficiency anaemia, haemangioma, neuroblastoma and osteosarcoma.

4. Thalassaemia major is an inherited disorder of haemoglobin synthesis. Normal adult haemoglobin has two α and two β chains. In α-thalassaemia there is a deficiency of α chains and in β-thalassaemia there is a deficiency of β chains. Thalassaemia major is the major form and is homozygous. Clinical presentation is retarded growth, retarded secondary sexual characters, pigmented skin, high bilirubin, high uric acid, hypochromic/microcytic anaemia, thrombocytopenia and leukopenia.

5. Radiological features of thalassaemia:

   Skull: the diploic spaces are widened with thinned cortex, coarse trabeculations, hair-on-end appearance in frontal bones, frontal bossing, opacified maxillary sinuses caused by marrow hyperplasia, narrow nasal cavity

   Appendicular skeleton: expansion of marrow, cortical thinning, osteopenia and premature epiphyseal fusion; bone lesions are less with systemic blood transfusion (secondary haemosiderosis is a complication); pathological fracture is a complication

   Chest: cardiomegaly, posterior mediastinal mass caused by extramedullary haematopoiesis

   Ribs: widening of ribs, rib-within-rib appearance

   Abdomen: hepatosplenomegaly, gallstones.

Case 4.52: Answers

1. The X-ray of the cervical spine shows discontinuity of the base of the odontoid process from the rest of the C2 vertebral body.

2. Odontoid fracture, type 2.

3. Odontoid fractures constitute 15% of all cervical spinal fractures. They are caused by a combination of flexion, extension and rotation. Types of odontoid fractures (Anderson and D'Alonzo classification):

   Type 1: fracture of tip of the odontoid – 5% – stable; avulsion of alar ligament; unstable if associated with occipitoatlantal dislocation

   Type 2: transverse fracture of the base of the odontoid at the attachment to body of C2 – most common type – 60%; when the dens is displaced, C1–dens– transverse ligament complex is intact

   Type 3: subdental fracture extending through the body of C2 – 30% – unstable.

   Other types are a vertical fracture through the odontoid and the body of the axis, which is a variant of C2 spondylolisthesis.

   Pain, inability to move the neck, sensation of instability and quadriplegia are the presenting features. They can be associated with injuries to the atlas, transverse ligament or pharynx.

4. Type 1 is difficult to detect; type 2 can be missed on axial CT. Hence CT is usually done in an axial plane and images are reconstructed in sagittal and coronal planes to assess fractures in all planes. Non-union is common in type 2 and is more common if there is comminution at the base of the odontoid, older age, displacement > 2 mm, posterior displacement, delay in diagnosis and redislocation. Prognosis is good for type 3. Type 1 is treated with a semi-rigid collar. Type 2 fractures are managed with a halo vest if it is mild. Posterior atlantoaxial arthrodesis or anterior screw fixation can be done. Type 3 is unstable and heals well with immobilisation. Anterior screw fixation can be done.

5. Differential diagnoses: os odontoideum, ossiculum terminale, hypoplastic odontoid process and aplastic odontoid process.

Case 4.53: Answers

1. The X-ray shows massively deformed bones in both legs. The bones are osteopenic and there are multiple fractures with callus formation.

2. Osteogenesis imperfecta tarda.

3. Osteogenesis imperfecta is a connective tissue disorder, which is characterised by micromelic dwarfism, bone fragility, blue sclera and abnormal dentition. The clinical types are osteogenesis imperfecta congenita (at birth, autosomal dominant, type II, lethal) and osteogenesis imperfecta tarda (not at birth, sporadic, types I and IV, non-lethal).

   Sillence classification

Type	Features	Inheritance
I	Normal stature, minimal deformity, blue sclera, hearing loss, dentition abnormal	AD
II	Perinatal, osteopenic calvaria, beaded ribs, compressed femurs, long bone deformities, platyspondyly; lethal	AD, mosaic
III	Progressively deforming, sclera lightens with age, hearing loss, abnormal dentition, short stature	AD, AR, mosaic
IV	Mild deformity, variable short stature, hearing loss, abnormal dentition, variable sclera	AD, mosaic
V	Similar to type IV, hypertrophic callus, dense metaphyseal bands, interosseus membrane ossification; unique histology	Unknown
VI	Similar to type IV; unique histological features	Unknown

4. The characteristic radiological features are decreased skull ossification, wormian bones, normal vertebrae, normal pelvis, short and bowed long bones, progressive deformities of limbs and spine into adulthood, rib fractures and multiple fractures with exuberant callus formation.

5. Complications are hearing loss and death from intracranial haemorrhage. Differential diagnoses are achondrogenesis, congenital hypophosphatasia and campopelic dysplasia.

Case 4.54: Answers

1. The X-ray of the spine shows narrowing of the disc space at T9–10 with irregular end-plates. There is paravertebral soft-tissue swelling on both sides. MRI shows narrowing of the disc space with irregular end-plates and there is soft tissue in the epidural space. In the axial plane, the soft-tissue mass is seen in the paravertebral region.

2. Tuberculous spondylitis.

3. Tuberculous spondylitis is caused by *Mycobacterium tuberculosis.* The infection reaches the vertebrae usually by haematogenous spread via Batson's plexus. Infection spreads to adjacent vertebrae in the subligamentous space beneath the anterior and posterior longitudinal ligaments. Contiguous spread occurs through the subchondral plate into the disc space.

4. Spinal TB is common in the lower thoracic and upper lumbar vertebrae, with L1 being the most common vertebra. In the vertebrae, it starts in the anterior aspect of the body adjacent to the superior or inferior end-plate, from where it spreads to the other parts. Clinically TB spine presents with backache, stiffness and tenderness. No chest lesion is seen in 50% of individuals.

5. The characteristic features of tuberculous spondylitis are narrowing of disc space and irregular end-plates. Collapse of a vertebral body leads to gibbus, kyphotic deformity and vertebra plana. Paravertebral extension causes widening of the paravertebral soft-tissue opacity. Calcification can be seen. Bone density is decreased in chronic cases. Ivory vertebrae are seen during the healing phase. A CT scan shows a destructive, stippled bone pattern in the vertebrae, with calcified paravertebral soft tissue. MRI is very sensitive and accurate in characterising and evaluating the disease extent. The lesion is centred in the subchondral region, with end-plate irregularity. The lesion is low in T1 and high in T2. Abscess can be seen in the epidural space or paravertebral space, which shows rim enhancement and calcification. Differential diagnoses are **pyogenic spondylitis** (rapid destruction, no calcification of abscess rim, posterior elements not involved, little new bone formation), **tumour** (multiple lesions, non-contiguous, no disc destruction, no soft-tissue abscess), **brucellosis** (minimal paraspinal mass, lower lumbar spine, gas within disc) and **sarcoidosis**.

Case 4.55: Answers

1. The X-ray of the legs shows extensive bilateral lamellated periosteal reaction with soft-tissue swelling. There is also narrowing of the medulla.

2. Caffey's disease (infantile cortical hyperostosis).

3. Infantile cortical hyperostosis is an inflammatory disorder of the periosteum and soft tissues, of unclear aetiology. There are familial and sporadic forms. Pathologically there is proliferation of osteoblasts and connective tissue cells with deposition of immature bony trabecula. It is seen before the age of 6 months, with the familial form presenting at or soon after birth. Clinically there is irritability, sudden onset of hard bone swellings and fever. ESR, ALP and WBC count are raised. Anaemia is found. The disease is usually self-limiting with complete recovery by 30 months. The chronic form persists or recurs for years, resulting in delayed muscular development and deformities.

4. The mandibles, clavicle, ulna and long bones are affected. Phalanges, vertebrae, and round bones of wrists and ankles are not affected. The tibia is the most common bone in familial involvement. The disease is multifocal and asymmetrical. In long tubular bones, there is hyperostosis affecting the diaphysis of tubular bones asymmetrically, with sparing of the epiphysis. X-rays show massive lamellated periosteal reaction with focal soft-tissue swelling. Endosteal proliferation leads to medullary narrowing. Eventually the density of periosteal new bone increases and becomes homogeneous with the underlying cortex; the bone remodels and resumes a normal appearance.

5. The classic feature of Caffey's disease is the triad of irritability, swellings and bone lesions with mandibular involvement. Differential diagnoses for extensive periosteal reactions in children include hypervitaminosis (< 1 year), healing rickets, scurvy (< 4 months), syphilis, leukaemia, osteomyelitis, neuroblastoma metastasis, periostitis of prematurity, non-accidental injury, prostaglandin therapy and hereditary hyperphosphatasia.

Case 4.56: Answers

1. The X-ray of the pelvis shows a deformed and destroyed head of right femur. The left femoral head and the rest of the pelvic bones are normal.

2. Septic arthritis of the right hip.

3. Septic arthritis of the hip in neonates and infants is usually caused by *Staphylococcus aureus*. Infection can reach the hip from femoral metaphysis directly (as the growth plate is intra-articular) or into the epiphysis through vascular channels crossing the growth plate and from there into the joint. Other mechanisms of spread are haematogenous seeding of the synovium or direct implantation. Clinical features are fever, loss of appetite, irritability, pain, swelling and limping, with leukocytosis. Swelling and the hip held in abduction, flexion and external rotation are noted. Intravenous antibiotics or surgical drainage at the early stages is essential for preventing joint destruction. Residual deformity becomes apparent as the child develops. Deformities include coxa magna, dissolution of femoral head and neck with the lesser trochanter articulating with the acetabulum, and dislocation of the femoral head/shaft. Complications in older child include limb length discrepancy as a result of leg shortening or overgrowth, fibrous or bony ankylosis, and avascular necrosis of the femoral head.

4. X-rays are usually normal in the early stages. The earliest finding is soft-tissue swelling, which is seen as displacement of the fat stripes around the hip joint. With accumulation of joint fluid, the joint space is increased and there might be subluxation/dislocation of the femoral head. Lateral displacement of the epiphysis is an early finding. Bone changes include lysis, sclerosis and periosteal reaction. Loss of joint space and subchondral osseus defects develop. If osteonecrosis develops, there is increased density, fragmentation and collapse of the femoral head. When diagnosis is in doubt, ultrasonography of the hip is done and, if there is fluid, it is aspirated to confirm the diagnosis of septic arthritis.

5. Differential diagnoses for displacement of the femoral head: developmental dysplasia of the hip, neurological deficits and traumatic epiphyseal separations. Differential diagnoses for late changes: Perthes' disease and juvenile chronic arthritis. Joint aspiration is essential to differentiate it from other conditions and to decide on the appropriate antibiotics for treatment.

Case 4.57: Answers

1. The X-ray of the knee shows multiple exostoses around the knee joint, which point away from it. There is also abnormal bone modelling, with expansion of the metaphysis and epiphysis.

2. Diaphyseal aclasis.

3. Diaphyseal aclasis (hereditary multiple exostoses) is an autosomal dominant condition, which is characterised by multiple bony exostoses and associated with abnormal bone modelling. Clinical presentation is with multiple bony masses, deformities and joint restriction. It is common in the proximal and distal femur, tibia, fibula and proximal humerus. Other bones can also be affected.

4. The X-ray shows multiple exostoses, which are bilaterally symmetrical. These are commonly seen around the knee joint. They are pedunculated or broad based, and grow away from the joints. They have a cartilaginous cap, which is not completely ossified. It is associated with abnormal bone modelling. Differential diagnoses include Ollier's disease (multiple enchondromas), polyostotic fibrous dysplasia and metaphyseal dysplasia.

5. Complications are pain, fracture, deformities (pseudo-Madelung, coxa valga), neurological complications, bursa formation, mechanical complications and malignant conversion.

Case 4.58: Answers

1. The lateral view of the lumbar vertebrae shows complete flattening of the L3 vertebral body. The X-ray of the skull shows a well-defined, geographical, lucent defect in the parietal bone, close to the vertex.

2. This abnormality is called vertebra plana, where there is complete collapse of the vertebra. The diagnosis in this case is eosinophilic granuloma.

3. The causes of vertebra plana are eosinophilic granuloma, neuroblastoma metastases, Ewing's sarcoma, aneurysmal bone cyst, leukaemia, lymphoma, infection and trauma. Causes of multi-level platyspondyly are osteogenesis imperfecta, Morquio syndrome, Cushing syndrome, lymphoma, leukaemia, Gaucher's disease and metastasis

4. Eosinophilic granuloma is characterised by expanding erosive accumulations of histiocytes, usually within the medullary cavity. It can be a single or multiple skeletal lesions, and it predominantly affects children, adolescents or young adults. Solitary lesions are more common. Any bone can be involved, but the most common sites include the skull, mandible, spine, ribs and long bones. In the skull, it produces a well-defined, geographical, lytic lesion. In the spine, it is most common at the thoracic level and it may present with progressive bone pain. The highest frequency is seen between age 5 and 10 years. Scoliosis can be seen. Pathological fracture can occur. Eosinophilic granuloma can produce expansile lytic lesions of the vertebral bodies and the posterior vertebral elements. A paraspinal soft-tissue mass may occasionally occur. Involvement of the second cervical vertebra is an extremely rare occurrence, but it may cause atlantoaxial instability. MRI shows low signal intensity in T1 and high intensity in T2, and can show extradural soft-tissue space exquisitely. Contrast enhancement may be seen. Bone scan appearance is variable. It can be hot, cold or cold with a ring of reparative activity. If the diagnosis is uncertain, a biopsy is required.

5. The lesion is usually self-limiting and at least 50% reconstitution of vertebral height may be expected. Lesions with no neurological deficit or mild non-myelopathic signs are followed up or treated with bracing, which prevents progressive kyphosis. Chemotherapy is used for the systemic form of the disease. Surgical decompression is done in severe lesions. Low-dose radiotherapy is used if surgery is not possible.

5

NEURORADIOLOGY QUESTIONS

Case 5.1

A 2-year-old boy presents with recurrent generalised tonic–clonic seizures and delayed milestones.

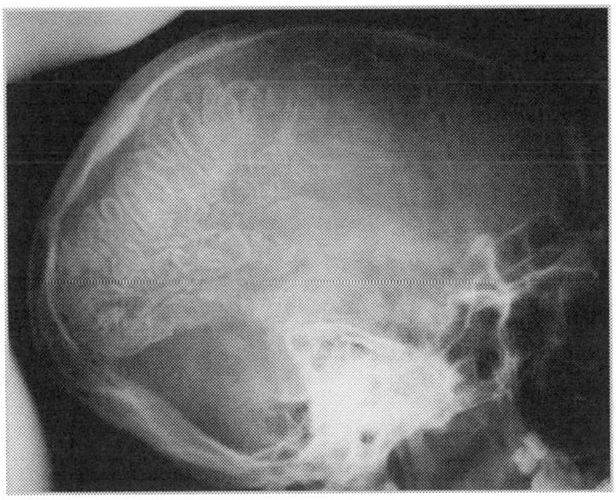

Fig 5.1a

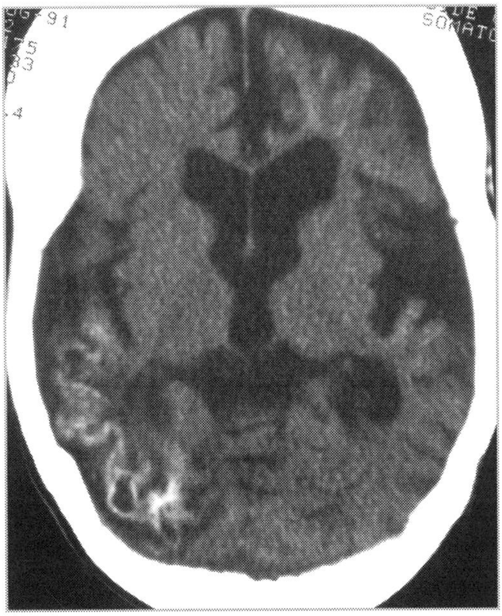

Fig 5.1b

1. What do you see on the skull X-ray?
2. What do you note on the CT scan of the brain?
3. What is the diagnosis?
4. What is the development of this condition?
5. What are the radiological features and the differential diagnosis?

Answers *on pages 375–410*

Case 5.2

A 6-year-old boy presents with backache. Clinical examination did not reveal any obvious abnormality, except for tenderness in the lower lumbar spine.

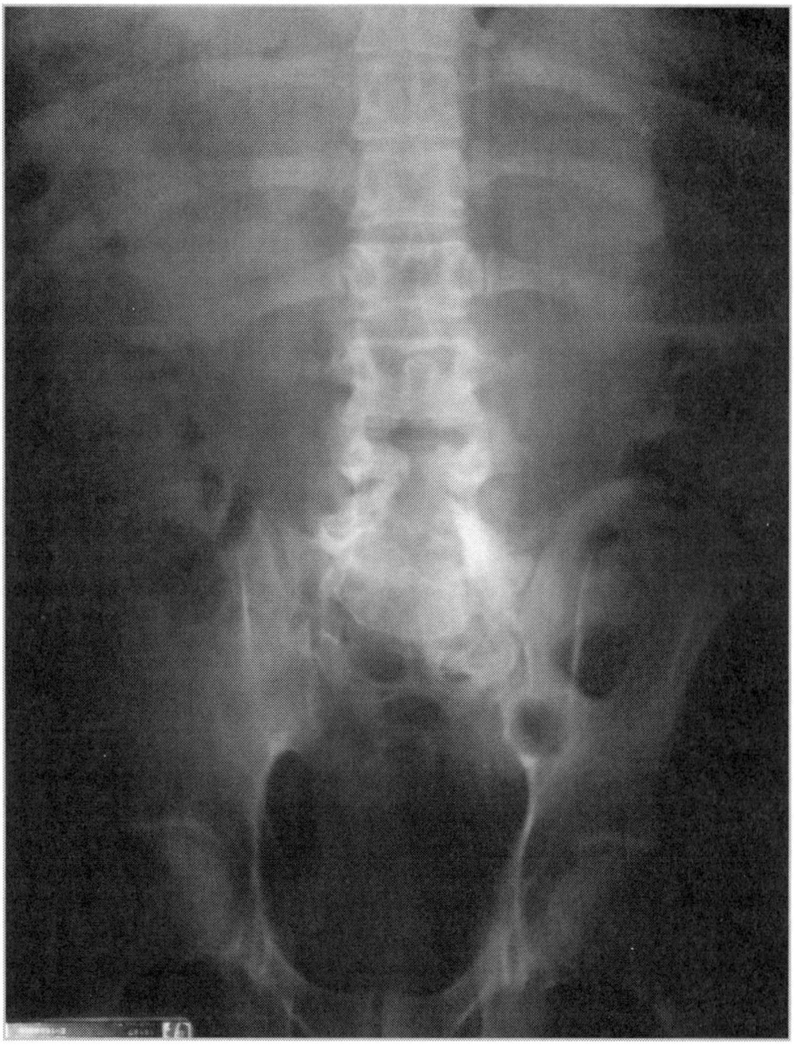

Fig 5.2

1. What are the radiological findings?
2. What is the diagnosis?
3. What is the development of this condition?
4. What are the clinical presentations and the associations?
5. What are the radiological features?

Answers *on pages 375–410*

Case 5.3

An 8-year-old boy presents with headache, drowsiness and loss of consciousness. On examination he is disoriented and does not respond to oral stimuli. His BP is low, and pulse and respiratory rate are normal.

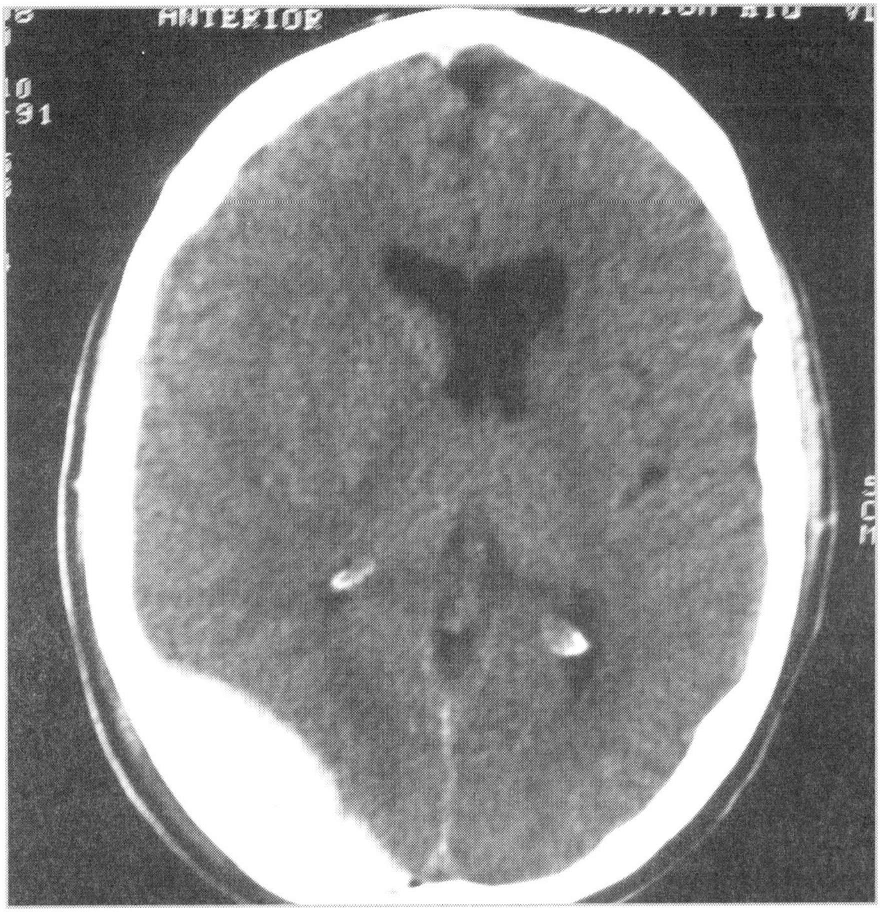

Fig 5.3

1. What are the findings on the CT scan?
2. What is the diagnosis?
3. What is the mechanism?
4. What are the clinical and the radiological features?
5. What is the treatment of this condition?

Answers *on pages 375–410*

Case 5.4

A 2-year-old baby was brought to A&E with a history of a fall, feeding difficulties and poor arousability

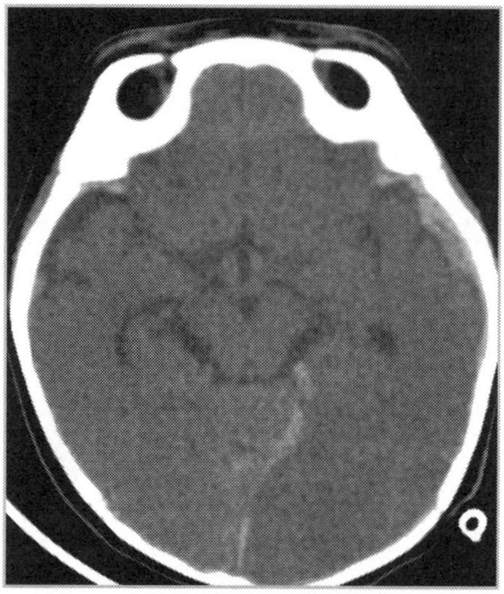

Fig 5.4a

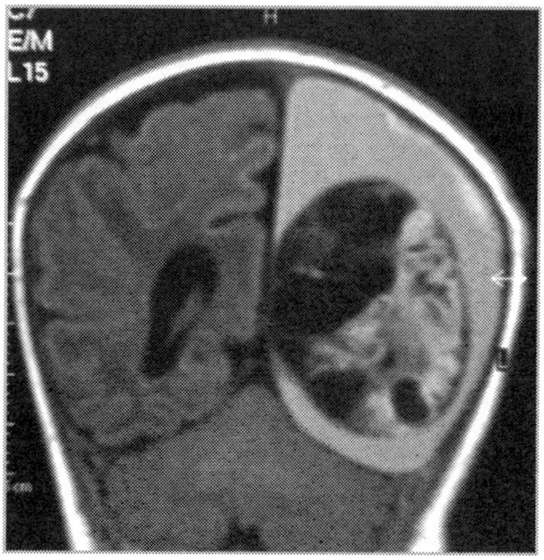

Fig 5.4b

1. What are the findings in the CT scan of the brain? Waht do you observe in the MRI scan, done two weeks after the CT scan?
2. What is the diagnosis?
3. What is the mechanism of this disease?
4. What are the characteristic radiological findings?
5. What are the long-term complications?

Answers *on pages 375–410*

Case 5.5

A 2-year-old girl presents with failure to thrive and delayed milestones.

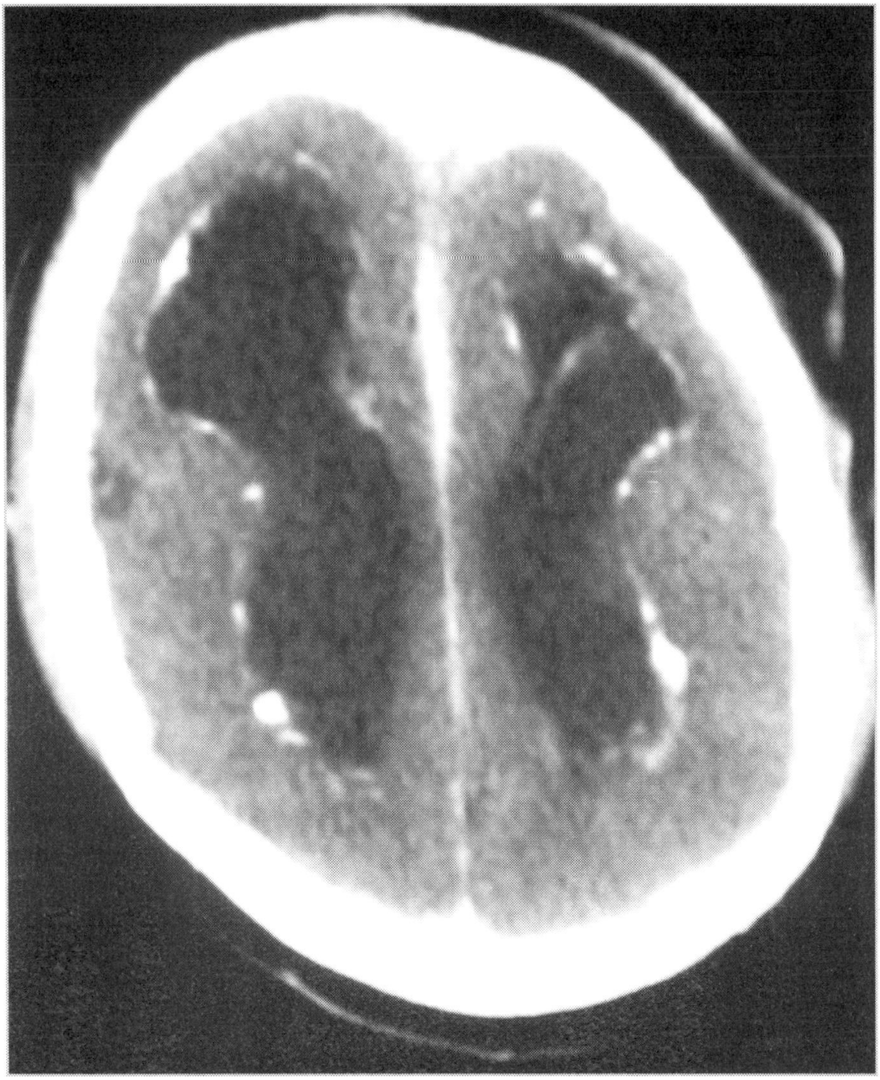

Fig 5.5

1. What do you see on the CT scan?
2. What is the diagnosis?
3. What are the clinical features?
4. What are the radiological features?
5. What is the differential diagnosis?

Answers *on pages 375–410*

Case 5.6

A 12-year-old boy presents with fever, headache, vomiting and seizures. On examination he is febrile with left-sided weakness and brisk reflexes.

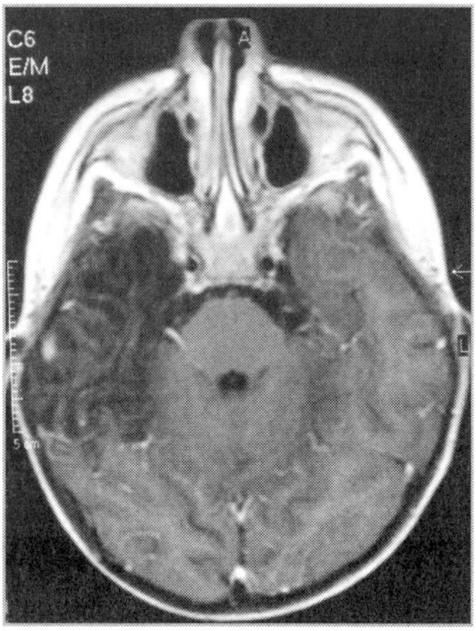

Fig 5.6a

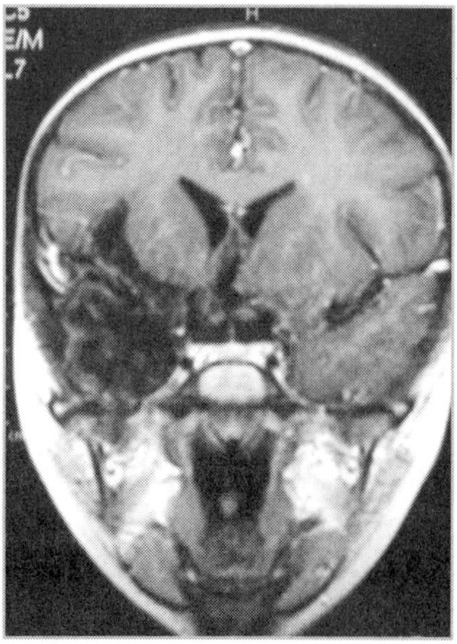

Fig 5.6b

1. What are the findings on the MR scan?
2. What is the diagnosis?
3. What are the aetiology and the clinical features?
4. What are the radiological findings and the differential diagnosis?
5. What is the management of this disease?

Answers *on pages 375–410*

Case 5.7

A 5-year-old boy presents with headache, vomiting and frequent falls. Clinical examination revealed brisk reflexes and ataxia.

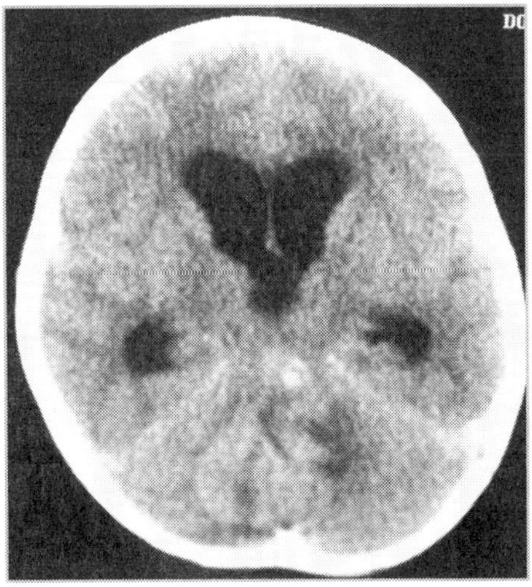

Fig 5.7a

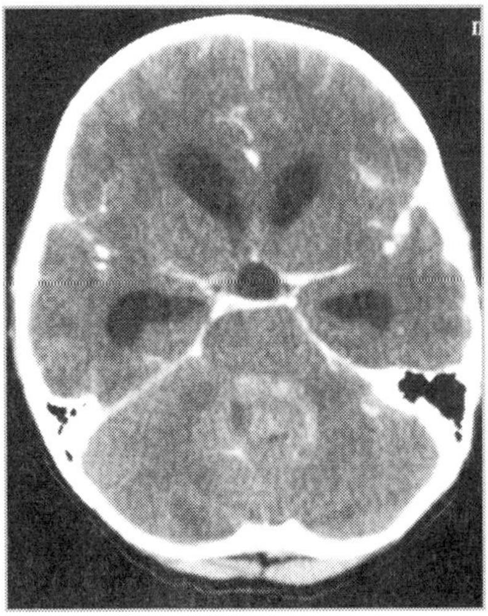

Fig 5.7b

1. What do you observe on the CT scan of the brain?
2. What is the diagnosis?
3. What are the clinical features?
4. What are the radiological findings?
5. What is the differential diagnosis?

Answers *on pages 375–410*

Case 5.8

A 4-year-old boy presented with an abnormally shaped head and seizures. Radiological tests were ordered.

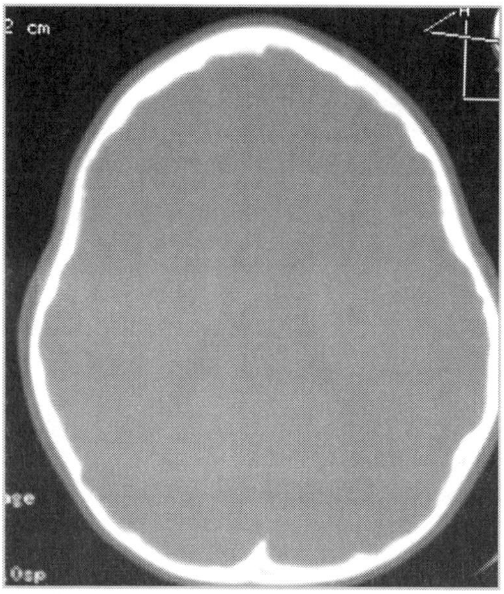

Fig 5.8a

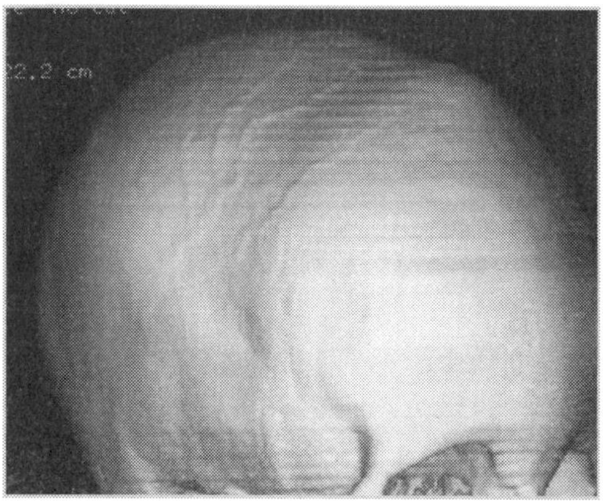

Fig 5.8b

1. What are the findings on the first picture?
2. What is the second investigation and what do you observe?
3. What is the diagnosis?
4. What are the types and development?
5. What are the associations of this condition?
6. What are the clinical features and prognosis?

Answers *on pages 375–410*

Case 5.9

A 13-year-old girl presents with pain in the neck and both arms. Clinical examination showed increased reflexes, and loss of power and sensation in all four limbs.

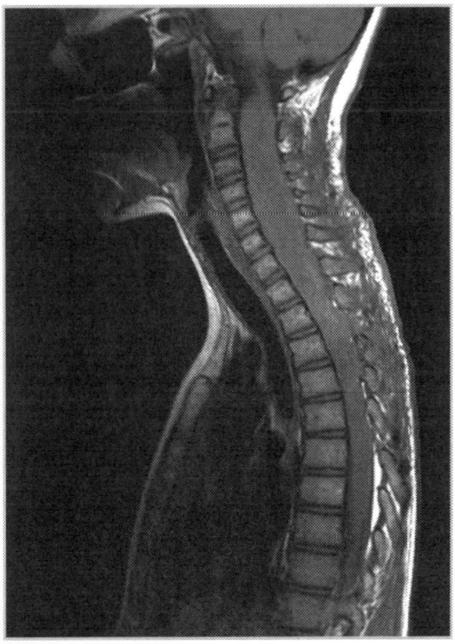

Fig 5.9a

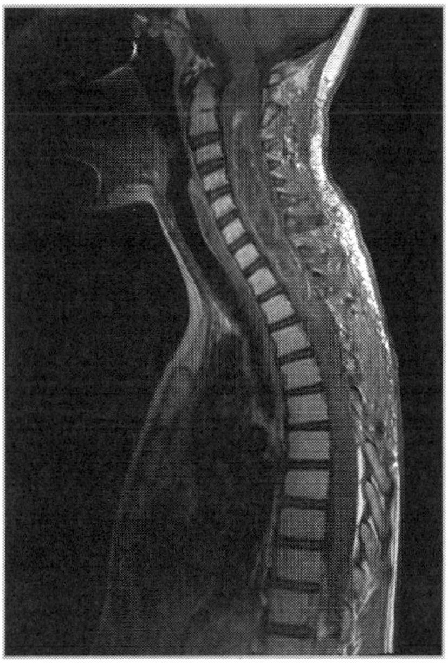

Fig 5.9b

1. What do you see on MRI of the spine?
2. What is the diagnosis?
3. What are the different types of this disease?
4. What are the radiological features?
5. What is the differential diagnosis?

Answers *on pages 375–410*

Case 5.10

A 2-year-old boy presents with a large swelling in the lower back. On examination the swelling is cystic and mobile.

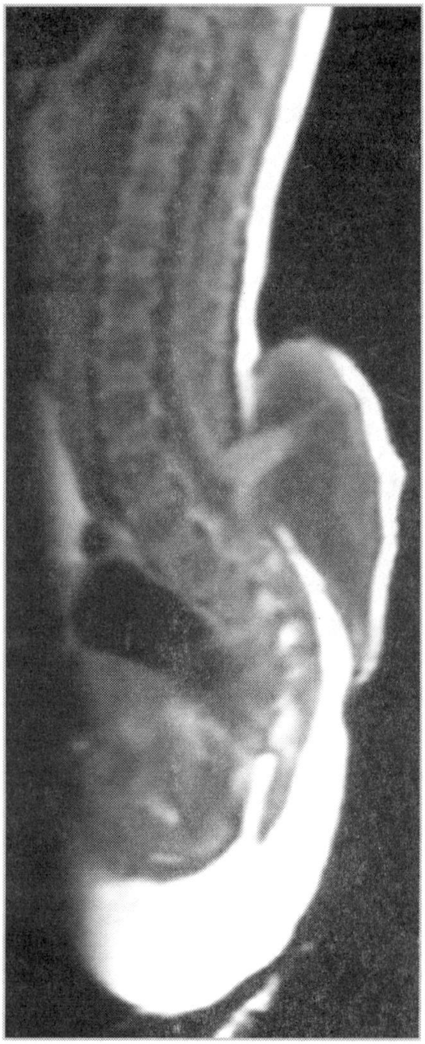

Fig 5.10a

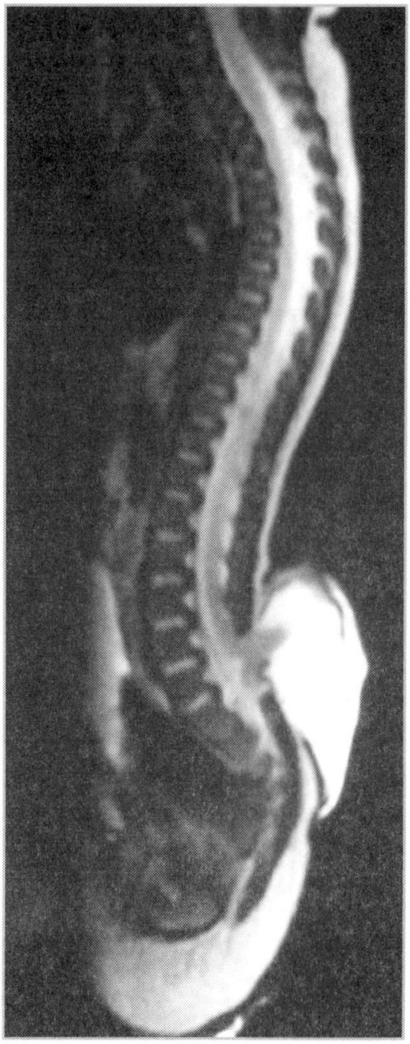

Fig 5.10b

1. What are the findings on the MR scan?
2. What is the diagnosis?
3. What are the types of disease?
4. What are the clinical presentations?
5. What are the radiological features?

Answers *on pages 375–410*

Case 5.11

A 12-year-old boy presented with intermittent headache, nausea and vomiting. Clinical examination did not reveal any neurological deficit. Power, tone and reflexes were normal.

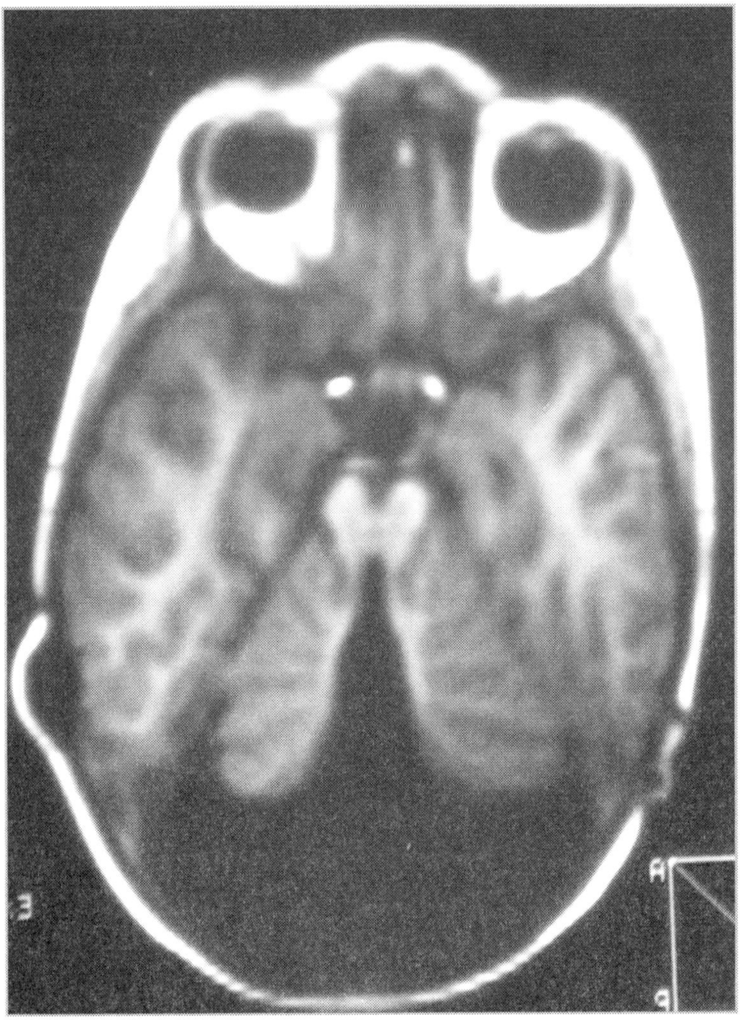

Fig 5.11

1. What are the findings on the MR scan?
2. What is the diagnosis?
3. What are the aetiology, development and clinical features of this disease?
4. What are the radiological features?
5. What is the differential diagnosis?

Answers *on pages 375–410*

Case 5.12

A 10-year-old boy presented with headache. Clinical examination was unremarkable.

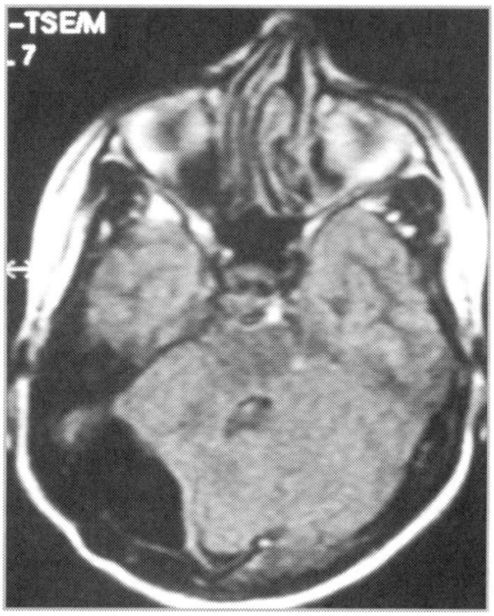

Fig 5.12a

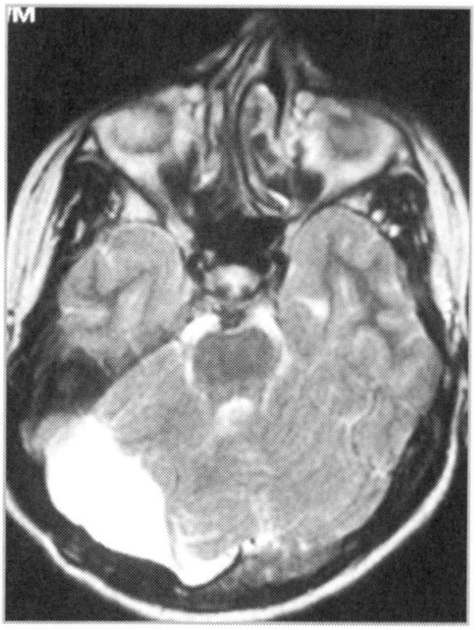

Fig 5.12b

1. What do you observe on MRI of the brain?
2. What is the diagnosis?
3. What are the development and the clinical features?
4. What are the radiological findings?
5. What is the differential diagnosis?

Answers *on pages 375–410*

Case 5.13

A 7-year-old girl with developmental delay presents with sudden-onset diffuse headache and seizures. Clinical examination showed mild decreased power in all limbs with increased reflexes. A skin nodule was noted on her face.

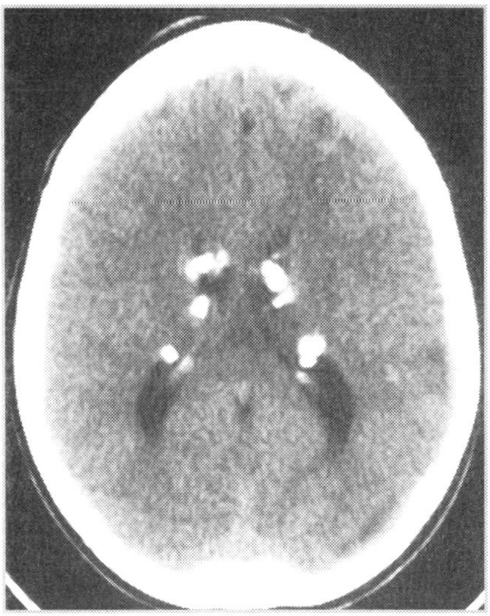

Fig 5.13a

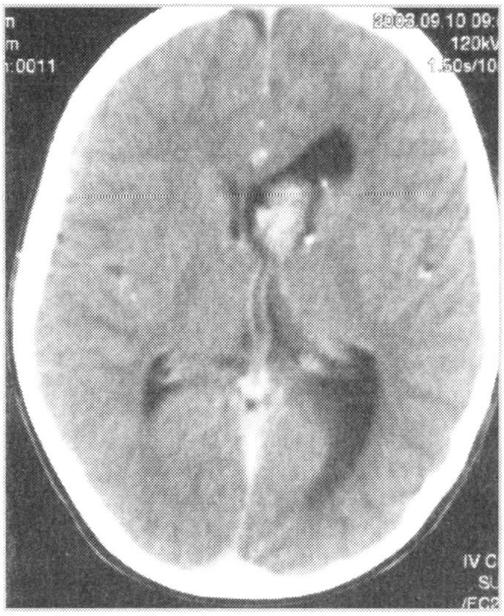

Fig 5.13b

1. What do you observe on the CT scans of the brain?
2. What is the cause for the developmental delay and seizures?
3. What are the clinical features?
4. What is the cause of the sudden onset of headache? What are the other complications?
5. What are the radiological features of this condition?

Answers *on pages 375–410*

Case 5.14

A 1-year-old baby boy, who was delivered preterm, presents with seizures, spastic quadriparesis and delayed milestones.

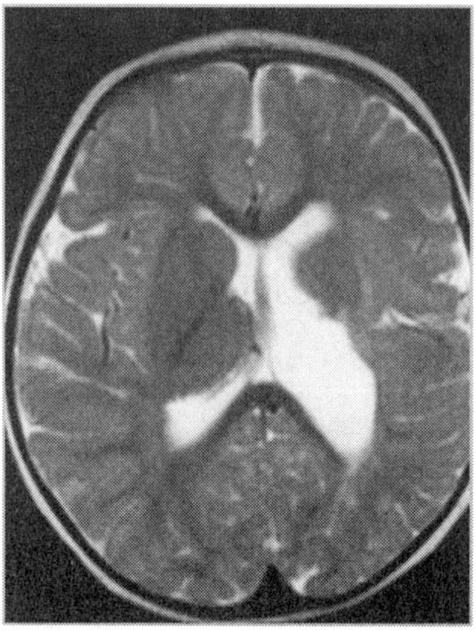
Fig 5.14a

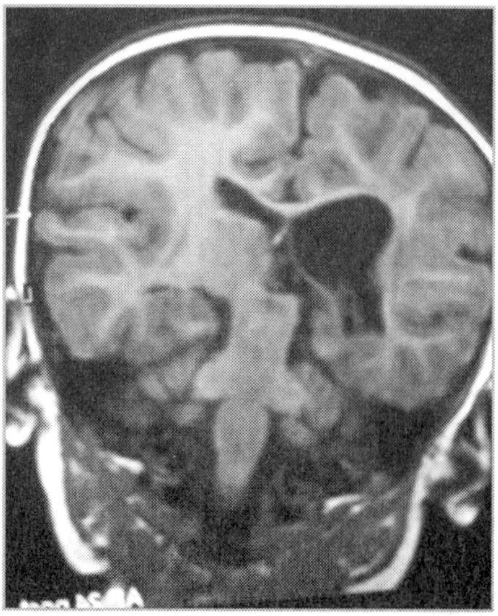
Fig 5.14b

1. What do you find on MRI?
2. What is the diagnosis?
3. What is the aetiology?
4. What are the radiological features?
5. What are the prognosis and the differential diagnosis?

Answers *on pages 375–410*

Case 5.15

A 7-year-old boy presented with seizures. No focal neurological deficit was identified on clinical examination. Laboratory and CSF tests were normal.

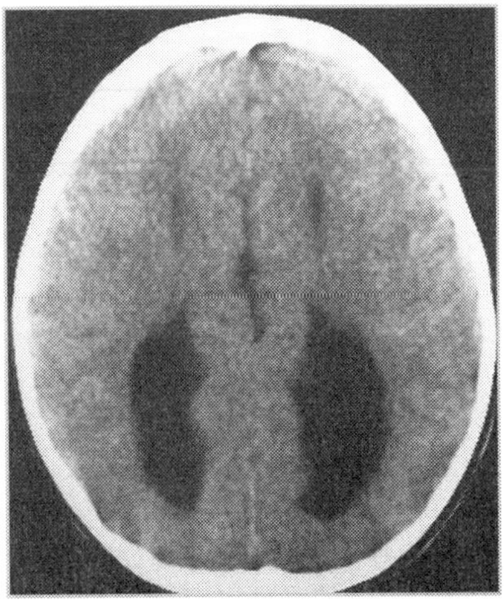

Fig 5.15a

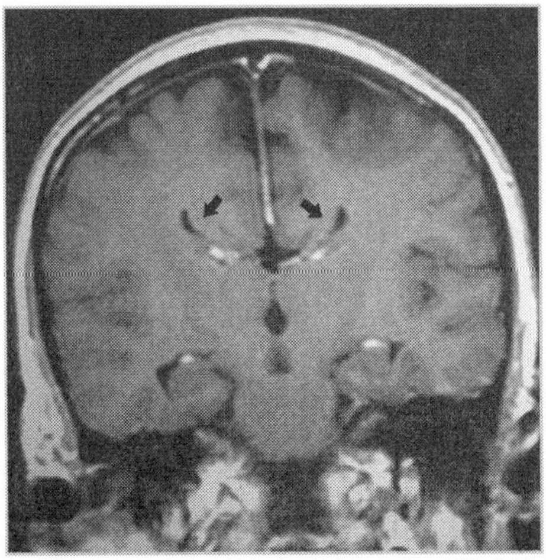

Fig 5.15b

1. What are the findings on the CT and MR scans?
2. What is the diagnosis?
3. What are the types and embryological development?
4. What are the associations of this condition?
5. What are the radiological features?
6. What is the management?

Answers *on pages 375–410*

Case 5.16

A 6-month-old baby is investigated for an enlarging head and seizures.

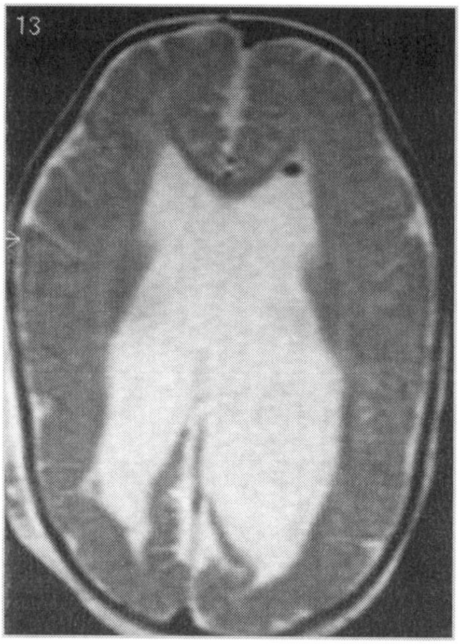

Fig 5.16a

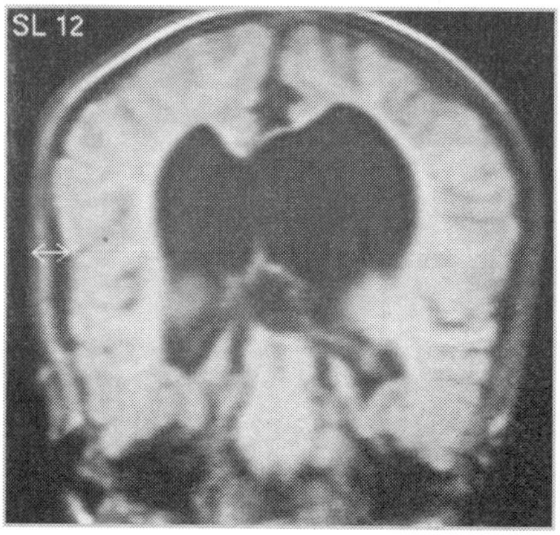

Fig 5.16b

1. What are the findings on the MR scan?
2. What is the diagnosis?
3. What are the types?
4. What are the radiological findings?
5. What are the associations?
6. What is the differential diagnosis?

Answers *on pages 375–410*

Case 5.17

An 11-year-old girl presents with loss of pain and temperature sensation in the upper limbs and muscle weakness.

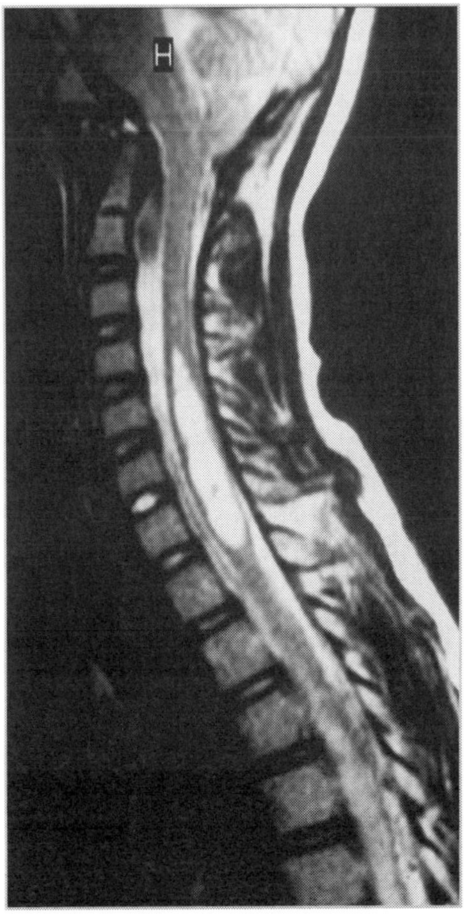

Fig 5.17a

1. What are the findings on MRI?
2. What is the diagnosis?
3. What are the types of disease?
4. What are the clinical presentations?
5. What are the radiological features and the differential diagnosis?

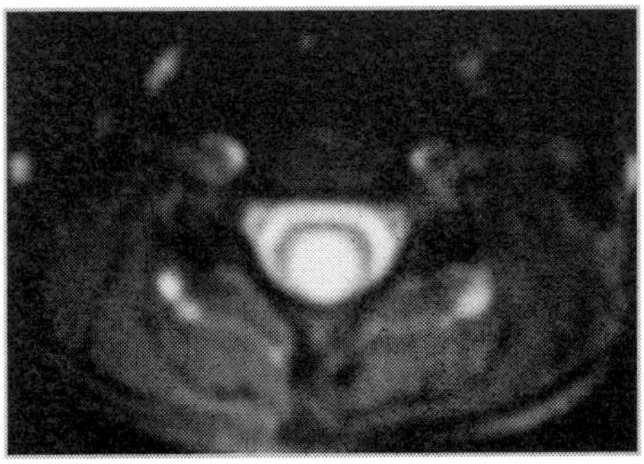

Fig 5.17b

Answers *on pages 375–410*

Case 5.18

A 6-month-old baby presents with a large head, vomiting and seizures.

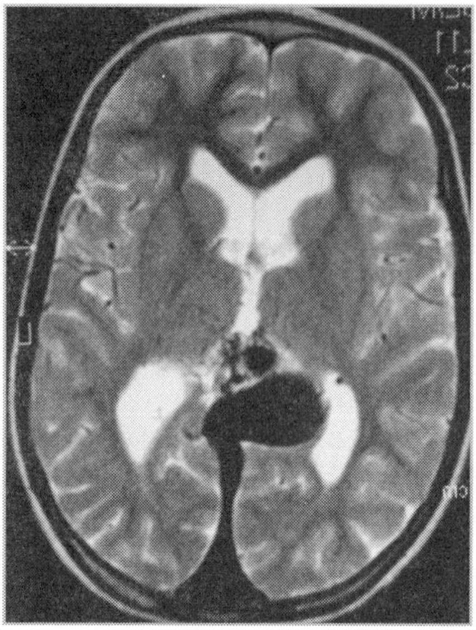

Fig 5.18a

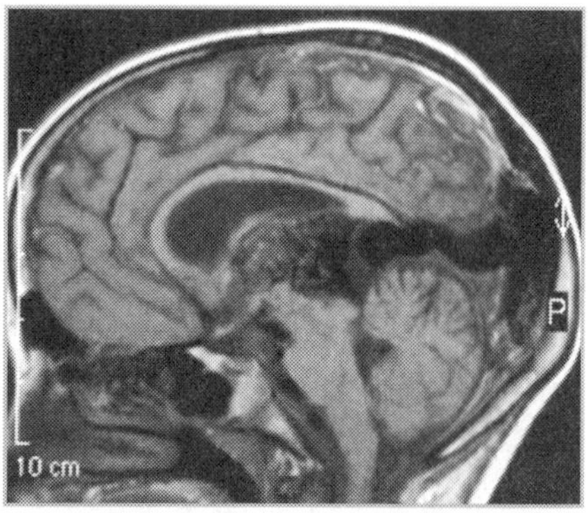

Fig 5.18b

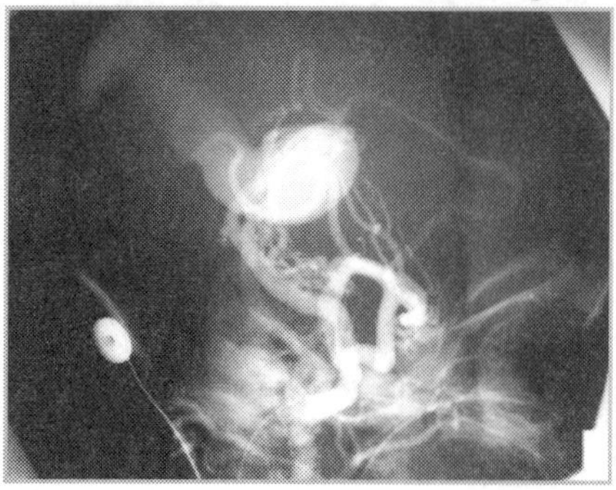

Fig 5.18c

1. What are the findings on the MR scan?
2. What is the diagnosis?
3. What are the types?
4. What are the radiological findings?
5. What are the feeding vessels?
6. What is the differential diagnosis?

Answers *on pages 375–410*

Case 5.19

A 10-year-old girl presented with weakness and back pain. Clinical examination showed decreased power in the lower limbs with exaggerated reflexes.

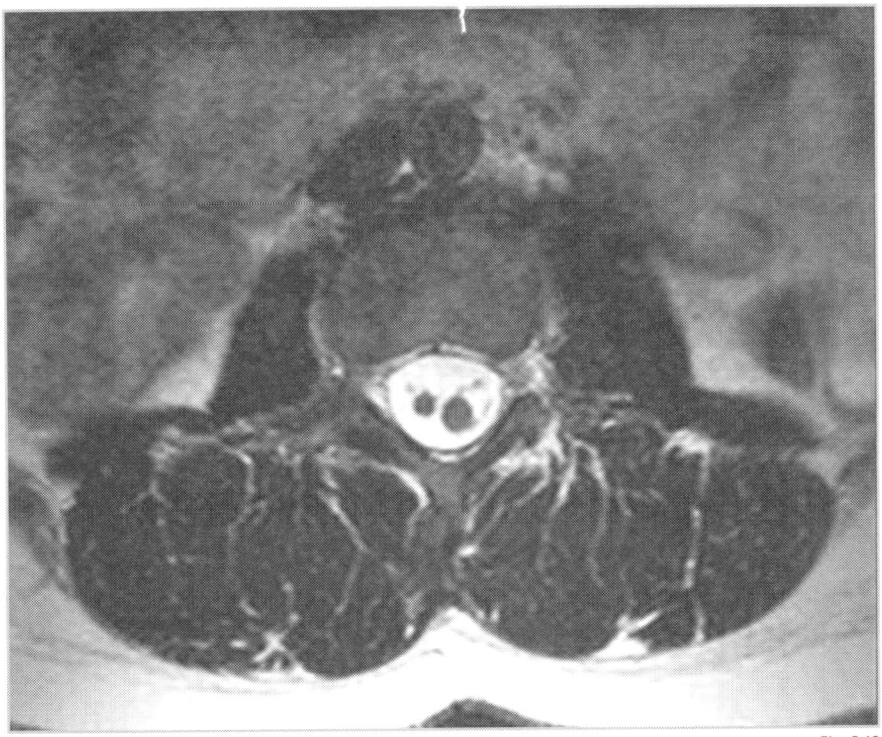

Fig 5.19

1. What are the findings on MRI?
2. What is the diagnosis?
3. What are the types of disease?
4. What are the clinical presentations?
5. What are the radiological features?

Answers *on pages 375–410*

Case 5.20

A 14-year-old boy presents with headache and focal seizures. On examination he does not have any neurological deficit.

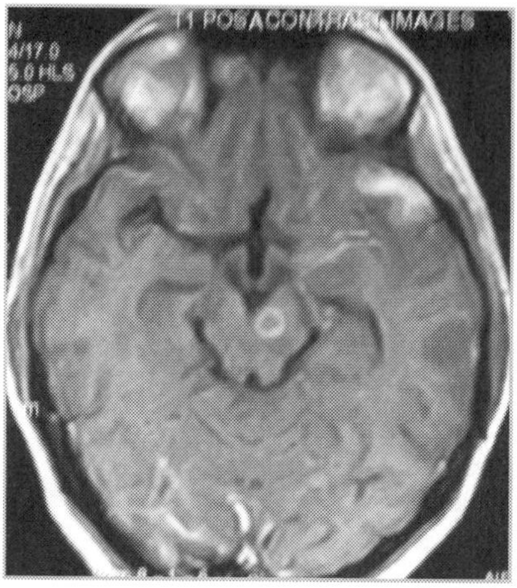

Fig 5.20a

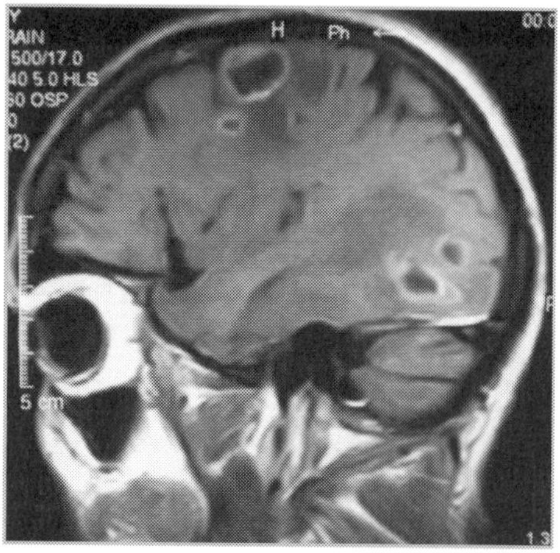

Fig 5.20b

1. What are the findings on the MR scan?
2. What is the diagnosis?
3. What is the mode of spread to the brain?
4. What are the clinical features?
5. What are the radiological findings? What is the differential diagnosis?

Answers *on pages 375–410*

Case 5.21

A 5-year-old boy presents with headache, growth retardation and visual disturbances. On examination he has bitemporal hemianopia.

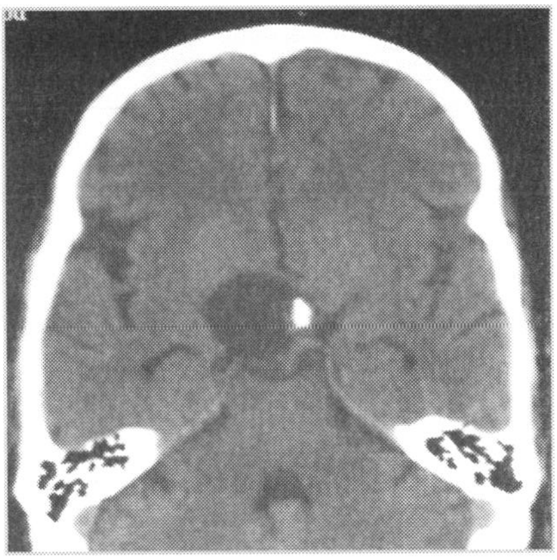

Fig 5.21a

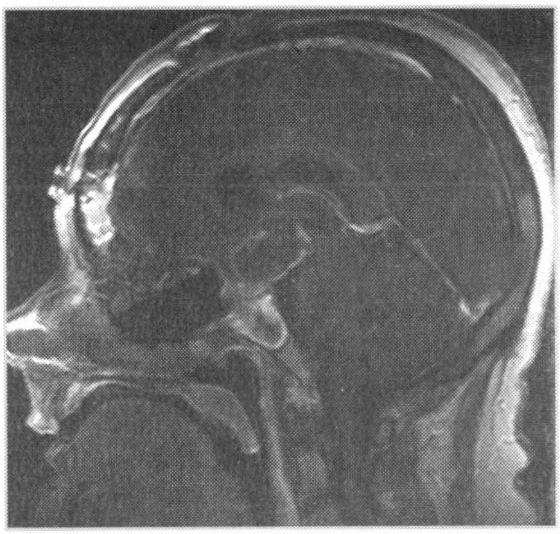

Fig 5.21c

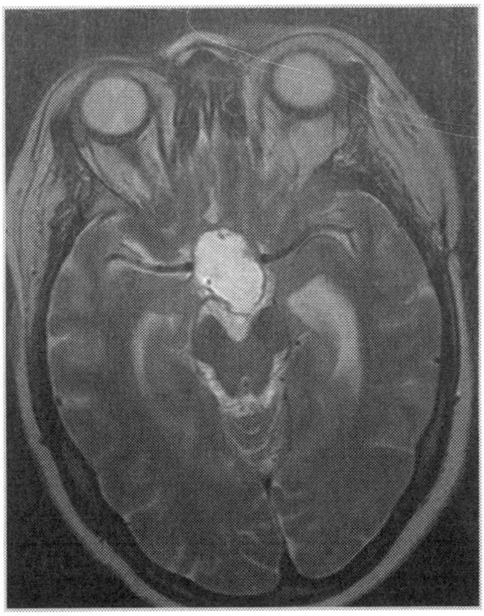

Fig 5.21b

1. What are the findings on the CT scan?
2. What do you observe on the MR scan?
3. What are the diagnosis and the differential diagnosis?
4. What are the clinical presentations?
5. What are the radiological features?

Answers *on pages 375–410*

Case 5.22

An 11-year-old girl presents with headache, gait disturbance and nystagmus. On examination cerebellar signs are positive.

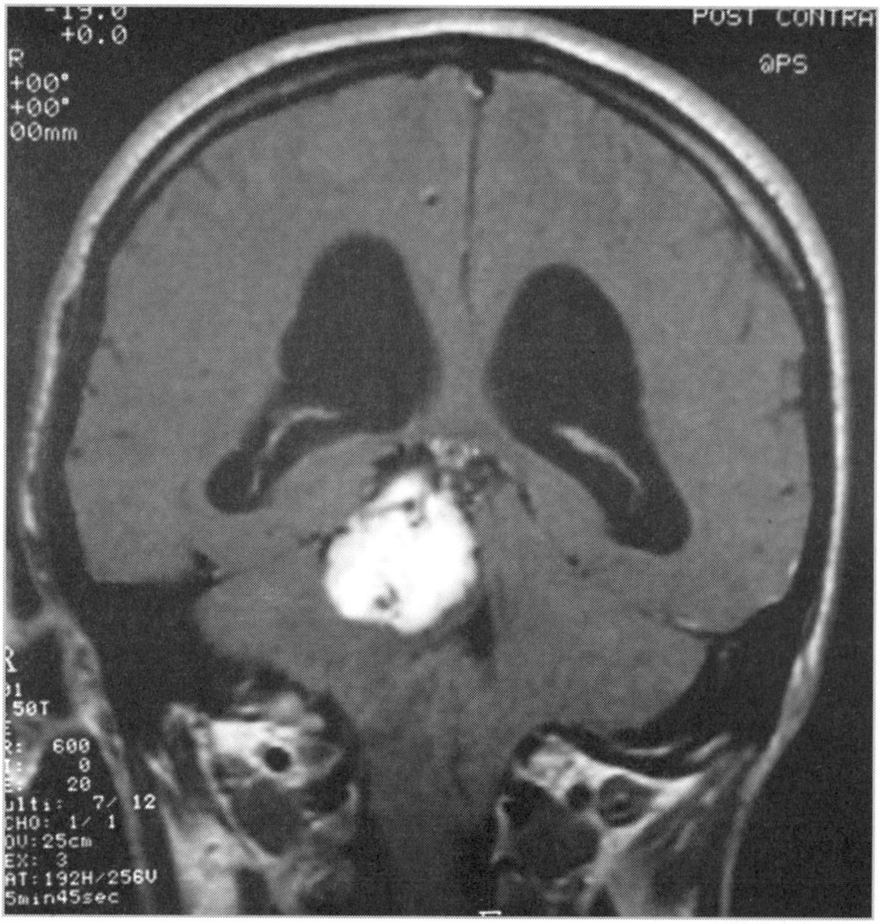

Fig 5.22

1. What do you observe on MRI of the brain?
2. What is the diagnosis?
3. With what syndrome is this associated?
4. What are the radiological findings?
5. What is the differential diagnosis?

Answers *on pages 375–410*

Case 5.23

A 4-year-old girl presented with recurrent bouts of projectile vomiting and generalised tonic–clonic seizures. Clinical examination showed normal power, tone and reflexes.

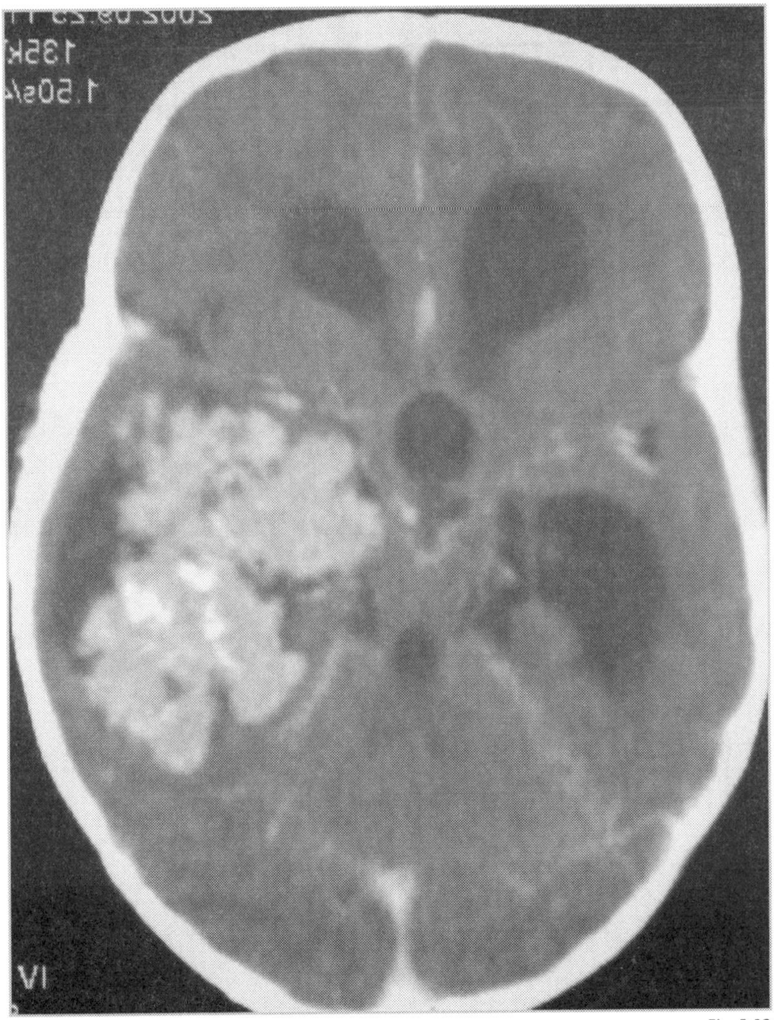

Fig 5.23

1. What are the findings on the CT scan?
2. What are the diagnosis and the differential diagnosis?
3. What are the clinical presentations?
4. What is the most common location?
5. What are the radiological features?

Answers *on pages 375–410*

Case 5.24

A 3-year-old girl presents with headache, seizures, nausea, vomiting and fever.

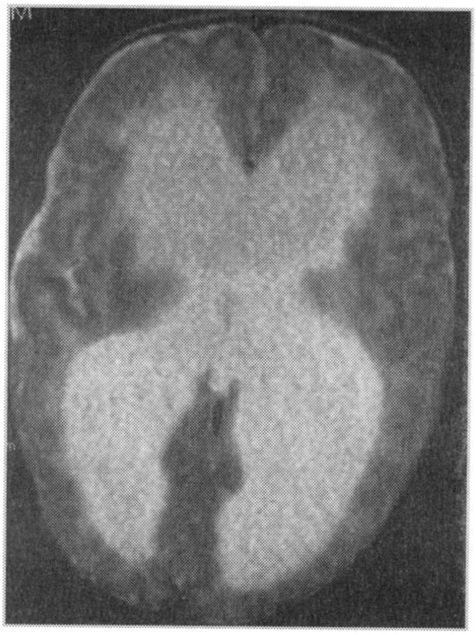

Fig 5.24a

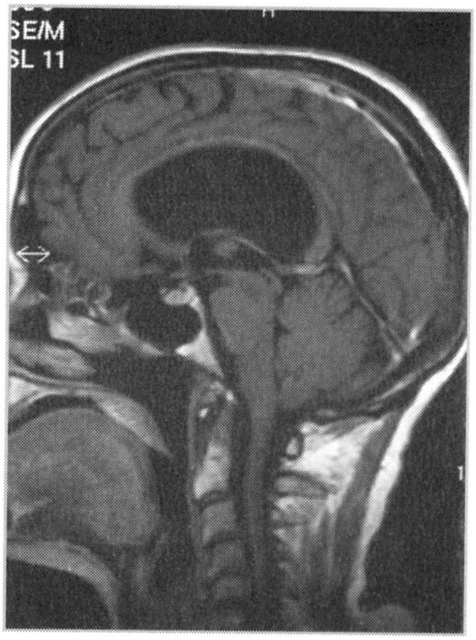

Fig 5.24b

1. What are the findings on the MR scan?
2. What is the diagnosis?
3. What is the cause for this appearance?
4. What are the radiological findings?
5. What is the differential diagnosis?

Answers *on pages 375–410*

Case 5.25

A 13-year-old boy, who had a recent bone marrow transplantation, presents with severe headache, nausea, vomiting, fever and seizures. On examination, he is febrile. There is left hemiparesis.

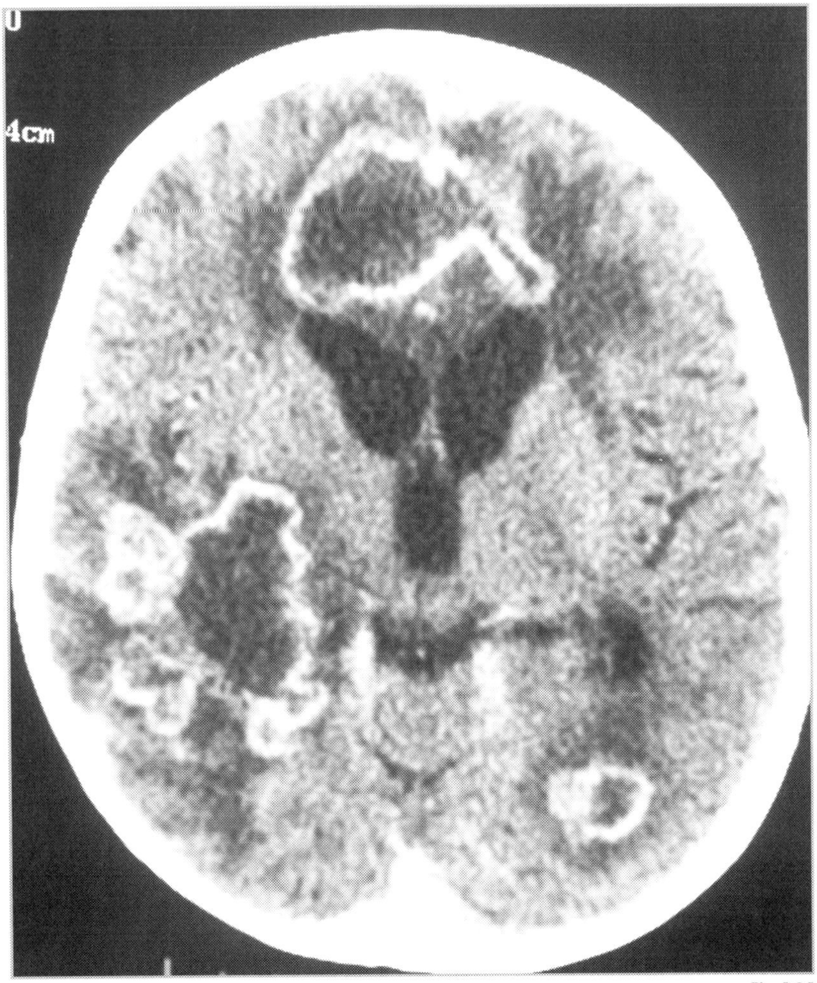

Fig 5.25

1. What are the findings on the CT scan?
2. What is the diagnosis?
3. What are the causative agents and how is the brain affected?
4. What are the clinical features and the complications?
5. What are the radiological findings?
6. What is the differential diagnosis?

Answers *on pages 375–410*

Case 5.26

A preterm male neonate is on an ICU and underwent a scan of his head.

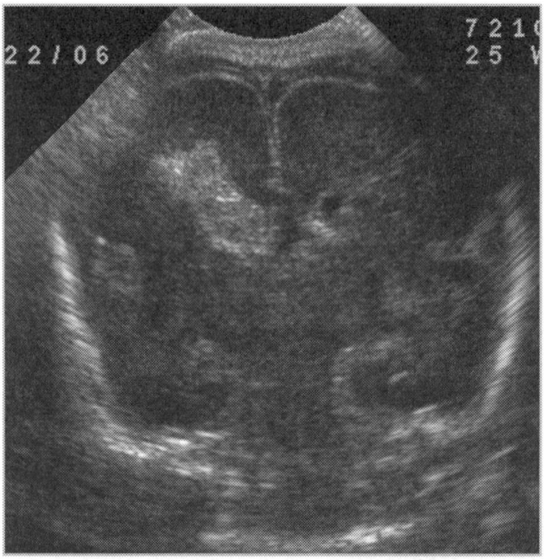

Fig 5.26a

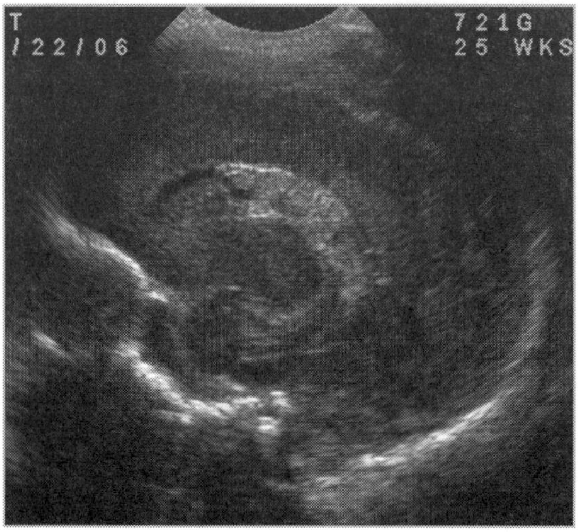

Fig 5.26b

1. What do you see on the ultrasound scan of the head?
2. What is the diagnosis?
3. What are the risk factors for this disease?
4. What is the pathophysiology of this disease?
5. What are the grades and ultrasound features?

Answers *on pages 375–410*

Case 5.27

A 9-year-old boy presented with nystagmus, headache and frequent falls. Clinical examination showed dysdiadochokinesia and left hemiparesis.

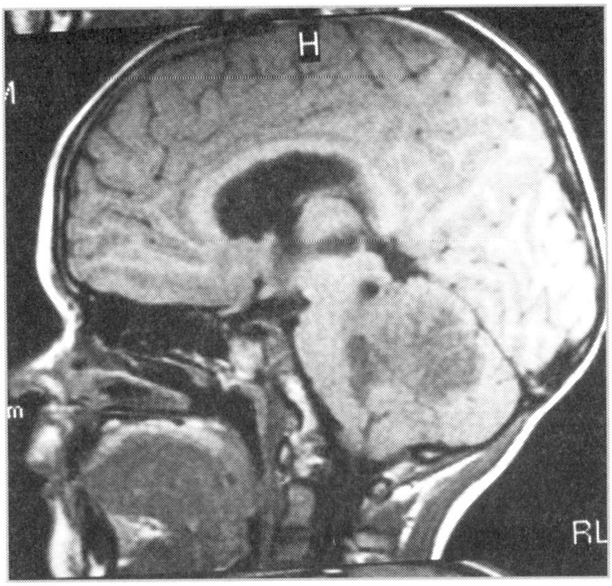

Fig 5.27a

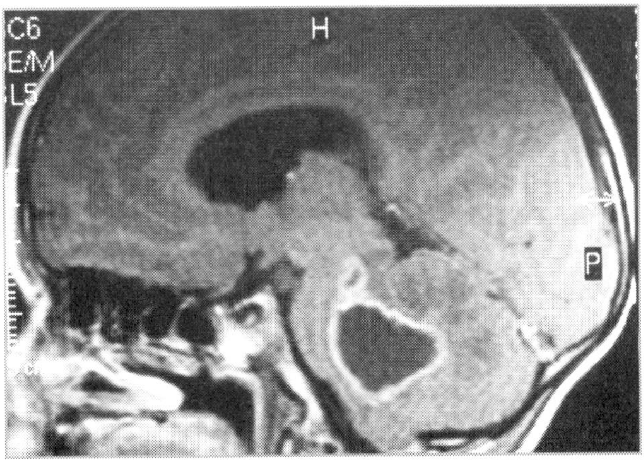

Fig 5.27b

1. What do you observe on MRI of the brain?
2. What is the diagnosis?
3. What are the clinical features?
4. What are the radiological findings?
5. What is the differential diagnosis?

Answers *on pages 375–410*

Case 5.28

A 4-year-old girl presented with nystagmus, syncopal episodes and weakness of the upper limbs. On examination, there was decreased power in the upper extremities. The reflexes were exaggerated.

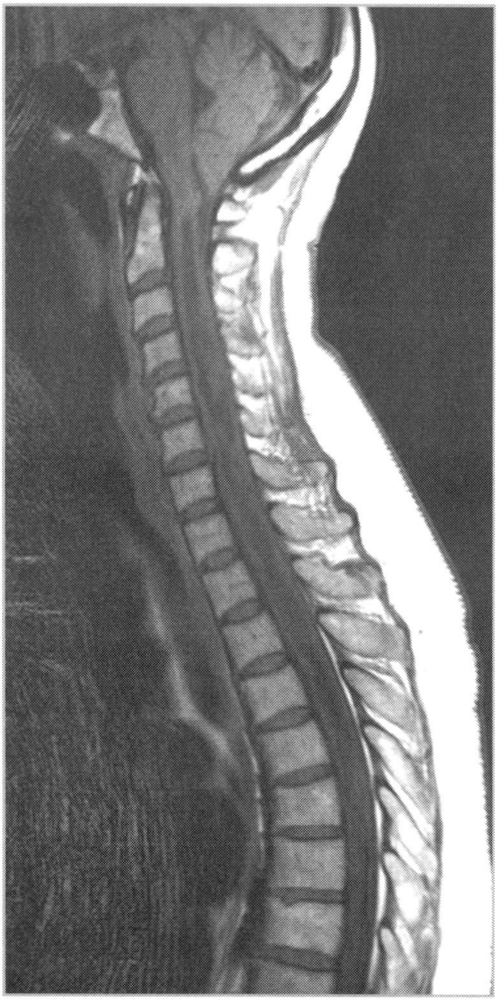

Fig 5.28

1. What are the findings on the MR scan?
2. What is the diagnosis?
3. What are the types of the disease?
4. What are the radiological features?
5. What are the clinical and associated features?

Answers *on pages 375–410*

Case 5.29

A 7-year-old boy was involved in an accident. He presents with brief loss of consciousness, amnesia, headache and vomiting. On examination he is slightly drowsy. His pupils are normal.

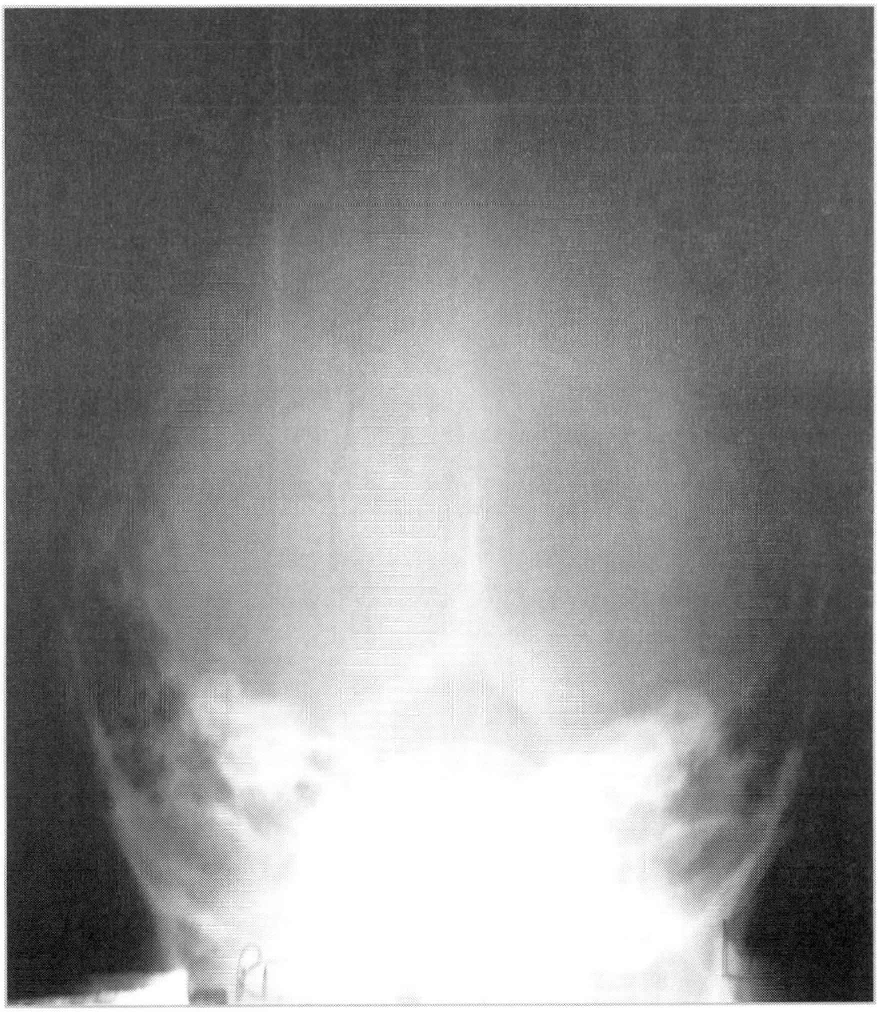

Fig 5.29

1. What are the findings on the X-ray?
2. What is the diagnosis?
3. What is the classification of this finding?
4. What is a growing fracture?
5. What is the role of imaging?

Answers *on pages 375–410*

Case 5.30

A 14-year-old boy presents to the hospital with intractable seizures for a year. His seizures begin with a feeling of déjà vu followed by a motionless stare and fumbling, indicating a complex, partial type. Clinically no neurological deficit was observed.

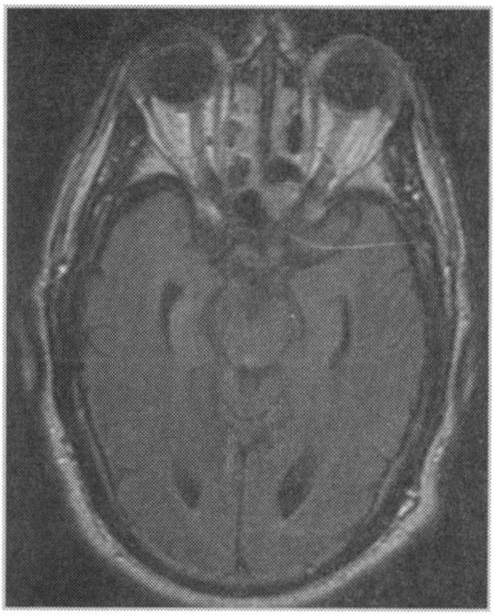

Fig 5.30a

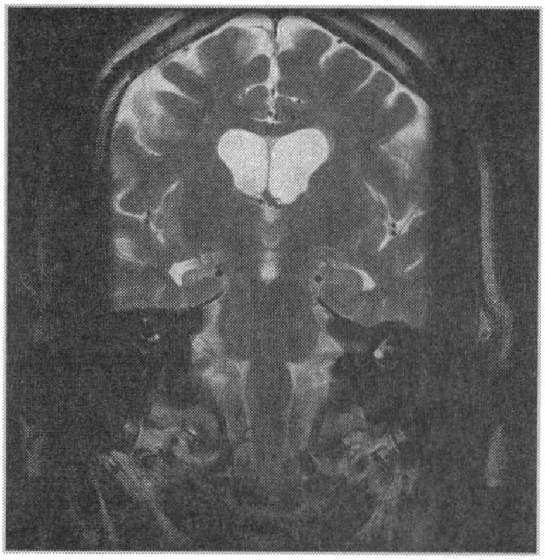

Fig 5.30b

1. What is this investigation and what do you observe?
2. What is the diagnosis?
3. What are the causes of epilepsy?
4. What is the relationship of this lesion to epilepsy?
5. What is the role of MRI in diagnosis of epilepsy?

Answers *on pages 375–410*

Case 5.31

A 5-year-old boy presents with right eye swelling, visual problems, headache and vomiting.

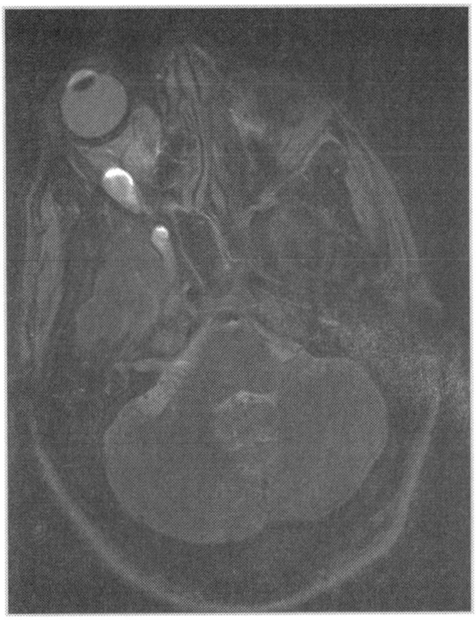

Fig 5.31a

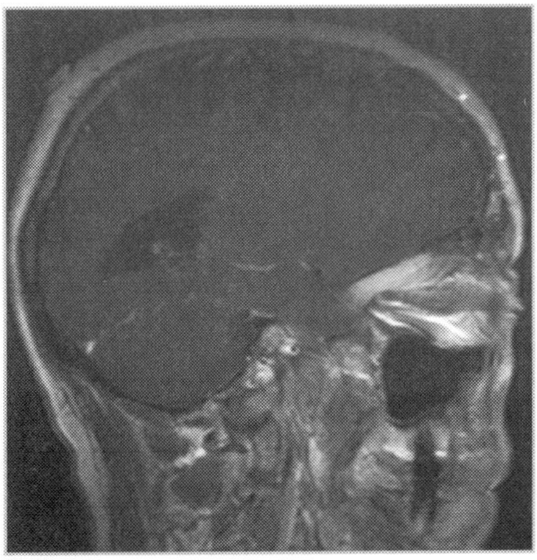

Fig 5.31b

1. What do you observe on MRI of the brain?
2. What is the diagnosis?
3. What is the important condition associated with it?
4. What are the radiological findings?
5. What is the differential diagnosis?

Answers *on pages 375–410*

Case 5.32

A 12-year-old girl presents with a swelling and pain in the left side of the neck. On examination, there is a well-defined, smooth mass along the anterior border of the left sternomastoid, which becomes prominent on contraction of the muscle.

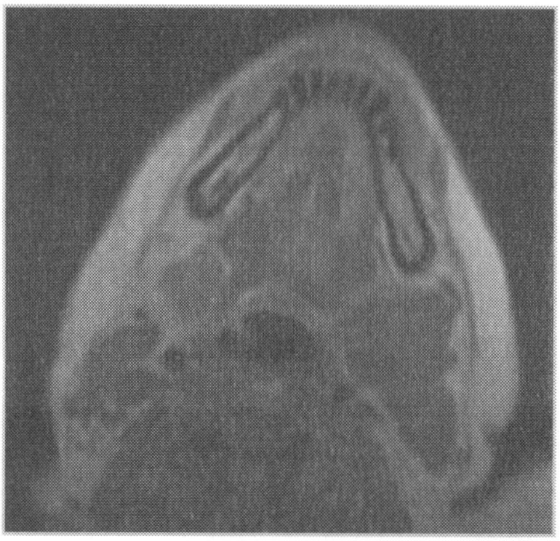

Fig 5.32a

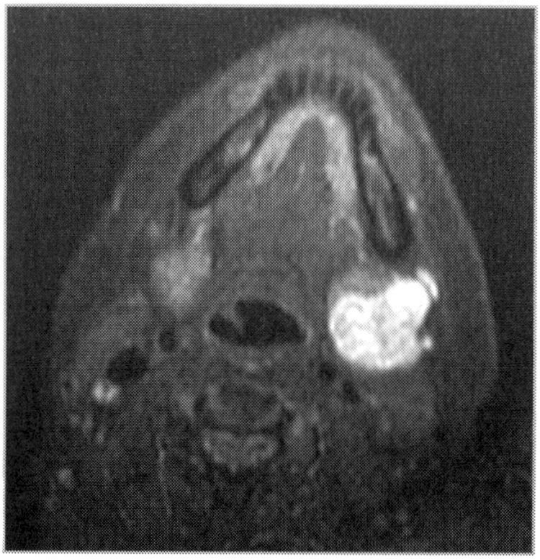

Fig 5.32b

1. What do you observe on the MR scan?
2. What is the diagnosis?
3. What is the development of this lesion?
4. What are the classification and the radiological features?
5. What are the differential diagnosis and the management?

Answers *on pages 375–410*

Case 5.33

A 13-year-old girl presents with swelling and discomfort in the right eye. On examination there is limitation of movement in the superior direction and diplopia is elicited when using the superior oblique muscle.

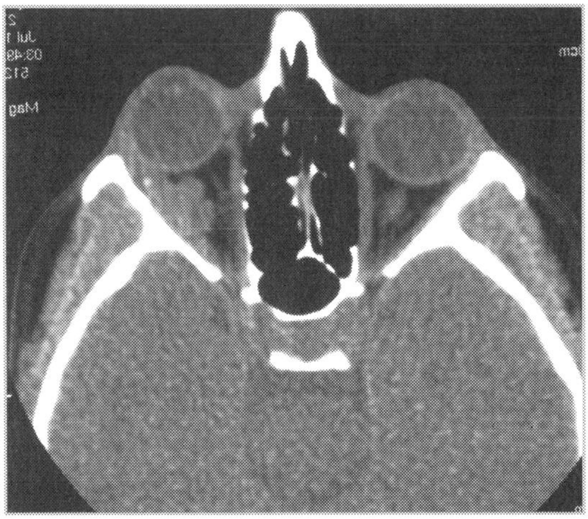

Fig 5.33a

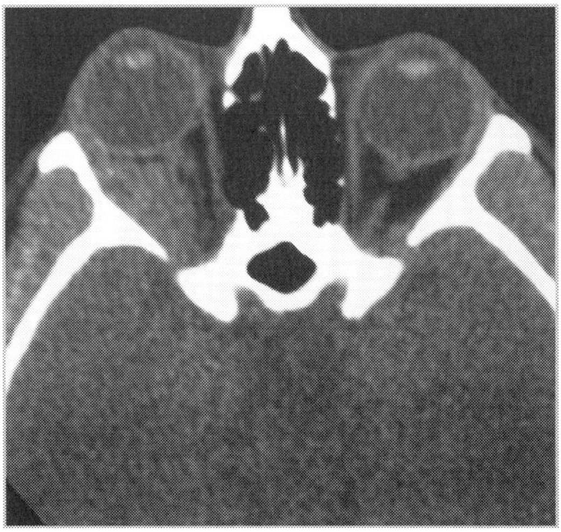

Fig 5.33b

1. What do you find on the first CT scan?
2. The second CT scan has been done after a Valsalva manoeuvre. Do you notice any change in the appearance on the scan?
3. What is the diagnosis?
4. What are the radiological features?
5. What is the differential diagnosis?

Answers *on pages 375–410*

Case 5.34

A 5-year-old boy presents with rapid development of swelling and pain in the right eye. Clinical examination shows a tender mass in the right eye, associated with proptosis. There is limitation of upward rotation of the eye.

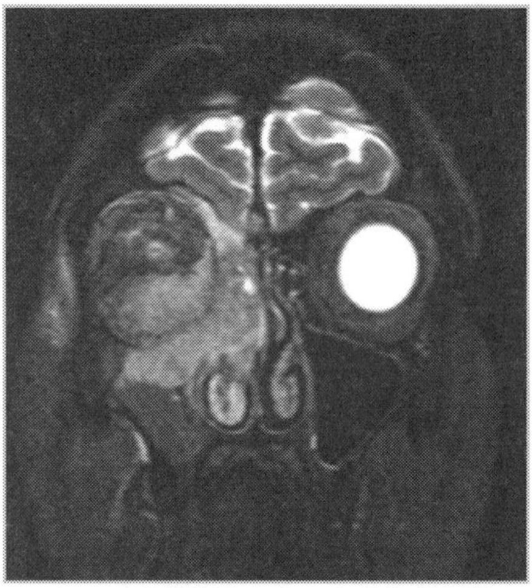

Fig 5.34a

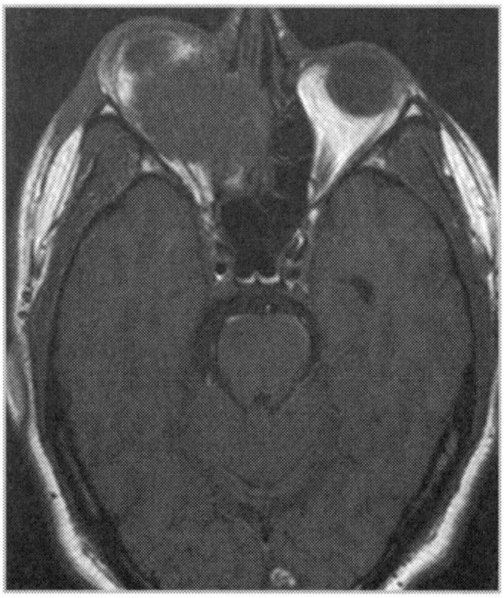

Fig 5.34b

1. What are the findings on the MR scan of the orbits?
2. What is the diagnosis?
3. What are the pathological features of this disease?
4. What are the radiological features?
5. What is the differential diagnosis?

Answers *on pages 375–410*

Case 5.35

A 14-year-old boy presents with epistaxis, headache and nasal obstruction.

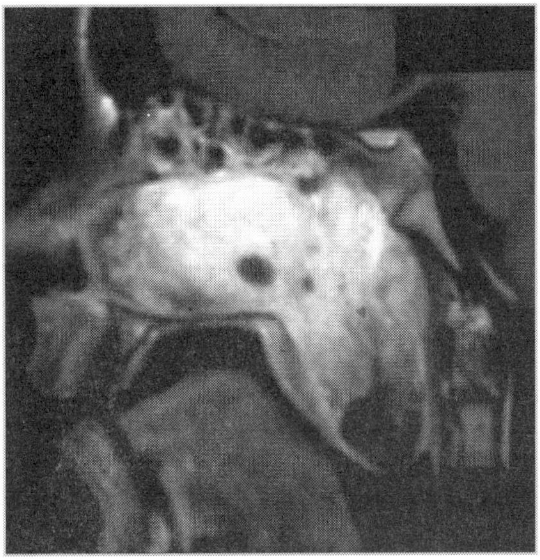

Fig 5.35a

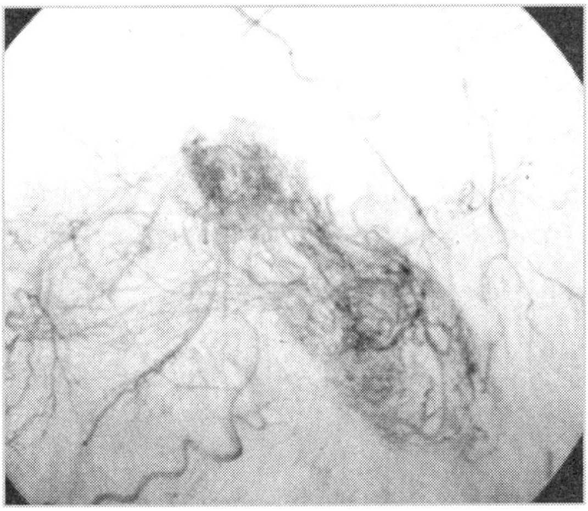

Fig 5.35b

1. What do you see on the plain MR scan of the neck?
2. What do you see on the second investigation?
3. What is the diagnosis?
4. What are the pathology and the clinical features?
5. What are the radiological features and the differential diagnosis?
6. What is the role of radiology in treatment?

Answers *on pages 375–410*

Case 5.36

A 9-year-old girl presents with severe headache, weakness of the left arm, fever and vomiting. On examination she is febrile, and has neck stiffness and left hemiparesis.

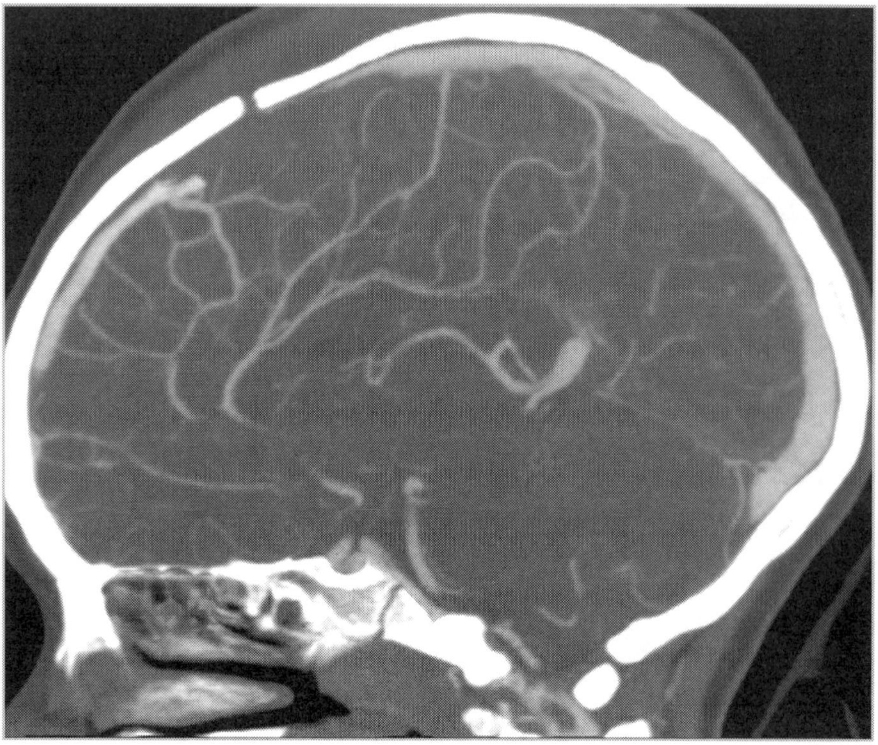

Fig 5.36

1. What is this investigation and what do you observe?
2. What is the diagnosis?
3. What are the predisposing factors?
4. What are the clinical features?
5. What are the imaging features?

Answers *on pages 375–410*

Case 5.37

A 9-year-old girl presents with difficulty in swallowing and a lump in the neck. On examination, there is a mobile, lump in the midline of neck, extending to the right side.

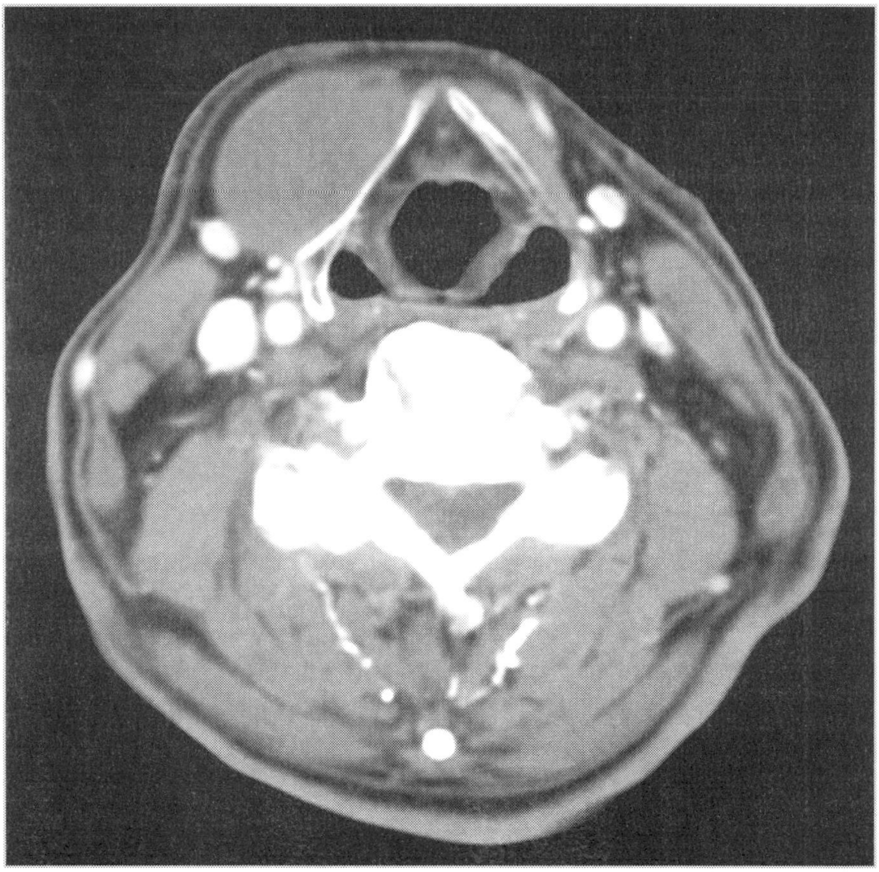

Fig 5.37

1. What do you observe on the CT scan?
2. What is the diagnosis?
3. What is the development of this lesion?
4. What are the clinical features?
5. What are the radiological features
6. What is the management?

Answers *on pages 375–410*

Case 5.1: Answers

1. The skull X-ray shows extensive tram-track calcifications on the surface of the brain.

2. The CT scan shows an area of calcification along the gyrus in the right parieto-occipital lobe and there is generalised brain atrophy.

3. Sturge–Weber syndrome.

4. Sturge–Weber syndrome is a vascular malformation that is caused by persistence of the primordial sinusoidal plexus stage of brain development. Clinically there is a port wine stain on the face in the trigeminal nerve distribution, seizures/hemiatrophy opposite to the side of the naevus, learning disability and homonymous hemianopia. In the brain leptomeningeal vascular malformation is seen. Glaucoma, choroidal haemangioma and buphthalmos are also seen. Angiomatous malformation can be seen in viscera, such as the kidneys, spleen, ovaries, thyroid, pancreas, lungs and intestines.

5. The X-ray shows characteristic tram-track cortical calcification of the gyri underlying the pial angioma, most commonly in the pariteo-occipital region. The CT scan shows the calcification and contrast enhancement of the angioma, with atrophy of the underlying brain. There is enlargement of the choroid plexus and thickening of the skull. MRI shows areas of gliosis with hypointensity in T1 and hyperintensity in T2. Angiography shows capillary blush, deep medullary draining veins and large subependymal veins. Differential diagnoses include Klippel–Trenauney syndrome and Wyburn–Mason syndrome.

Case 5.2: Answers

1. The X-ray shows a defect in the L4 and L5 vertebrae, which do not appear to be fused midline.

2. Spina bifida occulta.

3. Spina bifida is a type of spinal dysraphism. Spinal dysraphism is caused by abnormal/incomplete fusion of midline embryological, mesenchymal, neurological, bony structures. During development, the neural tube is formed by deepening of the neural groove, with infolding of its edges. The neural tube closes at 26–28 days. Failure of closure at the top end causes anencephaly. Failure of closure at the lower end results in a meningomyelocele with pilonidal sinus. The lumen of the tube forms the central canal of the spinal cord and expands with budding of the cephalic end of the nervous system, and makes the ventricles in the brain. The tissues around the neural tube are induced to make supporting structures.

4. Spina bifida occulta – a normal variant, incomplete ossification of lamina of vertebrae. There is no skin opening. There is no herniation of spinal cord. The skin may be normal or have hair/dimple/lipoma/dermal sinus. Tethered cord or lipoma can be associated.

   Spinal dysraphism: defect in neural tube closure

   Myelocele: protrusion of spinal cord through the spinous defect.

   Meningocele: protrusion of meningeal membranes through a bony defect; can be posterior or lateral

   Myeloschisis: exposure of neural contents of vertebral canal, without the meninges

   Myelomeningocele: protrusion of spinal cord and meningeal membranes through the spinous defect.

5. X-rays show a defect in the bony fusion. MRI is useful for assessing the spinal canal and its contents. Herniation of the meningeal membranes and spinal cord can be assessed. The cord is tethered if it extends below its normal level. The presence of lipoma or epidermoid cyst is identified. In children, ultrasonography can also be used to detect occult spina bifida and tethered cord.

Case 5.3: Answers

1. The CT scan shows a well-defined, lentiform, bright haematoma in the right occipital region, overlying the right occipital cortex. There is oedema in the underlying brain and compression of the left lateral ventricle.

2. Acute extradural haematoma.

3. Extradural haematoma is an accumulation of haematoma between the dura mater and the inner table of the skull. Direct trauma results in laceration of arteries, usually a middle meningeal artery. Occasionally, meningeal veins, dural venous sinuses or diploic veins are lacerated. It is more common in younger children.

4. Patients present early after injury with loss of consciousness. There might be a lucid interval, in which the patient is normal, and then he or she deteriorates. Focal neurological signs, such as hemiparesis, and seizures might develop. Venous bleed is slow and presents late. The CT scan is the main test used for diagnosis. Acute haematoma is hyperdense, subacute is isodense and chronic is hypodense. If there is a hypodense swirl within the haematoma, it indicates active bleeding. The most common location is the temporoparietal region. It is usually associated with skull fractures in 85%. The haematoma is in the extradural compartment and appears lentiform in shape (a subdural haematoma is crescenteric). The venous sinuses are separated from the skull. The haematoma produces a mass effect with effacement of underlying gyri and sulci, displacement of the ventricles and herniation. MRI shows signal intensity depending on the stage of haemorrhage. It shows displacement of venous sinuses away from the inner table.

5. Complications of haematoma are mass effect, herniation and brain damage. Emergency surgical decompression is indicated for evacuation of the haematoma.

Case 5.4: Answers

1. The CT scan shows a subdural haematoma in the left temporal region. There is also dense blood in the midline, in the subfalcine region. MRI of the same patient done a day later shows a large, bright, subdural collection.

2. Non-accidental injury (NAI) of the head with subdural haematomas.

3. Non-accidental injury of head is seen in 12% of abused children and accounts for 80% of all deaths. When the baby is shaken, sudden changes in rotational motion produce relative movement between the brain and the skull, and shearing strains within the brain. This rotational acceleration results in stretching and tearing of bridging veins causing subdural and subarachnoid haemorrhages. Axons running between the superficial and deeper areas of the brain are also stretched, resulting in axonal injury. The same mechanism explains retinal haemorrhages

4. Characteristic findings:

Fractures: contact injuries, multiple fractures, fractures crossing suture lines, bilateral fractures; diastasis > 3 mm likely to be abuse; there is no correlation between skull fracture and underlying brain injury

Subdural haemorrhage: interhemispherical extra-axial haemorrhage (subarachnoid or subdural haematoma [SAH or SDH]) is caused by shearing of bridging veins to sagittal sinuses and has a high specificity for NAI. It indicates rotational movement of the brain. SDH usually does not produce a mass effect as sit does in adults. It is seen as a crescenteric hyperdense collection in the convexity or an interhemispherical hyperdense collection, and becomes iso- and hypointense as it ages. Layering may be seen. A membrane is seen in an old SDH. Differential attenuation is seen in active bleeding. MRI detects small SDHs. Ultrasonography can be useful. Rebleeding can happen from the outer membrane

Subarachnoid haemorrhage: shearing injuries of bridging veins

Extradural haemorrhage: not specific

Haemorrhage: intraparenchymal

Axonal injury: shearing at grey–white junction; CT scan is abnormal only if it is haemorrhagic; MRI is hyperintense in T1 and hypointense in T1 if haemorrhagic; FLAIR is better

Contusion: focal haemorrhage

Oedema: diffuse, loss of grey–white matter, hypodensity, bright cerebellum, thalamus, brain stem, basal ganglia and reversal sign.

5. Long-term sequelae are brain atrophy, porencephaly, encephalomalacia, infarction and microcephaly. Learning disability is seen clinically.

Case 5.5: Answers

1. A CT scan of the brain shows dilated ventricles that are surrounded by dense calcifications. There is no soft-tissue mass in the periventricular region or in the rest of the brain parenchyma.

2. TORCH infection.

3. TORCH infection (**t**oxoplasmosis, **o**ther [syphilis, hepatitis, zoster], **r**ubella, **c**ytomegalovirus, **h**erpes simplex) is a congenital infection. TORCH infection is infection of a fetus or newborn by one of the organisms involved in the above. Symptoms are fever, feeding difficulty, purplish or reddish spots caused by bleeding, hepatosplenomegaly, jaundice, hearing impairment and ocular changes.

4. Periventricular calcification and dilated ventricles are features of TORCH infection.

5. The main differential diagnosis is **tuberous sclerosis**, which has periventicular, subependymal tubers and calcifications. **Cytomegalovirus** produces punctate/stippled/curvilinear periventricular calcifications with hydrocephalus. **Rubella** produces punctate or nodular calcifications. Porencephaly and microcephaly are other features.

Case 5.6: Answers

1. MRI of the brain shows a hypointense area occupying the entire right temporal lobe with areas of patchy enhancement. The second picture, which is a post-contrast coronal scan, also shows a patchily enhancing temporal lobe lesion. There is a mass effect in the right temporal lobe, with effacement of the sulci.

2. Herpes simplex encephalitis.

3. Herpes simplex encephalitis is caused by herpes simplex virus type 1 (HSV-1) infection, or HSV-2 in neonates from transplacental spread. Initial symptoms are related to systemic viral illness, such as fever, arthralgia, fatigue, weakness followed by confusion, headache, disorientation and seizures.

4. The characteristic location is the inferomedial temporal lobe. Occasionally it is seen in frontal or parietal lobes. The CT scan is normal initially, but a lateral one shows patchy areas of hypodensity, which spares the putamen. Areas of haemorrhage are seen as high density. Contrast enhancement is seen. A mild mass effect is seen with compression of the ventricles and herniation. MRI shows high signal in T2 and low signal in T1, with areas of haemorrhage, mass effect and contrast enhancement. Increased signal is seen in diffusion-weighted images. Differential diagnoses include abscess, venous infarction and tumour. The clinical features and characteristic location help in diagnosis.

5. Diagnosis is confirmed by identification of the virus in the CSF. If in doubt, a brain biopsy is done. Treatment is with antiviral drugs such as adenine arabinoside.

Case 5.7: Answers

1. The CT scan shows a hyperdense mass in the vermis, which is causing compression of the fourth ventricle anteriorly, resulting in hydrocephalus. There is intense enhancement after contrast administration.

2. Medulloblastoma.

3. Medulloblastoma is the most common malignant tumour of posterior fossa in childhood. It originates from the external granular layer of inferior medullary velum, and 75% present in the first decade. Symptoms are nausea, vomiting, headache and ataxia.

4. Medulloblastoma is located in the vermis. The lesion is seen in cerebellar hemispheres in older children. Usually the lesion is well defined and hyperdense, with shift of the fourth ventricle. The tumour is aggressive and extends into the cerebellar hemisphere, brain stem, cisterna magna, upper cervical cord and cerebellopontine angle. The tumour enhances homogeneously on contrast. Occasionally it may be cystic. Haemorrhage and calcification are rare. MRI shows iso- or hypointense lesion on T1, hypo-, iso- or hyperintense on T2, with homogeneous enhancement. The tumour spreads through the CSF to the spinal cord and cauda (drop metastasis). Metastases can be seen outside the CNS.

5. Differential diagnoses:

Midline tumours: ependymoma, astrocytoma

Eccentric: astrocytoma, meningioma, acoustic neuroma.

Case 5.8: Answers

1. The first image is an axial CT image that shows an abnormally shaped skull, which appears more pointed anteriorly. The intracranial contents appear normal. The ventricles are not dilated.

2. This is a three-dimensional reconstruction of CT images, which shows the abnormal skull shape and fused coronal suture.

3. This is plagiocephaly, which is a type of craniosynostosis, caused by premature fusion of the coronal suture.

4. Craniosynostosis refers to a premature fusion of one or more cranial sutures, resulting in an abnormal skull shape. The normal skull has many sutures at the junction of bones. They are: metopic (separates frontal bones), coronal (frontal and parietal bones), sagittal (parietal bones) and lambdoid (occipital and parietal bones). Normal growth of the brain keeps the sutures open. There are two types of craniosynostosis:

Primary where there is defect in skull ossification, which restricts growth perpendicular to the suture, and there might be raised intracranial pressure (ICP)

Secondary: defect in brain growth (endocrine – rickets, renal osteodystrophy, hypercalcaemia, hypophosphataemia, hyperthyroidism; haematological – sickle cell, thalassaemia; inadequate brain growth – microcephaly and other causes). In secondary type, ICP is normal.

Another classification is:

Simple: premature closure of one suture

Complex: premature closure of more than one sutures

Syndromic: associated with syndromes.

Location – sagittal 50–58%, coronal 20–29%, metopic 4–10%, lambdoid 2–4%.

---

5. **Trigonocephaly**: premature fusion of metopic suture

Scaphocephaly: premature fusion of sagittal suture

Brachycephaly: premature fusion of both coronal sutures

Anterior plagiocephaly: premature fusion of one coronal suture

Posterior plagiocephaly: premature fusion of one lambdoid suture

Oxycephaly (turricephaly): fusion of all sutures including those at skull base

Kleeblattschädel (cloverleaf skull): fusion of all sutures except metopic and squamosal sutures.

---

5. Crouzon syndrome, Carpenter syndrome, Apert syndrome, Chozen syndrome and Pfeiffer syndrome are syndromes associated with craniosynostosis.

---

6. Surgery is usually cosmetic for infants with fusion of one to two sutures resulting in a misshapen head. For infants with microcephaly, surgery is not usually required. In microcephaly, the cause is investigated and brain development monitored. The head circumference is measured longitudinally to monitor development of normal brain in primary craniosynostosis. Signs of elevated ICP are assessed. Surgery typically is indicated for increased ICP or cosmetic reasons.

Case 5.9: Answers

1. Sagittal views on MRI of the cervical spine show a large hypointense mass in the spinal cord, which expands the cord. There is intense enhancement after contrast administration.

2. Spinal cord tumour – astrocytoma.

3. Spinal tumours can be divided into **intramedullary** (within the cord), **intradural extramedullary** (within the thecal sac, outside the cord) and **extradural** (outside the thecal sac):

Intramedullary: astrocytoma, ependymoma, haemangioblastoma, metastasis

Intradural extramedullary: eurofibroma, meningioma, lipoma, dermoid, drop metastasis

Extradural: metastasis, lymphoma, myeloma, sarcoma, chordoma – DD – disc prolapse, haematoma, abscess, neurofibroma, osteochondroma, vertebral body tumours.

4. Spinal cord tumours are diagnosed with MRI. Most of the tumours are gliomas. Ependymomas are common in the filum terminale, especially in children. Astrocytomas are seen in the cervical cord. Haemangioblastomas are seen in the posterior columns and can be associated with other haemangioblastomas in the brain, especially in von Hippel–Lindau syndrome. These tumours are usually associated with cysts. The cyst can be intratumoral or peritumoral (above and below the tumour) and syringomyelic, extending the whole length of the cord. On MRI the tumour can be of same signal intensity as the cord or lower signal in T1 and brighter in T2. Cysts are low signal in T1 and higher in T2. Good contrast enhancement is seen.

5. Differential diagnoses for intramedullary lesions are syringomyelia, abscess, myelitis and haematomyelia.

Case 5.10: Answers

1. MRI shows a large fluid-filled lesion in the posterior aspect of the sacrococcygeal lesion. There is a posterior spinal defect and the CSF is communicating with the spinal canal.

2. Myelomeningocele.

3. Myelomeningocele is a CSF-containing space lined by leptomeninges with variable amounts of neural tissue, herniating through a defect in the spine. It is a neural tube closure defect. Types:

Posterior: lumbosacral, below L2, dorsally, tethered cord seen

Anterior sacral: neurofibromatosis 1, Marfan syndrome, imperforate anus, anal stenosis, tethered cord, genitourinary anomalies

Lateral thoracic: through intervertebral foramen, right side, scoliosis, expanded spinal canal, eroded posterior surface, thinned neural arch, enlarged neural foramen

Lateral lumbar: enlarged neural foramen, Marfan syndrome, Ehler–Danlos syndrome, neurofibromatosis

Traumatic: avulsion of spinal nerve roots secondary to meningeal nerve root sheath.

Cranial.

4. If the spinal bifida is open, there is a prominent swelling. If the defect is covered, pigmented naevus, skin dimple, tuft of hair or angioma can be seen. Reddish neural tissue can be seen in the middle of back. α-Fetoprotein (AFP) is elevated. It is associated with hydrocephalus, Chiari II malformation, scoliosis, vertebral anomalies, diastomatomyelia, duplication of central canal, hydromyelia, chromosomal anomalies, tethered cord and arachnoid cyst.

5. MRI shows a large fluid-filled cyst, low signal in T1, high signal in T2, communicating through a defect in the spinal canal with the cord. The spinal cord is abnormally low and tethered. MRI is very useful in assessing the spinal cord and detecting the presence of other spinal cord and spinal anomalies. Ultrasonography of the spine can be done for assessing a meningomyelocele and communication with the cord. Tethered cord can also be demonstrated.

Case 5.11: Answers

1. Axial view of the brain shows a large cyst in the posterior fossa, which is seen communicating anteriorly with the fourth ventricle. The inferior cerebellar vermis is not seen where it should be

2. Dandy–Walker malformation.

3. The exact aetiology of the Dandy–Walker malformation is not known. A possible theory is insult to the developing cerebellum and fourth ventricle, which leads to developmental arrest in the formation of the hindbrain, with lack of fusion of the cerebellum in the midline between gestational weeks 7 and 10. This results in persistence of the anterior membranous area, which extends and herniates posteriorly. Another theory is congenital atresia of the foramina of Magendie and Luschka. It is frequently associated with agenesis of corpus callosum, lipoma, heterotopias, holoproscencephaly, cephaloceles, cleft palate, polydactyly and cardiac abnormalities. Patients with Dandy–Walker malformation present with developmental delay, enlarged head circumference, or signs and symptoms of hydrocephalus. The clinical presentation depends to some extent on the combination of the developmental anomalies in the infant. Treatment consists of ventriculoperitoneal or cystoperitoneal shunt

4. MRI shows a large posterior fossa cyst that enlarges the posterior fossa, with thinning and bulging of the occipital bones. The inferior cerebellar vermis is absent or hypoplastic and this vermian remnant is elevated by the cyst. The torular herophili, tentorium and straight sinus are elevated above the level of the lambdoid sutures (torular lambdoid inversion). Hypoplastic cerebellar hemispheres that are winged anterolaterally are also seen. Falx cerebelli is absent. Hydrocephalus, aqueductal stenosis and other associated lesions can be seen, as well as brain-stem compression or hypoplasia.

5. **Dandy–Walker variant** is a milder variation of the malformation, where there is a small cyst in the cisterna magna that communicates through a keyhole-shaped deformity with a partially formed fourth ventricle and mild vermian hypoplasia. The fourth ventricle is not as dilated as the malformation, because it communicates freely with the basal cistern through a patent foramen of Magendie. There is no enlargement of the posterior fossa. Hydrocephalus is not a feature. **Megacisterna**

magna is a large cisterna magna, which is a CSF cistern seen posterior to the cerebellum communicating with the fourth ventricle. There is no hypoplasia of the vermis. **Arachnoid cyst**: occasionally a large arachnoid cyst can be seen posterior to the cerebellum. The fluid attenuation value is the same as for the CSF and it can cause smooth scalloping of the skull as a result of chronic pressure. The posterior fossa can be enlarged. There is no communication with the forth ventricle. **Epidermoid cyst**: high signal in T1 and T2 as a result of fat content.

Case 5.12: Answers

1. MRI shows a lesion in the right occipital region, which is hypointense (dark) on the T1-weighted image and hyperintense (bright) on the T2-weighted image, with no mass effect. The ventricles are normal.

2. Arachnoid cyst.

3. Arachnoid cyst is a CSF-containing cyst in the arachnoid space. It may be congenital as a result of splitting of arachnoid membrane with expansion through CSF secretion by arachnoid cells or acquired after trauma, surgery, subarachnoid haemorrhage, infection or tumours. The cyst is lined by ependymal cells and filled with CSF. Most cysts are asymptomatic. The symptoms are non-specific, such as headache, seizures, hydrocephalus, big head, developmental delay, visual loss and precocious puberty.

4. CT shows a hypodense mass with CSF values. MRI has low signal in T1 and high in T2, with signal characteristics of CSF in all sequences. Diffusion images are not positive. The common locations are near the tip of the temporal lobe, suprasellar cistern, posterior fossa, interhemispherical fissure and convexity. There is no calcification or enhancement. There might be erosion of the inner table. There is forward bowing of the anterior wall of the cranial fossa.

5, Differential diagnoses: **epidermoid cyst** (signal slightly lower than CSF, high signal in diffusion-weighted images), **dermoid cyst** (fat signal within the lesion) and **porencephaly** (associated with atrophy, infarction and subdural hygroma). Complications are hydrocephalus and subdural haemorrhage.

Case 5.13: Answers

1. A pre-contrast scan shows dense calcified nodules in the subependymal region of the ventricles on both sides. A post-contrast scan shows a densely enhancing mass in the region of foramen of Monro, which expands the frontal horn of the left lateral ventricle.

2. The patient has tuberous sclerosis. Calcified subependymal nodules are characteristic of this condition.

3. Tuberous sclerosis is an autosomal dominant disease with multisystem involvement including neurological, cutaneous, ocular, renal, cardiac, pulmonary and other organs. Deletions in chromosomes 9 and 11 are identified. The classic clinical triad is seizures, learning disability and adenoma sebaceum, which is found in less than 50% of patients. Diagnosis is made on finding one of the following: adenoma sebaceum, ungual or subungal fibromas, cortical or subependymal harmatomas, or giant cell tumours. Hypopigmented macules, shagreen patches, infantile spasm, retinal hamartomas, renal hamartomas, cysts, cardiac rhabdomyomas or a first-degree relative favours a presumptive diagnosis. Of cases of tuberose sclerosis, 90% have skin and brain lesions. Seizures start before age 2 years and there is some degree of learning disability.

4. The child has developed subependymal giant cell astrocytoma as a complication of tuberous sclerosis. This is the cause of the headache. Renal angiomyolipomas, cysts, cardiac rhabdomyomas, pulmonary lymphangioleiomyomatosis and cutaneous changes are the other complications.

5. In the CNS, the characteristic features are cortical tubers, white matter abnormalities, subependymal nodules and subependymal giant cell astrocytoma, which are caused by a migration abnormality of dysgenetic neurons. Subependymal nodules are the hallmark of this lesion and seen as dense, calcified nodules along the ventricular margins. Cortical tubers are hypointense in T1 and hyperintense in T2. White matter lesions are seen as straight or curvilinear bands extending from the ventricles towards the cortex. Subependymal astrocytomas occur near the foramen of Monro and cause obstructive hydrocephalus. Regular follow-up is done with MRI of the brain and ultrasonography of the abdomen.

Case 5.14: Answers

1. MRI shows atrophy of the brain parenchyma (note the prominent sulci on both sides, which indicates loss of brain substance). The periventricular white matter is thinned, especially on the left side, which results in dilatation of the left occipital horn. In the coronal image, normal white matter is seen on the right side, but there is paucity of white matter on the left side, with a dilated ventricle. There are prominent sulci extending close to the ventricles as a result of loss of white matter on this side.

2. Periventricular leukomalacia.

3. Periventricular leukomalacia is caused by hypoxic ischaemic encephalopathy in a preterm infant. In a preterm infant the watershed territory is located in the periventricular region, and in periventricular leukomalacia there is coagulative necrosis in this region. Clinical presentation of periventricular leukomalacia is cerebral palsy with spastic diplegia, quadriparesis, ataxia, chorea, ataxia, learning disability, delayed milestones, seizures, and visual and motor disturbances.

4. Periventricular leukomalacia changes are seen in the periventricular white matter, particularly adjacent to the trigones, centrum semiovale, optic radiation and acoustic radiation. Ultrasonography or MRI can be used for diagnosis. In ultrasonography, at the earlier stages there is increased echogenicity in the periventricular regions, which subsequently evolves into cystic changes. MRI shows hypointense areas in T1 and hyperintense areas in T2, indicating gliosis. There is white matter loss with dilatation of the ventricles. The sulci run from the surface of the ventricles to the brain surface (normally sulci are separated from the ventricular margins by the periventricular white mater). There is thinning of the posterior body and splenium of the corpus callosum.

5. Severe neurological deficits are seen. If periventricular leukomalacia is localised to the frontal lobe, development may be normal. Differential diagnoses include ventriculitis, metabolic disorders and ischaemia.

Case 5.15: Answers

1. This is a CT scan in an axial plane. The two lateral ventricles are parallel to each other and there is wide separation between them. The second image is an MR scan acquired in the coronal plane. The corpus callosum is not visualised. There is increased distance between the bodies of the lateral ventricles. Note the antler-horn appearance of the frontal horn of the lateral ventricles.

2. Agenesis of corpus callosum.

3. The corpus callosum begins to form in week 10. Initial formation of the corpus callosum occurs in the genu and the body, progressing posteriorly. The anterior genu and rostrum develop last, folding back under the genu. The corpus callosum thickens with increasing myelination. The adult form is reached by week 17. In hypogenesis of the corpus callosum, the parts of it that develop early are still seen, but the rostrum, which develops last, is never seen.

4. Agenesis of corpus callosum is associated with other CNS anomalies (85%), Dandy–Walker cyst, interhemispherical cysts, hydrocephalus, lipoma, Arnold–Chiari, encephalocele, porencephaly, holoprosencephaly, hypertelorism, polymicrogyria, heterotopia, and cardiovascular, gastrointestinal and genitourinary anomalies. Associated syndromes are Dandy–Walker syndrome, Aicardi syndrome, fetal alcohol syndrome and trisomies.

5. Sagittal T1-weighted images are the most accurate for diagnosis of agenesis of corpus callosum. Complete or partial agenesis can be differentiated. Coronal images show a high-riding third ventricle interposed in the interhemispherical fissure. The third ventricle may be high riding and interposed between the bodies of the lateral ventricles. An interhemispherical cyst or lipoma can be associated. The lateral ventricles are widely separated and medially concave with superomedial indentation by the longitudinal callosal bundles of Probst, which gives a batwing or bull's horns appearance on coronal images. The cingulate gyri are not rotated and the cingulate sulcus is absent with the resultant radial pattern of sulci in the medial surface of the cerebral hemisphere. Keyhole dilatation of the temporal horns, secondary to incomplete inversion of the hippocampal formation, is often present. These findings can also be seen on antenatal ultrasonography.

6. Agenesis is often asymptomatic, but it is generally considered a potential marker for neurological impairment. The prognosis is frequently related to other associated abnormalities. The corpus callosum allows sharing of learning and memory between the two cerebral hemispheres. Patients may present with learning disability or delayed development, seizures and cerebral palsy. Macrocephaly can be seen as a result of hydrocephalus associated with interhemispherical cysts.

Case 5.16: Answers

1. MRI shows a single ventricular chamber anteriorly (instead of the normally seen two separate lateral ventricles), with a thin rim of brain tissue. There is separation of the two posterior horns of the lateral ventricles. The thalami are fused. Septum pellucidum is absent.

2. Lobar holoprosencephaly.

3. Holoprosencephaly is a migration anomaly that is characterised by lack of cleavage of the prosencephalon. Cortical brain tissue develops to cover a monoventricle. The posterior part of the monoventricle is enlarged and becomes cystic. There are three types: alobar, semilobar and lobar. The septum pellucidum is absent in all the three.

4. In the **alobar** form there is no hemispherical development. Associated facial anomalies are seen. There is no septum pellucidum, but a third ventricle, falx, interhemispherical fissure, corpus callosum, crescent-shaped monoventricle, and a large dorsal cyst occupying most of the skull. A horseshoe configuration of cortex is seen.

   In the **semilobar** form, there is some hemispherical development. Partially formed occipital and temporal horns, partially fused thalami, absent septum, corpus callosum and olfactory tract are seen. A rudimentray falx cerebri and interhemispherical fissure and hippocampus are also seen.

   In the **lobar** form there is frontal and temporal lobation and a small monoventricle. Also seen are holpocephaly, box-shaped frontal horns caused by unseparated frontal horns, dysplastic anterior falx and an absence of septum pellucidum.

5. Holoprosencephaly is associated with septo-optic dysplasia, aplastic pituitary gland, anophthalmia, microphthalmia, polyhydramnos, renal and cardiac anomalies, and trisomy 13 or 18.

6. Differential diagnoses: severe hydrocephalus – septum pellucidum present, symmetrically thinned cortex; agenesis of corpus callosum with midline cyst – wide separation of lateral ventricles; hydranencephaly – frontal and parietal cortex affected more; Dandy–Walker cyst – posterior fossa cyst, normal lateral ventricles; large arachnoid cyst.

Case 5.17: Answers

1. The sagittal view of MRI shows a long cavity, which has high signal intensity in T2-weighted images, extending through cervical and upper thoracic levels. Axial T2-weighted image shows a bright fluid-containing space in the centre of the cervical spinal cord.

2. Syringomyelia.

3. Syringomyelia is a cavity in the spinal cord that may communicate with the central canal, not lined by ependymal tissue. Although many mechanisms for syrix formation exist, the exact pathogenesis is not yet known. It is caused by interrupted flow of CSF through the perivascular space of the cord between the subarachnoid space and the central canal. The causes are trauma, postinflammatory, tumours, vascular insufficiency and idiopathic. Hydromyelia is dilatation of the central canal of the spinal cord. This is associated with a Chiari malformation, Dandy–Walker syndrome, spinal dysraphism, myelocele, scoliosis, diastomatomyelia, Klippel–Feil syndrome, segmentation defects and tethered cord.

4. Loss of pain and temperature, trophic changes in the skin, muscle weakness, spasticity, hyperreflexia and abnormal plantar reflexes are seen. It is usually seen in the cervical cord, and can extend into the thoracic level or the brain stem. Treatment options are suboccipital/cervical decompression, laminectomy with syringotomy, ventriculoperitoneal/lumboperitoneal/syringoperitoneal shunt, fourth ventriculostomy, terminal ventriculostomy, percutaneous needling and neuroendoscopic surgery.

5. MRI is the imaging procedure of choice. It shows a longitudinal CSF-filled cavity, low signal in T1 and high signal in T2. Usually the wall is smooth, but it may be beaded with metameric haustrations in syringomyelia secondary to tumour. Traumatic syringomyelia has septations, irregular borders and arachnoid loculations. Serial examinations are required to evaluate changes in cavity size over time. Phase contrast MRI can be used to analyse the CSF flow dynamics. CT shows low-density areas, with no contrast enhancement. The cord is enlarged. A CT myelogram will demonstrate delayed filling of the cysts. In hydromyelia, the central canal is dilated with CSF. Differential diagnoses for syringomyelia include other intramedullary lesions such as tumours, infarcts, demyelination and infections, and vascular malformations.

Case 5.18: Answers

1. The MR scan shows a large area of signal void in the posterior fossa compressing the third ventricle, which is dilated. On contrast angiography there is a large vascular structure with multiple feeding vessels.

2. Vein of Galen malformation.

3. A vein of Galen aneurysm is actually an AVM that drains into an enlarged vein of Galen. There are three types:

   Type I: AV fistula fed by enlarged arterial branches, leading to dilated vein of Galen, straight sinus and torular herophili

   Type II: angiomatous malformation involving basal ganglia, thalami, midbrain draining into the vein of Galen

   Type III: transitional AVM with both features; a high output cardiac failure can be seen.

4. Transcranial ultrasonography shows an anechoic lesion in the posterior fossa with associated hydrocephalus and high flow within the lesion. CT shows a smooth and well-defined midline mass posterior to the third ventricle, with a dilated straight and transverse sinus with torcular herophili. CT shows a well-defined homogeneous hyperdense mass in the region of the third ventricle, which shows homogeneous enhancement of serpentine structures, vein of Galen and straight sinus.

5. The malformation is usually supplied by the posterior cerebral artery or posterior choroidal artery and occasionally by the anterior cerebral artery, anterior choroidal artery, middle cerebral artery, lenticulostriate artery and perforating arteries.

6. Pineal tumour, colloid cyst, arachnoid cyst and porencephalic cyst are the other differential diagnoses of tumours in the posterior aspect of the third ventricle. However, the appearance of the vein of Galen malformation is characteristic with its vascular appearance and feeding arteries.

Case 5.19: Answers

1. Axial view of the MR scan reveals a cleft in the middle of the spinal cord, showing two hemicords, with the left larger than the right. No bony septum is seen in between the cords.

2. Diastomatomyelia.

3. Diastomatomyelia is a sagittal division of the spinal cord into two hemicords, each of which has a central canal, a dorsal horn and a ventral horn. It is a congenital malformation caused by adhesions between the endoderm and ectoderm. There are two types of cord:

   Type **1**: no spur/fibrous band, single dural sac and subarachnoid space, with two hemicords, each having its own pial layer

   Type **II**: less common, bony spur or fibrous band; two hemicords each with its own pial, subarachnoid and dural sac; common in the lower thoracic and upper lumbar regions.

4. Muscle wasting, weakness, clubfoot and hypertrichosis are the clinical features.

5. MRI shows a sagittal cleft, with a bony spur arising from the posterior aspect of **centra**, and two hemicords reuniting caudal to the cleft. Occasionally there are two coni medullaris. The filum terminale is thick and there is a tethered cord. The vertebrae show scoliosis, spina bifida, anteroposterior narrowing of the vertebral bodies, a wide interpeduncular distance, a narrow disc space with hemivertebra and thick adjacent lamina.

Case 5.20: Answers

1. MRI shows multiple, small, ring-enhancing lesions in the brain. In the first scan, it is seen in the midbrain. In the second, there are multiple lesions in the cerebral and cerebellar hemispheres.

2. Tuberculoma of the brain.

3. TB spreads by haematogenous dissemination to the subependymal or subpial focus (**Rich's** focus) and subsequent seeding of the brain parenchyma

4. Tuberculoma is granuloma formation within the brain parenchyma. It is common in the cerebellar hemispheres and may be associated with tuberculous meningitis. It is common in children and young adults, and solitary in 70%. Clinical features are headache, seizures and focal neurological deficits.

5. The imaging findings of tuberculoma are variable, because it is an evolving granuloma. In the acute phase, a CT scan may be normal or hypodense. After the inflammation is established, it is usually isodense or hypodense with ill-defined margins caused by minimal surrounding oedema and shows marked contrast enhancement. When the granuloma caesates, it is hypo-, iso- or hyperdense, with occasional calcifications. Contrast enhancement can be homogeneous, nodular or rim enhancement (target sign – central calcification in isodense lesion with rim enhancement). Calcification can be seen. In the early stages, MRI shows a hypointense lesion in T1, hyperintense in T2, and homogeneous nodular enhancement. After a granuloma is formed, the lesion is iso- to hyperintense on T2 with rim enhancement. The core is hypointense in T1 and hyperintense in T2. Differential diagnoses: cysticercosis, toxoplasmosis, bacterial abscess, fungal infections, lymphoma, glioma, metastasis and vasculitis.

Case 5.21: Answers

1. The axial view on the CT scan shows a cystic lesion with circumferential calcification in the sellar and suprasellar regions. The adjacent structures are normal.

2. The sagittal view from an MR scan shows a lesion of low signal intensity in T1-weighted images in the suprasellar region. There is superior displacement of the optic chiasma and hydrocephalus.

3. Craniopharyngioma. A suprasellar mass in a child is considered to be a craniopharyngioma unless proven otherwise. Differential diagnoses of a cystic lesion in the suprasellar region include necrotic pituitary adenoma (no calcification), dermoid cyst (fatty component seen), epidermoid cyst (high signal in diffusion images, minimal enhancement), arachnoid cyst (angular margins, no solid component/enhancement), Rathke's cleft cyst (no solid component, calcification rare), cystic optic chiasma/hypothalamic glioma (solid with necrotic areas, calcification rare, enhancement seen) and thrombosed aneurysm.

4. Craniopharyngioma is a benign tumour that arises from squamous epithelial remnants along Rahke's duct/pouch. Pathologically the tumour has a cyst with a solid component. The cyst has fluid similar to motor oil, containing blood products, protein products and cholesterol. It is lined with stratified squamous epithelium. This is the most common tumour of the suprasellar cistern, and is commonly seen between age 5 and 10 years, with a second peak at 40–50 years. Most are combined sellar and suprasellar, with variable clinical findings. Growth retardation (compression of hypothalamus), diabetes insipidus (pituitary compression), bitemporal hemianopia (optic chiasma compression), headaches, nausea, vomiting, seizures, cranial nerve palsies (cavernous sinus involvement), growth delay, obesity and hydrocephalus are some of the clinical features. In children growth delay is a common manifestation. Diabetes insipidus is more commonly seen with eosinophilic granuloma of the stalk and precocious puberty is more common with hypothalamic hamartomas.

5. CT and MRI are useful in the diagnosis. The three characteristic features are a cyst, calcification and contrast enhancement. CT shows a hypodense cyst, with a mural nodule. Calcification is seen in 90%. The solid component shows rim enhancement but there is no enhancement

of the cystic component. The MRI signal is variable depending on the content of the cyst, which can be protein, blood or cholesterol. It can be hypointense in T1 and hyperintense in T1 – especially if the contents are proteinaceous or cholesterol. The solid component is isointense and enhances on contrast. The cystic component extends anteriorly or laterally and typically wraps around the solid component. MRI also demonstrates compression of adjacent structures. Hydrocephalus is seen as a result of compression of the foramen of Monro.

Case 5.22: Answers

1. Coronal MRI of the brain reveals a well-defined lesion in the right cerebellar hemisphere, which shows intense contrast enhancement.

2. Haemangioblastoma.

3. Von Hippel–Lindau syndrome.

4. Haemangioblastoma is a benign tumour of vascular origin, commonly seen in the cerebellar hemispheres. It can also be seen in the spinal cord, cerebral hemispheres and brain stem. The lesion can be solid, cystic with a mural nodule or cystic. A CT scan shows a well-defined cyst, a cyst with an enhancing nodule or a solid, enhancing lesion. MRI shows a cyst with a low signal in T1 and a high signal in T2, with a solid nodule within that shows intense enhancement. Flow voids are seen in the solid component. Haemorrhage is high signal in both T1- and T2-weighted images. Oedema is seen around the tumour. Angiography shows a vascular nidus in the cyst. Draining veins are seen. It is associated with von Hippel–Lindau syndrome, other features of which are cerebellar, spinal cord haemangioblastomas, cysts of the pancreas or kidneys, endolymphatic sac tumour, rhabdomyoma of the heart, renal carcinoma, phaeochromocytoma, cystadenoma of the epididymis, pancreatic cyst, islet cell tumour, liver adenoma and paraganglioma. Renal carcinomas in von Hippel–Lindau syndrome are often bilateral, multiple and seen at a younger age than conventional renal carcinomas.

5. Differential diagnoses: pilocytic astrocytoma (cerebellar hemisphere, large cyst > 5 cm, thick wall, mural nodule that is not as vascular, medulloblastoma (solid, vermis), arachnoid cyst (no mural nodule) or metastasis (more oedema)

Case 5.23: Answers

1. The axial view in a CT scan shows a lobulated papillary mass with specks of calcification in the right lateral ventricle, which is expanded. There is no extension outside the ventricle into the surrounding brain parenchyma. The rest of the ventricles are also dilated.

2. Choroid plexus papilloma. The characteristic appearance is a papillary lobulated tumour in the trigone of lateral ventricle with calcifications in a child < 5 years. It is difficult to differentiate from choroid plexus carcinoma radiologically, because both invade the surrounding brain parenchyma and produce drop metastasis. Differential diagnoses include xanthogranuloma, glioma, metastasis, epidermoid, haematoma, ependymoma (more common in fourth ventricle), pilocytic astrocytoma, haemangioblastoma (cystic with mural nodules), choroid plexus lipoma and choroid plexus cyst.

3. Choroid plexus papilloma is a benign tumour that arises from the epithelium of the choroid plexus. The tumour has papillary fronds and fibrovascular connective tissue. The peak incidence is < 5 years. Of these tumours 90% represent choroids plexus papillomas and 10% are choroid plexus carcinomas. The most common location in children is the trigone of the lateral ventricle (in adults it is seen in the fourth ventricle). Clinical presentation is non-specific with vomiting, seizures, visual field defects and cranial nerve palsies.

4. Complications are choroid plexus carcinoma (10–30%), hydrocephalus (caused by obstruction at outlet and at arachnoid granulations and increased CSF production). Drop metastasis in subdural space, intraventricular extension, extraventricular extension to brain parenchyma and bony invasion (indicates malignancy) are other complications.

5. CT and MRI show a solid, lobulated papillary intraventricular mass, in the trigone of a child's lateral ventricle. Calcification is seen in 25%. The mass shows intense contrast enhancement. The tumours are supplied by anterior and posterior choroidal arteries. MRI is isointense in T1 and hyperintense in T2. It shows drop metastasis and extension to adjacent structures.

Case 5.24: Answers

1. The MR axial image shows massively dilated lateral ventricles. The sagittal image shows dilated lateral ventricles and third ventricle with collapsed fourth ventricle.

2. Hydrocephalus.

3. Aqueduct stenosis. This is the most common cause of congenital hydrocephalus. In aqueduct stenosis, there is focal narrowing of the cerebral aqueduct, which connects the third and fourth ventricles, at the level of the superior colliculi. Aqueductal stenosis results from postinflammatory changes (TORCH, TB) or developmental (septum, narrowing, forking), neoplastic (tectal glioma, pinealoma) or subarachnoid haemorrhage. It can be associated with other congenital anomalies and thumb deformities.

4. The lateral and third ventricles are enlarged, but the fourth is normal sized. There are periventricular hypodensities with indistinct margins. An absence of CSF pulsation is seen in CSF flow studies.

5. Other causes of congenital hydrocephalus are postinfectious, communicating hydrocephalus, Chiari II malformation, superior vena cava (SVC) obstruction, Dandy–Walker malformation, tumour, haemorrhage, choroid plexus papilloma and vein of Galen malformation.

Case 5.25: Answers

1. The CT scan shows multiple ring-enhancing lesions. The larger lesions are seen in the midline frontal region and right parietal region, and a small lesion in the left occipital region. The lesions are surrounded by perilesional vasogenic oedema.

2. Cerebral abscesses caused by *Aspergillus* spp.

3. Streptococci, anaerobic organisms, *Bacteroides* spp., staphylococci and fungi are common causative organisms. The infection can extend from the adjacent sinuses/middle ear/mastoid or by penetrating trauma, surgery or septicaemia, or may be cryptogenic. Predisposing factors are immunosuppressive drugs, HIV, steroid use and trauma, lung infections (bronchiectasis, empyema, bronchopleural fissural, pneumonia) and cardiac conditions (AVM, endocarditis, right-to-left shunt).

4. Headache, drowsiness, confusion, seizures, focal neurological deficit, fever and leukocytosis are the clinical features. Complications are daughter abscesses and rupture into the ventricular system.

5. The most common location of an abscess is the corticomedullary junction. It is more common in the frontal and temporal lobes. A CT scan reveals a hypodense area with mass effect, which shows rim enhancement. The wall is thin and smooth, with relative thinning of the medial wall. Gas can be seen within the lesion. There is extensive perilesional oedema that can produce mass effect and compression of the ventricles. Satellite nodules can be seen. MRI shows a hypointense lesion in T1 and hyperintense in T2, with the rim appearing hypointense in T2. Contrast enhancement of the rim is seen. There is a high-signal perilesional oedema.

6. Differential diagnoses: cystic glioma, metastasis, ganglioglioma, pilocytic astrocytoma, haemangioblastoma, haematoma, infarct and cyst.

Case 5.26: Answers

1. The ultrasound scan shows high echogenicity in the right caudothalamic groove (shown in the sagittal view), which is extending medially into the lateral ventricle. The right lateral ventricle is expanded with this echogenic material.

2. Periventricular haemorrhage – grade III.

3. Risk factors for neonatal haemorrhage are preterm delivery, low birthweight, being male, multiple gestations, birth trauma, prolonged labour, hypocoagulation, PDA, pneumothorax and hyperosmality.

4. Neonatal haemorrhage commonly happens in the germinal matrix, which is a vascular gelatinous subependymal tissue adjacent to the lateral ventricles. The neuronal cells originate here. The matrix involutes by 32–34 weeks. The matrix is prominent above the caudate nucleus in the floor of the lateral ventricle and tapers as it sweeps from the frontal horn posteriorly into the temporal horn – roof of third and fourth ventricles. It is supplied by Heubner's artery from the anterior cerebral artery, striate branches of the middle cerebral artery, the anterior choroidal artery and perforating branches from the meningeal artery. Causes of haemorrhage are rupture of this vascular bed as a result of fluctuating cerebral blood flow in preterm infants with respiratory distress or increased cerebral blood flow, such as rapid volume expansion, hypercapnia, systemic hypertension, increased cerebral venous pressure, decreased flow resulting from systemic hypotension and coagulation disturbance.

5. It is seen in preterm infants < 32 weeks and < 1500 g. Ultrasonography is the most useful modality for diagnosing and monitoring periventricular haemorrhage. There are four grades:

   Grade I: germinal matrix haemorrhage

   Grade II: subependymal haemorrhage, intraventricular haemorrhage with no hydrocephalus

   Grade III: intraventricular haemorrhage, with hydrocephalus

   Grade IV: intraparenchymal haemorrhage.

   Germinal matrix haemorrhage is seen as a hyperechoic area in the caudothalamic groove in the region of the caudate nucleus and thalamostriate groove. As the haemorrhage resolves, it becomes lucent. It can completely involute or leave a scar or cyst. The normal choroid plexus can be bright too, but it is attached to the inferomedial aspect of the ventricular floor, tapers towards the caudothalamic groove and is never anterior to the foramen of Monro.

Case 5.27: Answers

1. MRI done in the sagittal plane shows a well-defined hypointense mass in the cerebellar hemisphere. The post-contrast scan shows a cystic lesion with peripheral solid enhancement. There is mild anterior compression of the fourth ventricle.

2. Cerebellar pilocytic astrocytoma.

3. Pilocytic astrocytoma is the second most common posterior fossa tumour in children. It is common in children and there is no specific age distribution. It usually originates midline with extension to the cerebellar hemispheres. The vermis, tonsils and brain stem are also affected. It is a benign tumour, and malignant transformation is very rare. It presents with truncal ataxia and dysdiadochokinesia.

4. The lesion is usually cystic with a mural nodule. Hemispherical astrocytomas are cystic in most cases. Some lesions are purely solid with a cystic necrotic centre or a purely solid tumour. Calcification is seen in 20%. CT shows a cyst with a value for CSF with enhancement of the wall. The tumour can be purely solid with heterogeneous enhancement or solid with areas of necrosis. MRI is hypointense on T1 and hyperintense on T2.

5. Differential diagnoses for cystic cerebellar tumour are haemangioblastoma (< 5 cm, vascular nodule), arachnoid cyst, trapped fourth ventricle, megacisterna magna and Dandy–Walker cyst. Differential diagnoses for solid astrocytoma are medulloblastoma (hyperdense mass, non-calcified) and ependyoma (fourth ventricle, 50% calcification).

Case 5.28: Answers

1. Sagittal views of the brain stem and upper cervical spine show herniation of the cerebral tonsil below the level of the foramen magnum. There is also an abnormal, long segment of low signal intensity in the cervical and thoracic spinal cord.

2. Arnold–Chiari I malformation associated with syringohydromyelia of the upper cervical cord.

3. Arnold–Chiari malformation is a congenital malformation resulting from defective neural tube closure. There are four types:

   I: downward herniation of the cerebellar tonsils below the level of the foramen magnum

II: caudal herniation of the tonsils and vermis, small posterior fossa, towering cerebellum, beaked tectum

III: Chiari II findings + encephalocele

IV: severe cerebellar hypoplasia.

4. In the normal sagittal pictures of the craniocervical junction, the cerebellar tonsils are above the level of the foramen magnum. If they extend below the foramen magnum, they do not extend > 5 mm. Any descent > 5 mm is considered to be tonsillar herniation and is a feature of Arnold–Chiari I malformation. The fourth ventricle can be elongated, but remains in a normal position. It is associated with syringomyelia in 50% of cases. Syringomyelia is seen as a lesion of low signal intensity on T1- and high signal intensity on T2-weighted images.

5. Arnold–Chiari I malformation is associated with intermittent compression of the brain stem, which manifests as nerve palsies, atypical facial pain, respiratory depression and long tract signs. Associated features are syringomyelia (50%), hydrocephalus (25%), basilar invagination (30%), Klippel–Feil anomaly (10%) and atlanto-occipital fusion (5%).

Case 5.29: Answers

1. The X-ray shows a long, linear lucency in the right occipital bone.

2. Fracture of the skull.

3. Skull fractures can be linear, depressed, comminuted, growing or skull base fractures. Linear fractures are the most common and require two views for diagnosis. A CT scan might miss this fracture if not taken in the proper plane. This should be differentiated from a vascular marking that is in the expected location of an artery, branches and has smooth margins. A depressed fracture is palpable. In plain film there is a bone-on-bone appearance, with a sclerotic area surrounded by a lucent rim. A CT scan is required for confirmation and to assess underlying brain damage. A basilar skull fracture usually presents with CSF rhinorrhoea, otorrhoea, haemotympanum, racoon eyes and pneumocephalus. A fracture can be seen in temporal bone and the skull base.

4. A growing skull fracture is also called a leptomeningeal cyst, and is seen in children. The fracture ends separate and there is a cystic fluid collection because of skull growth. The X-ray shows well-defined lucency with a rim of sclerosis.

5. The X-ray is not routinely indicated. If the patient had a head injury and has a neurological deficit, an X-ray is indicated. CT is indicated if there is loss of consciousness, amnesia, neurological deficit, persistent headache or vomiting, depressed skull fracture or symptoms of basilar skull fracture.

Case 5.30: Answers

1. This is high-resolution MRI of the brain. The coronal image through the temporal lobe shows a normal appearance of the left temporal lobe, including the hippocampus. There is slight atrophy of the right hippocampus, with dilatation of the temporal horn. There is also high signal in the right hippocampus (compare with the left side, which has a signal similar to the normal brain parenchyma).

2. Mesial temporal sclerosis.

3. Epilepsy is a common neurological disorder characterised by recurrent, unprovoked seizures. Causes are mesial temporal sclerosis, developmental venous anomaly, tuberous sclerosis, heterotopias/cortical dysplasias, perinatal hypoxia, infections, traumatic scarring, tumours and vascular malformations.

4. Temporal lobe epilepsy manifests with complex partial seizures. The most common cause of complex partial seizures is mesial temporal sclerosis (35–65%), in which the hippocampus is small. It is usually unilateral, but can be bilateral in 10–15% of cases. The epileptogenic focus involves structures in the mesiotemporal lobe such as hippocampus, amygdala and parahippocampal gyrus. Mesial temporal sclerosis is seen in 65% of temporal lobectomy specimens obtained in temporal lobe epilepsy. Whether mesial temporal sclerosis is the cause or the result of temporal lobe epilepsy is controversial. Patients present with complex partial seizures that can become generalised.

5. MRI is the best imaging modality to detect and delineate brain lesions in partial seizures, especially temporal lobe lesions. Thin-section, high-resolution, coronal MR images are the most useful for detecting these lesions. In T1-weighted images, the affected side is small as a result of hippocampal atrophy, with associated dilatation of the temporal horn of the lateral ventricle. In T2-weighted images, a high signal is seen in the affected hippocampus, as a result of gliosis and increased free water content. A FLAIR sequence (**fl**uid **a**ttenuation **i**nversion **r**ecovery) suppresses the fluid in the surrounding temporal horn of the lateral ventricle and makes the high signal in hippocampus conspicuous. Quantitative three-dimensional volume measurements can be used. MRI is also useful in diagnosing other causes of epilepsy. MR spectroscopy shows reduced *N*–acetylaspartate. Tumours produce a mass effect and show contrast enhancement. Cortical dysplasias are similar to tumours, without the enhancement and have a signal similar to that of the brain's grey matter. Cavernous angiomas are the most common vascular malformations associated with seizures. Post-traumatic scarring produces a high signal.

Case 5.31: Answers

1. In axial MRI, there is proptosis of the globe. There is an elongated, bright tumour arising from the optic chiasma and extending through the optic canal into the right orbit. In the sagittal view, the bright tumour can be seen extending along the superior aspect of the right orbit.

2. Optic chiasma glioma. Optic nerve glioma is the most common primary neoplasm of the optic nerve, constituting 7% of all childhood gliomas. It is a grade I astrocytoma (pilocytic astrocytoma) because it is slow growing and does not metastasise.

3. Neurofibromatosis I is associated with optic chiasma glioma in 20–50% of cases. Optic chiasma glioma is a low-grade glioma that arises from the optic chiasma and might extend to the hypothalamus. It is seen in 2–9 year olds, with a peak at 4 years. Clinical features are decreased visual acuity, pallor, emaciation, precocity, obesity and diabetes insipidus.

4. An X-ray of the skull shows the characteristic omega/cottageloaf sella, which is caused by erosion of chiasmatic sulcus/anterior half of sella turcica and undercutting of planum sphenoidale. The optic

canal is enlarged, measuring > 5 mm, and becomes rounded. A CT scan shows a hypodense lobulated mass in the chiasmatic cistern with inhomogeneous enhancement. MRI shows expansion of the optic chiasma, with hypointensity in T1 and high signal in T2 with inhomogeneous enhancement. Cyst formation, necrosis and calcifications are seen. The tumour may extend anteriorly into the optic nerve, and posteriorly into the optic tracts and hypothalamus. Hydrocephalus may develop in large tumours.

5. Differential diagnoses: hypothalamic glioma and hypothalamic hamartoma.

Case 5.32: Answers

1. MRI shows a well-defined cystic lesion, with internal septations, located along the anterior border of sternocleidomastoid, deep to the platysma. On the T1-weighted image, the lesion is dark and on the T2-weighted image it is bright, indicating that the lesion is filled with fluid. There is no solid component inside the cyst, no lymphadenopathy and no vascular invasion.

2. Branchial cyst.

3. Branchial cleft anomalies are formed as a result of failure of involution of the branchial cleft. The anomalies can be cysts, fistulae or sinuses. The most common type is a cyst of the second branchial cleft, which results from incomplete obliteration of the second branchial cleft tract. It is seen between age 10 and 40 years.

4. There are four types:

Type I: along the anterior surface of sternomastoid deep to the platysma

Type II: along anteromedial surface of sternomastoid, lateral to the carotid space, posterior to the submandibular gland

Type III: medial extension between the internal and external carotid branches to the pharyngeal wall

Type IV: within the pharyngeal mucosal space.

Pathologically, the cyst is lined by stratified squamous epithelium and filled with yellowish fluid and cholesterol crystals. Clinically there is a history of multiple parotid abscesses not responding to treatment, otorrhoea, pain, redness and tenderness. It is located anywhere along a line from the tonsillar fossa to the supraclavicular region. Type II is the most common. The cyst is round or oval at the mandibular angle, with displacement of the sternocleidomastoid muscle posteriorly, carotid vessels posteromedially and submandibular gland anteriorly. The mass shows internal debris caused by haemorrhage or infection. The mass is compressible. MRI and CT might show a curved rim of tissue between the internal and external carotid arteries.

5. Differential diagnoses: necrotic lymph node, abscess, cystic lymphangioma, submandibular gland cyst and necrotic metastasis. Large, symptomatic cysts are surgically resected.

Case 5.33: Answers

1. The first CT scan shows a well-defined, smooth, hypodense mass, with a speck of calcification in the superior and lateral aspects of the right orbit.

2. The second CT shows that the mass has now increased in size.

3. Orbital varix. This is a malformation involving the orbital veins. It can be congenital (venous malformation/venous wall weakness) or acquired (AVM – intraorbital or intracranial). It presents with intermittent exophthalmos associated with straining, diplopia and blindness.

4. Orbital varix involves the superior or inferior ophthalmic veins. A non-contrast scan usually shows a phlebolith (calcification in walls of veins) and a small mass. The mass enlarges after a Valsalva manoeuvre or jugular compression. There is intense enhancement after contrast administration. Bony erosion can be seen without sclerotic reactions. Spontaneous thrombosis can be seen. Ultrasonography shows an anechoic tubular structure with venous flow increasing during a Valsalva manoeuvre. MRI shows flow void and flow-related enhancement.

5. Differential diagnoses for orbital mass in this age group include lymphoma, inflammatory pseudotumour, metastasis, haemangioma, lymphangioma, glioma, meningioma and metastasis. None of these tumours shows the characteristic changes with a Valsalva manoeuvre.

Case 5.34: Answers

1. There is a large tumour, dark in the axial T1 and bright in the coronal fat-suppressed sequences, which is seen in the medial and inferior aspects of the right orbit. The mass extends into the right nasal cavity and maxillary sinus.

2. Orbital rhabdomyosarcoma.

3. Rhabdomyosarcoma is the most common soft-tissue tumour in children under the age of 15 years and the third most common extracranial solid tumour after neuroblastoma and Wilms' tumour. Most are seen before 5 years of age. Orbital rhabdomyosarcoma is the most common orbital malignancy in children, and 10% of paediatric rhabdomyosarcomas occur in the orbit. Pathologically it can be alveolar, undifferentiated, embryonal, spindle cell or botryoid type. It is equally frequent in both sexes and both orbits.

4. Orbital rhabdomyosarcomas are non-invasive and confined to the bony orbit. At the time of presentation, the mass is of a similar size to the globe. It can cross the muscle cone and be inta-/extraconal. It is commonly seen in the supranasal quadrant of the globe and is rare in the lower outer quadrant. It presents with unilateral proptosis and usually has an insidious onset. It is also usually confined to the orbit. A CT scan shows a heterogeneously enhancing lesion. Stranding is seen in the orbital fat. On MRI the tumour is isointense to muscle on the T1-weighted image and heterogeneously hyperintense on the T2. Extension outside the orbit has a bad prognosis, especially if there is skull-base erosion and parameningeal spread. Regional lymph node extension is rare, as a result of a paucity of periorbital lymphatics. Lung metastasis is uncommon.

   The survival rate for orbital tumours is high (90%), with combined radiotherapy and radiation.

5. Orbital lesions can be differentiated based on the compartments of their location. The orbital muscles divide the orbit into conal (in muscles), intraconal (in between muscles) and extraconal (outside muscles).

Extraconal	Infection, neurofibroma, lymphoma, bone tumour, adenocarcinoma, mucoepidermoid, adenoid cystic carcinoma
Conal	Rhabdomyosarcoma, thyroid eye disease, orbital pseudotumour
Intraconal	Haemangioma, lymphangioma, venous malformation, AVM, optic nerve glioma, meningioma
Globe	Retinoblastoma, metastasis, melanoma

Case 5.35: Answers

1. Sagittal sections through the neck show a large, contrast-enhancing mass in the nasopharyngeal region, which extends anteriorly into the nasal cavity.

2. This is an angiogram of the carotid vessels, which shows a very vascular tumour in the nasopharyngeal region supplied by the internal maxillary branch of the external carotid artery.

3. Juvenile nasopharyngeal angiofibroma.

4. Juvenile nasopharyngeal angiofibroma is a locally aggressive tumour and is the most common nasopharyngeal tumour of children. It is seen exclusively in boys and usually seen in the second decade. Clinical presentation is with nasal obstruction, deformity, nasal speech, headache, facial swelling and epistaxis. It originates from the superior aspect of the sphenopalatine foramen. There are many theories about its origin: hormonal, desmoplastic response to nasopharyngeal periosteum and tumour of non-chromaffin paraganglionic cells of the internal maxillary artery that supplies the tumour are some of them.

5. A lateral view of the neck X-ray shows a nasopharyngeal mass, which causes anterior displacement and bowing of the posterior wall of the maxillary sinus (Holman–Miller sign) and maxillary sinus opacification. A CT scan shows a mass in the nasopharynx, which enhances on contrast examination. There is widening of the pterygopalatine fossa, and superior

and inferior orbital fissures. The tumour extends into the infratemporal fossa, sphenoid sinus, greater sphenoidal wing, pterygomaxillary space and skull base. MRI shows intermediate signal intensity on T1, with areas of signal void as a result of vascular channels. Angiography shows supply from an internal maxillary artery. Treatment is with hormonal therapy, radiation, embolisation and surgery. Differential diagnoses of nasopharyngeal mass in children are hypertrophied adenoids, nasal polyps, antrochoanal polyp, rhabdomyosarcoma, inverting papilloma, dermoids, encephalocele and squamous cell carcinoma.

6. The tumour is very vascular. Embolisation of the tumour is performed before surgery to devascularise the tumour and reduce the size.

Case 5.36: Answers

1. This is CT venography. Contrast is injected intravenously and images are acquired in the venous phase of cerebral vascular enhancement. MR venography is also performed in a similar way and can be done without administration of intravenous contrast. This is a sagittal view, which shows normal appearing superior sagittal sinus, anteriorly and posteriorly, although it is not visualised in the mid-portion, near the vertex.

2. Superior sagittal sinus thrombosis.

3. The causes of cerebral venous thrombosis are idiopathic, infections, tumour, trauma, dehydration, shock, cardiac failure, hypercoagulable states (antiphospholipid syndrome, protein C and S disease, polycythaemia vera, thrombocytopenia, thrombocytosis, sickle cell, disseminated intravascular coagulation), HIV, SLE, nephritic syndrome, chemotherapy (asparaginase) and Behçet's disease.

4. Clinical features are headache, nausea, vomiting, visual blurring, drowsiness, lethargy, seizures, stroke and fever.

5. A non-contrast CT scan shows a dense clot in the sinuses. On contrast scans, the clot does not enhance and is seen as a filling defect. One of the classic CT signs of sinus thrombosis is the **empty delta sign**, in which the walls of the dural sinus enhance and the clot does not enhance and

is seen as a filling defect. Focal haemorrhage in the brain and infarct can be seen. There is gyriform enhancement of the periphery of the infarct. MRI shows a thrombus of high signal intensity within the sinuses, which is isointense on T1 and hypointense on T2. Chronic thrombus is hyperintense on T1 and T2. MR or CT venography exquisitely demonstrates the venous anatomy and exact location of the thrombosis.

Case 5.37: Answers

1. The CT scan shows a hypodense cyst with no internal contents in the right side of the neck, anterior to the thyroid cartilage and inferior to the hyoid bone.

2. Thyroglossal duct cyst. This is the most common congenital neck mass. Although it is usually seen in midline, in 25% it can be seen laterally.

3. Thyroglossal duct is the duct along which the thyroid gland descends from the base of the tongue (foramen caecum) to its adult position, passing anterior and then posterior to the hyoid bone, by 7 weeks. Normally the thyroglossal duct involutes by weeks 8–10. In thyroglossal duct cyst, the duct persists and a cyst lined by stratified squamous/pseudostratified columnar epithelium is formed. Ectopic thyroid tissue can be present.

4. It is usually seen in the second and third decades. It presents as a painless mass in the midline, which moves with swallowing and tongue protrusion. Most are located in the infrahyoid location, but a few are located in the suprahyoid and hyoid location; 75% are located in the midline, whereas others are located within 2 cm of the midline.

5. Ultrasound shows a well-defined cyst, up to 3 cm, with clear internal contents and posterior acoustic enhancement. A CT scan also shows a well-defined cyst with peripheral enhancement. On MRI the cyst is hypointense in T1 and hyperintense in T2. Ectopic thyroid tissue is seen and uptake might be evident on the thyroid scan.

6. Complications are infection, squamous cell carcinoma and thyroid carcinoma. Treatment is by the Sistrunk procedure, which is resection of the cyst along with a core of the hyoid bone.

COLOUR IMAGES

Case 3.18

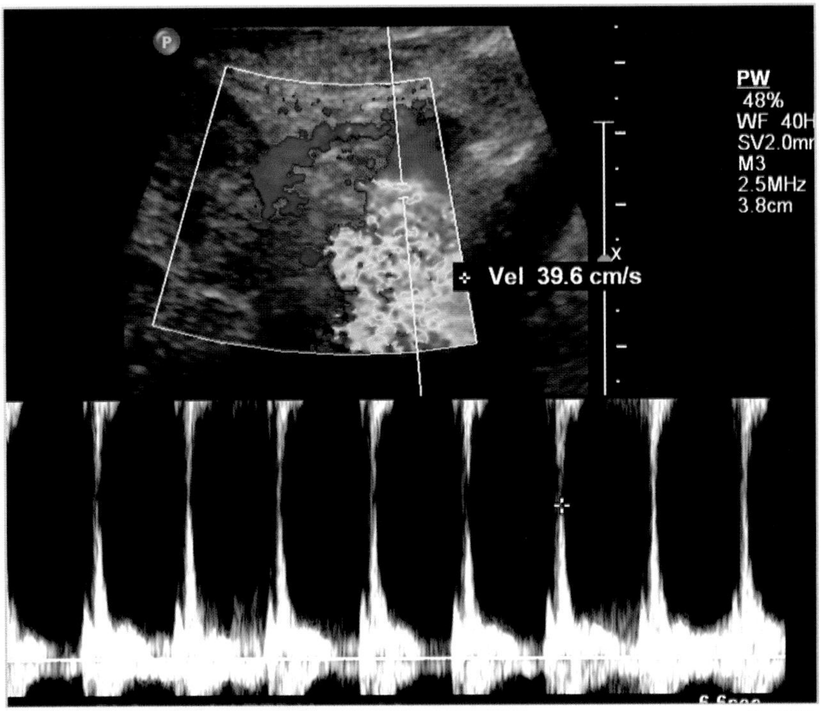

Fig 3.18b

Case 3.23

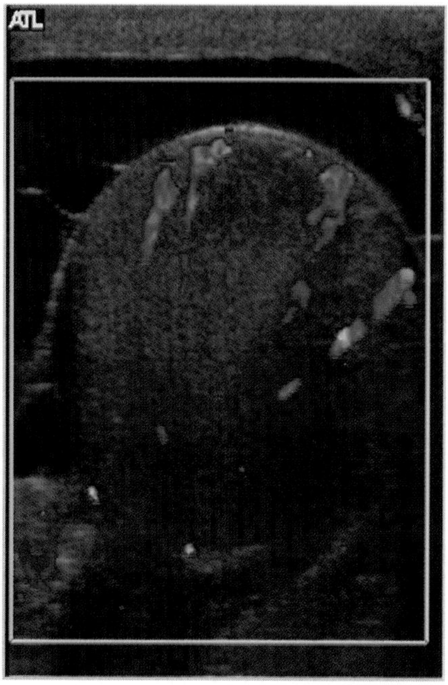

Fig 3.23b

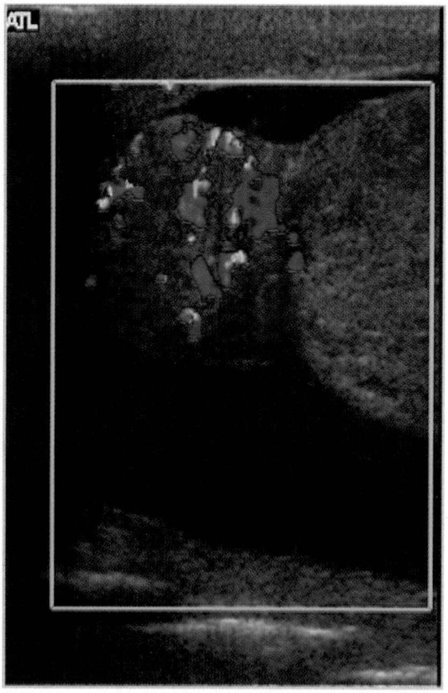

Fig 3.23c

Case 3.24

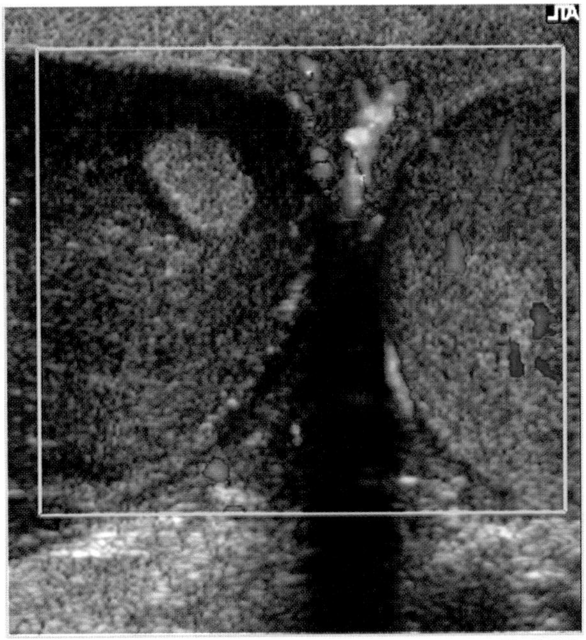

Fig 3.24b

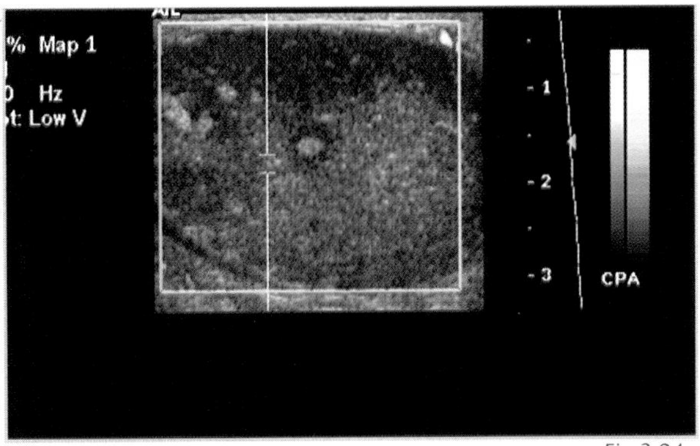

Fig 3.24c

INDEX